W9-BAW-573

INTRODUCTION TO
PHYSICAL
THERAPY

fifth edition

INTRODUCTION TO
PHYSICAL THERAPY

fifth edition

MICHAEL A. PAGLIARULO, PT, MA, EdD
Professor Emeritus
Department of Physical Therapy
Ithaca College
Ithaca, New York

ELSEVIER

ELSEVIER

3251 Riverport Lane
St. Louis, Missouri 63043

INTRODUCTION TO PHYSICAL THERAPY, FIFTH EDITION   ISBN: 978-0-323-32835-7

Notices

Knowledge and best practice in this field are constantly changing. As new research and experience broaden our understanding, changes in research methods, professional practices, or medical treatment may become necessary.

Practitioners and researchers must always rely on their own experience and knowledge in evaluating and using any information, methods, compounds, or experiments described herein. In using such information or methods they should be mindful of their own safety and the safety of others, including parties for whom they have a professional responsibility.

With respect to any drug or pharmaceutical products identified, readers are advised to check the most current information provided (i) on procedures featured or (ii) by the manufacturer of each product to be administered, to verify the recommended dose or formula, the method and duration of administration, and contraindications. It is the responsibility of practitioners, relying on their own experience and knowledge of their patients, to make diagnoses, to determine dosages and the best treatment for each individual patient, and to take all appropriate safety precautions.

To the fullest extent of the law, neither the Publisher nor the authors, contributors, or editors, assume any liability for any injury and/or damage to persons or property as a matter of products liability, negligence or otherwise, or from any use or operation of any methods, products, instructions, or ideas contained in the material herein.

Library of Congress Cataloging-in-Publication Data

Introduction to physical therapy / [edited by] Michael A. Pagliarulo, PT, MA, EdD, Professor Emeritus, Department of Physical Therapy, Ithaca College, Ithaca, New York. – Fifth edition.
  pages cm
  Includes bibliographical references and index.
  ISBN 978-0-323-32835-7 (pbk.: alk. paper) 1. Physical therapy. I. Pagliarulo, Michael A.
  RM700.P34 2015
  615.8'2–dc23   2015019314

Executive Content Strategist: Kathy Falk
Content Development Manager: Jolynn Gower
Senior Content Development Specialist: Brian Loehr
Publishing Services Manager: Hemamalini Rajendrababu
Project Manager: Umarani Natarajan
Design Direction: Ashley Miner

Printed in Canada

Working together
to grow libraries in
developing countries

www.elsevier.com • www.bookaid.org

Last digit is the print number: 9 8 7 6 5 4 3 2 1

This edition of the text is dedicated to my wife, Tricia, who is also a physical therapist. Our relationship began when we were both conducting clinical rotations at Rancho Los Amigos Hospital in Downey, CA as students from different programs. Our personal journeys soon aligned, while our professional journeys diverged a bit—I moved into academe and she continued with clinical practice. Over the decades of my academic career, her clinical perspectives were instrumental in ensuring I would apply the knowledge, skills, and attitudes I addressed in my courses into clinical applications. Her guest appearances in my classes and labs always added a clinical aspect to the content. I am grateful for her professional guidance and perspectives; caring for her patients/clients, family, friends, and complete strangers; and certainly her partnership through our 40 years of marriage.

Michael A. Pagliarulo
July 2015

Contributors

Barbara C. Belyea, PT, DPT, CSCS
Clinical Professor
Department of Physical Therapy
Ithaca College
Ithaca, New York

Katy Eichinger, PT, DPT, NCS
Physical Therapist
Department of Neurology
University of Rochester Medical Center
Rochester, New York

Hilary B. Greenberger, PT, PhD, OCS
Associate Professor
Department of Physical Therapy
Ithaca College
Ithaca, New York

Tiffany Hilton, PT, PhD
Associate Professor
Doctor of Physical Therapy Division
Duke University School of Medicine
Durham, North Carolina

Teresa A. Hoppenrath, PT, DPT
Physical Therapist
Cayuga Medical Center at Ithaca
Ithaca, New York

John E. Kelly, PTA, BS
Coordinator
Home Modification and Accessibility
Easter Seals Crossroads
Adjunct Professor in Aging Studies
University of Indianapolis
Center for Aging and Community
Indianapolis, Indiana

Helen L. Masin, PT, PhD
Associate Professor of Physical Therapy
Miller School of Medicine
University of Miami
Coral Gables, Florida

Karen W. Nolan, PT, DPT, PCS
Physical Therapist
Bright Start Pediatric Services
Fairport, New York

Michael A. Pagliarulo, PT, MA, EdD
Professor Emeritus
Department of Physical Therapy
Ithaca College
Ithaca, New York

Pamela D. Ritzline, PT, EdD
Chair, Division of Health Sciences
Professor
Physical Therapy
Walsh University
North Canton, Ohio

Laurie A. Walsh, PT, JD, MS
Associate Professor
Physical Therapy
Daemen College
Amherst, New York

R. Scott Ward, PT, PhD, FAPTA
Professor and Chair
Physical Therapy
University of Utah
Salt Lake City, Utah

Jennifer E. Green-Wilson, PT, MBA, EdD
Principal/Consultant
Institute for Business Literacy and Leadership
Rochester, New York

Cynthia M. Zablotny, PT, DPT, NCS
Associate Professor
Doctor of Physical Therapy Program
George Fox University
Newberg, Oregon

Preface

Our profession continues to evolve to meet the needs of society. Two examples of this are the revisions to the new Vision Statement of the American Physical Therapy Association and the Guide to Physical Therapist Practice 3.0. These documents and their predecessors have significantly influenced the three primary areas of the profession of physical therapy: practice, education, and research. Moreover, the ongoing changes in the legal and regulatory arenas, such as the Affordable Care Act, have also impacted the profession and practice of physical therapy. The current edition reflects these and other changes.

All contributors reviewed and revised their respective chapter in order to keep the content contemporary. This included updates to the information, references, photos, tables, and graphic material. We are pleased to publish the photos in full color, which more accurately displays the body area and therapist/patient interaction. Although content has been updated, the original purpose to serve as an introductory text remains the same. Part I addresses the Profession of physical therapy, and Part II provides an overview of primary practice areas with a consistent approach: General Description; Common Conditions; Principles of Examination; Principles of Evaluation, Diagnosis, and Prognosis; Principles of Intervention; and a Case Study to serve as an example of the application of the principles to that practice area. The comprehensive and current References and Additional Resources provide the opportunity to seek the advanced knowledge in the subject area.

It is now nearly 20 years since the first edition of this text was published. The success we have experienced across these 2 decades attests to the quality of the content and expertise of the contributors. I am pleased to maintain this level of quality in the 5th edition to describe the current status of the profession and practice of physical therapy.

Michael A. Pagliarulo

Acknowledgments

This text would not be possible without the efforts of the contributors to each chapter and personnel at Elsevier. Although personnel changes occur with each edition, including this one, the quality of the product remains outstanding, and for this, I am sincerely grateful.

In some cases, a contributor has moved from co-author to primary or sole author. Katy Eichinger now serves as the primary author for the Neuromuscular chapter and Cynthia Zablotny joins her as a co-author. Both have rich academic and clinical backgrounds in the area and provided an extensive update to the chapter. Karen Nolan (Pediatrics) and Teresa Hoppenrath (Older Adult) are now sole authors for their respective chapters. Having recently moved back to full-time clinical positions from academe, they ensure their chapters describe contemporary practice.

Changes have also occurred with the personnel at Elsevier. Christie Hart and Kathy Falk were instrumental in initiating the development of the current edition. Brian Loehr joined this project in 2014 and provided timely and excellent service in managing the content, revisions, and questions from contributors. This was welcomed given the extent of updates and number of contributors. Umarani Natarajan was helpful in the final stages of editing.

I continue to extend my gratitude to the students and faculty who use this text and provide helpful feedback. My commitment to this profession has not diminished over my 45 years of service, and I am thankful to have this opportunity to provide this learning material to students entering the discipline.

Michael A. Pagliarulo
July 2015

Contents

Part I

Profession

Physical therapy is knowledge. Physical therapy is clinical science. Physical therapy is the reasoned application of science to warm and needing human beings. Or it is nothing.[1]

Helen J. Hislop

1

The Profession of Physical Therapy: Definition and Development

Michael A. Pagliarulo

KEY TERMS

American Physiotherapy Association (APA)
American Women's Physical Therapeutic Association
Autonomous practice
Client
Core values
Evidence-based practice
Guide to Physical Therapist Practice 3.0
National Foundation for Infantile Paralysis ("the Foundation")
Patient
Physiatrist
Physical therapist
Physical therapy
Physiotherapist
Physiotherapy
Profession
Reconstruction aide
Vision 2020
Vision Statement for Physical Therapy 2020

LEARNING OBJECTIVES

After reading this chapter, the reader will be able to:
1. Define physical therapy.
2. Describe the characteristics of a profession.
3. Describe a brief history of the profession of physical therapy in the United States and the major factors that influenced its growth and development.
4. Identify issues that continue to impact the profession.

The profession of physical therapy continues to evolve to meet the needs of society. Although it has received substantial publicity, confusion remains regarding its unique characteristics. For example, how does physical therapy differ from occupational or chiropractic therapy? This chapter's first purpose, then, must be to present and define this profession.

To define physical therapy thoroughly, it is also important to present a brief history of its development. A review of the past will demonstrate how the profession has responded to societal needs and gained recognition as an essential component of the rehabilitation team. It will also link some current trends and practices with past events.

DEFINITION

Part of the confusion regarding the definition of **physical therapy** results from the variety of legal definitions seen from state to state. Each state has the right to define the profession of physical therapy and regulate its practice. Such definitions are commonly included in legislation known as *practice acts,* which pertain to specific professions (practice acts are further described in Chapter 5).

To limit the variety of definitions, the Board of Directors of the American Physical Therapy Association (APTA) created the Physical Therapist Scope of Practice (Box 1-1),[2] which was originally titled *Model Definition of Physical Therapy for State Practice Acts.* This definition identifies several activities inherent in the practice of physical therapy. It uses language and terminology based on the ***Guide to Physical Therapist Practice 3.0*** (the *Guide*),[3] a pivotal document describing the approach of the physical therapist (PT) to patient care. One of the fundamental concepts of the *Guide* is the five elements of the patient/client management model, and these are incorporated into the definition. (These are briefly described here. For more details on the elements of the model see Chapter 2.) First and foremost, physical therapy begins with an examination to determine the nature and status of the condition. An evaluation is then conducted to interpret the findings and establish a diagnosis and prognosis that includes a plan of care. Interventions are then administered and modified in accordance with the patient's responses. Interventions focus on musculoskeletal, neuromuscular, cardiovascular and pulmonary, and integumentary disorders. The definition of physical therapy also reflects the areas of prevention, and the promotion of health, wellness, and fitness, all of which occur across the life span. Other important activities in the role of the PT include consultation, education, and research. These may be separate from, but ultimately contribute to, effective practice.

Traditionally, PTs have provided care to **patients**—individuals who have disorders that require interventions to improve their function. **Client** is the term used to refer to an individual who seeks the services of a PT to maintain health or a business that hires a PT for consultation.[3] The latter area of involvement has become more significant in the recent development of the profession.

In addition to identifying the activities of a PT, the definition states that physical therapy is "provided by or under the direction and supervision of a physical therapist." This qualification is further stipulated in a section of another policy (adopted by the House of Delegates, the highest policy-making body of the APTA) specifying that PTs and physical therapist assistants (PTAs) working

BOX 1-1

Guidelines: Physical Therapist Scope of Practice

Physical therapy, which is limited to the care and services provided by or under the direction and supervision of a physical therapist, includes:

1. Examining (history, systems review, and test and measures) individuals with impairments, functional limitations, and disability or other health-related conditions in order to determine a diagnosis, prognosis, and intervention; tests and measures may include the following:
   - Aerobic capacity/endurance.
   - Anthropometric characteristics.
   - Arousal, attention, and cognition.
   - Assistive and adaptive devices.
   - Circulation (arterial, venous, and lymphatic).
   - Cranial and peripheral nerve integrity.
   - Environmental, home, and work (job/school/play) barriers.
   - Ergonomics and body mechanics.
   - Gait, locomotion, and balance.
   - Integumentary integrity.
   - Joint integrity and mobility.
   - Motor function (motor control and learning).
   - Muscle performance (including strength, power, and endurance).
   - Neuromotor development and sensory integration.
   - Orthotic, protective, and supportive devices.
   - Pain.
   - Posture.
   - Prosthetic requirements.
   - Range of motion (including muscle length).
   - Reflex integrity.
   - Self-care and home management (including activities of daily living and instrumental activities of daily living).
   - Sensory integrity.
   - Ventilation, and respiration/gas exchange.
   - Work (job/school/play), community, leisure integration or reintegration (including instrumental activities of daily living).

2. Alleviating impairment and functional limitation by designing, implementing, and modifying therapeutic interventions that include, but are not limited to:
   - Coordination, communication, and documentation.
   - Patient/client-related instruction.
   - Therapeutic exercise.
   - Functional training in self-care and home management (including activities of daily living and instrumental activities of daily living).
   - Functional training in work (job/school/play) and community and leisure integration or reintegration activities (including instrumental activities of daily living, work hardening, and work conditioning).
   - Manual therapy techniques (including mobilization/manipulation).

Continued

BOX 1-1

Guidelines: Physical Therapist Scope of Practice—cont'd

■ Prescription, application, and, as appropriate, fabrication of devices and equipment (assistive, adaptive, orthotic, protective, supportive, and prosthetic).
■ Airway clearance techniques.
■ Integumentary repair and protection techniques.
■ Electrotherapeutic modalities.
■ Physical agents and mechanical modalities.
■ Dry needling.
3. Preventing injury, impairment, functional limitation, and disability, including the promotion and maintenance of health, wellness, fitness, and quality of life in all age populations.
4. Engaging in consultation, education, and research.

From *Guidelines: Physical Therapist Scope of Practice*, BOD G03-01-09-29. Board of Directors Standards, Positions, Guidelines, Policies, and Procedures. Alexandria, VA, American Physical Therapy Association, 2009.

BOX 1-2

Provision of Physical Therapy Interventions and Related Tasks

Physical therapists are the only professionals who provide physical therapy interventions. Physical therapist assistants are the only individuals who provide selected physical therapy interventions under the direction and at least general supervision of the physical therapist.

From *Provision of Physical Therapy Interventions and Related Tasks*, HOD P06-00-17-28. House of Delegates Standards, Policies, Positions, and Guidelines. Alexandria, VA, American Physical Therapy Association, 2009.

under the direction of a PT are the only individuals who provide physical therapy (Box 1-2; see Chapter 3 for a comprehensive description of the background and role of the PTA.).[4]

PHYSICAL THERAPY AS A PROFESSION

The definition of physical therapy provides a broad description of the scope of practice of physical therapy. A companion document addresses physical therapy as a profession (Box 1-3).[5] This position was adopted by the House of Delegates of the APTA in 1983 and was subsequently revised to incorporate *Guide* language. Although the position states, "Physical therapy is a health profession...," it does not offer a spectrum of characteristic evidence to support this statement. Perhaps one reason is the difficulty in conclusively defining a profession.

Swisher and Page[6] presented a comprehensive review of the variety of descriptions of a profession. They addressed definitions based on a description of characteristics, stages of evolution, or power, but they focused on three qualities commonly held in high regard: autonomy, ethical standards, and accountability. Distinct applications of these qualities were made to physical therapy.

BOX 1-3   *Position on Physical Therapy as a Health Profession*

Physical therapy is a health profession whose primary purpose is the promotion of optimal health and function. This purpose is accomplished through the application of scientific principles to the processes of examination, evaluation, diagnosis, prognosis, and intervention to prevent or remediate impairments, functional limitations, and disabilities as related to movement and health.

Physical therapy encompasses areas of specialized competence and includes the development of new principles and applications to meet existing and emerging health needs. Other professional activities that serve the purpose of physical therapy are research, education, consultation, and administration.

From *Physical Therapy as a Health Profession*, HOD P06-99-19-23. House of Delegates Standards, Policies, Positions, and Guidelines. Alexandria, VA, American Physical Therapy Association, 2009.

Moore[7] also included autonomy in a description of a profession and positioned it at the peak of a hierarchy of characteristics (Figure 1-1). This description is particularly applicable to physical therapy. The first characteristic, a lifetime commitment requiring an individual's dedication to the profession, is formidable yet admirable. PTs and PTAs do not commonly leave this profession. The second

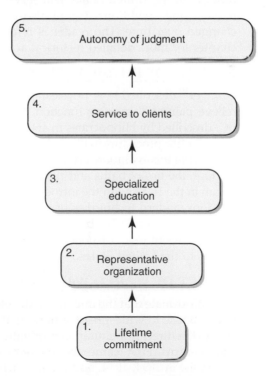

Figure 1-1 ■ Hierarchy of the criteria to define a profession.

characteristic, a representative organization, provides standards, regulations, structure, and a vehicle for communication. In physical therapy, this characteristic is fulfilled by the APTA. The third characteristic, specialized education, ensures competency to practice. For example, standards for the accreditation of physical therapist education programs (effective January 1, 2016) stipulate that the institution awards the Doctor of Physical Therapy (DPT) degree and standards for accreditation of PTA education programs stipulate that the institution awards the associate degree.[8,9] The fourth characteristic, service to clients, is obvious in physical therapy and provides a direct benefit to society. In this context, the term *patients* would also apply. The final feature, autonomy of judgment, applies regardless of whether the therapist practices in a jurisdiction where a physician's referral is required by law. Independent and accurate judgment is inherent in every evaluation, plan of care, and discharge plan conducted by the PT. This last criterion is frequently used to distinguish a professional from a technician (an individual who requires supervision).

As a profession, physical therapy is guided by the criteria listed in Figure 1-1. Such was not always the case, and evolution of the profession has entailed significant change and varying degrees of recognition from other professions. The next section provides a brief overview of the history of physical therapy, particularly as it developed in the United States.

HISTORICAL DEVELOPMENT

Examining the origin and development of the profession and practice of physical therapy in the United States will serve to explain some of the current characteristics and conditions. It will also demonstrate how certain positions have changed over time. The reader is referred to the resources at the end of this chapter for more detailed historical accounts.

ORIGINS OF PHYSICAL THERAPY

Granger[10] described how physical measures were used in ancient civilizations to relieve pain and improve function. Massage was used by the Chinese in 3000 BC, described by Hippocrates in 460 BC, modified by the Romans, and accepted as a scientific procedure in the early 1800s. Techniques of muscle reeducation developed from this evolution. Hydrotherapy was practiced by the Greeks and Romans through the use of baths and river worship. The development of electrotherapy began in the 1600s with the introduction of electricity and electrical devices.

More modern techniques of physical therapy were practiced extensively in Europe, particularly England and France, before being used in the United States. It took the outbreak of polio epidemics and World War I to bring these techniques to the United States.

IMPACT OF WORLD WAR I AND POLIO

It is unfortunate that the impetus to develop physical therapy in this country was the response to widespread suffering; at the same time, such an origin demonstrates the direct humanitarian motivation that serves as the foundation of physical therapy. First came the epidemics of polio (poliomyelitis or infantile paralysis) in 1894, 1914, and 1916, which left tens of thousands of children paralyzed and in need of "physical therapy." Then at the outbreak of World War I,

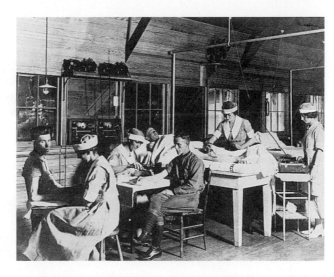

Figure 1-2 ■ Reconstruction aides treating soldiers wounded in World War I at Fort Sam Houston, Texas, in 1919. (From American Physical Therapy Association: Historical Photograph Packet.)

the Surgeon General of the United States sent a group of physicians to England and France to learn about physical therapy techniques for the better management of those wounded in war. As a result, the Division of Special Hospitals and Physical Reconstruction was created in 1917.[11] This division was responsible for training and managing **reconstruction aides** (exclusively women) who would provide physical reconstruction to those injured in war. These women were the forerunners of the profession and practice of physical therapy in the United States (Figure 1-2).

During this period, polio epidemics were occurring in Vermont. A statewide program known as the *Vermont Plan* was developed to study the cause and effects of the disease. Under this plan, health care teams conducted field visits to provide care for children with polio.[12] These teams consisted of orthopaedic surgeons, public health nurses, **physiotherapists** (commonly known as *physicians' assistants*), brace makers, and stenographers. The physiotherapists became involved in taking accurate measurements to determine muscle strength and providing therapy through exercise and massage (Figures 1-3 and 1-4).

POST-WORLD WAR I PERIOD

Even after the war, the need for physical therapy continued. Attention shifted from preserving a fighting force to maintaining a working force. Humanitarian interests and the labor requirements of an industrial society resulted in a focus on "crippled children."[13] As the reconstruction aides moved into civilian facilities to address these needs, their titles and practices were plagued by confusion and ambiguity. The time had come to establish a clear identity through a national organization.

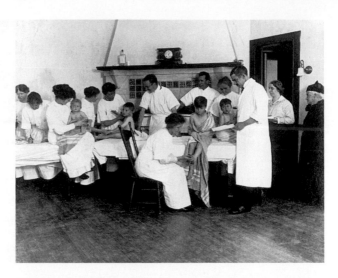

Figure 1-3 ■ Physical therapists and physicians working together to evaluate and treat children at a polio clinic in New England in 1916. (From American Physical Therapy Association: Historical Photograph Packet.)

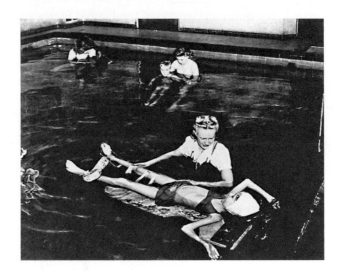

Figure 1-4 ■ Aquatic therapy was very effective for individuals who had polio. (From American Physical Therapy Association: Historical Photograph Packet.)

The origin of the first national organization representing "physical therapeutics" is traced to a meeting suggested by a military physician. This meeting, on January 15, 1921, at Keen's Chop House in New York City, was attended by 30 reconstruction aides and five physicians. Accomplishments of the first meeting included creation of a national organization, the **American Women's Physical Therapeutic Association**, and election of the first president, Mary McMillan.[14]

BOX 1-4	*Founding Objectives of the American Women's Physical Therapeutic Association*

1. To establish and maintain a professional and scientific standard for those engaged in the profession of physical therapeutics.
2. To increase efficiency among its members by encouraging them in advanced study.
3. To disseminate information by the distribution of medical literature and articles of professional interest.
4. To make available efficiently trained women to the medical profession.
5. To sustain social fellowship and intercourse on grounds of mutual interest.

Data from Beard G: Foundations for growth: A review of the first forty years in terms of education, practice, and research. *Phys Ther Rev* 41:843–861, 1961.

According to the first constitution, the organization was established to maintain high standards and provide a mechanism for sharing information (Box 1-4).

Mary McMillan was the overwhelming choice for president (Figure 1-5). Trained in England, she is credited with becoming the first "physical therapist" in the United States.[12] As a reconstruction aide she was stationed at Walter Reed

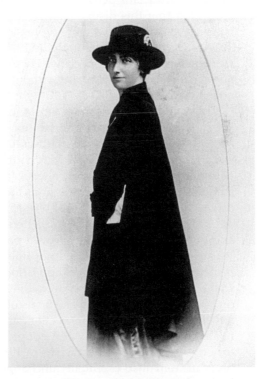

Figure 1-5 ■ Mary McMillan was elected in 1921 as the founding president of the American Women's Physical Therapeutic Association (precursor to the American Physical Therapy Association). (From American Physical Therapy Association: Historical Photograph Packet.)

General Hospital in Washington, DC, where she was appointed head reconstruction aide in 1918. Later, while at Reed College in Portland, Oregon, she participated in the largest (over 200 students) of seven emergency training programs for reconstruction aides.

Under the leadership of Miss McMillan, the new organization took immediate action. Two membership categories were established: charter members (reconstruction aides), and active members who "shall be graduates of recognized schools of **physiotherapy** or physical education, who have had training and experience in massage and therapeutic exercise, with some knowledge of either electrotherapy or hydrotherapy."[15] An official journal, *P.T. Review*, was established and first published in 1921. Annual meetings were initiated in conjunction with annual meetings of the American Medical Association (AMA) to capitalize on their programs and gain recognition. The name of the organization was changed in 1922 to the **American Physiotherapy Association** (APA). Two men were admitted in 1923. In 1926, the journal was retitled *Physiotherapy Review*. To honor the pioneering work of Mary McMillan, the organization eventually created in her name a lectureship (presented as a major opening event at the Annual Conference) and student scholarship programs that continue today.

Two issues involving physicians took decades to resolve. The first pertained to identity. Physicians perceived these practitioners to be technicians or aides and suggested that this distinction be reflected in their title. Members of the APA believed that they had a more professional status and objected to that reference. This issue was not settled until the 1940s, when physicians established physical medicine as a medical specialty. These physicians were known as **physiatrists**, and the term *physical therapist* (without adding *technician* or *aide*) became acceptable thereafter.[13]

The second issue was more substantive and involved education requirements. No standard educational program existed for a physiotherapist; therefore, the APA developed a suggested curriculum and published it in 1928. This was a 9-month program (1200 total clock hours). Entrance requirements included graduation from a school of physical education or nursing.[14] In contrast, most of the students in the 14 training programs for reconstruction aides were physical education teachers or graduates of physical education schools. A committee of the APA visited all institutions offering educational programs for physiotherapists and published a list of 11 approved programs in 1930.

The action by the APA did not fully resolve the issue of education requirements. Greater recognition of education programs and standards was required, so the APA sought assistance from the AMA in 1933. Consequently, the Council on Medical Education and Hospitals of the AMA inspected 35 schools of physiotherapy. Based on this inspection, as well as input from the APA and other related organizations, the AMA adopted the Essentials of an Acceptable School for Physical Therapy Technicians in 1936. Entrance requirements and length of program remained essentially unchanged; however, the curriculum was stated in detail, and other characteristics were stipulated (institutional affiliation, faculty, resources, and clinical facilities). Thirteen schools were approved by the AMA in 1936.[14]

IMPACT OF WORLD WAR II AND POLIO

Once again, national and global tragedies combined to expand the need for physical therapy, and, as before, the profession responded. To meet the demands of the war, eight emergency 6-month courses were authorized to be offered among the 15 approved full-length programs in physical therapy. These shortened courses were discontinued in 1946 when war-related demands for services dropped.

Unfortunately, polio continued to create a need for therapy. In response to repeated epidemics, the **National Foundation for Infantile Paralysis** (often referred to as "**the Foundation**") was established in 1938 for research, education, and patient services.[11] PTs continued to provide vital services for children affected by polio.

The Foundation was a source of substantial support for the profession and practice of physical therapy. Catherine Worthingham, a past president of the APA, accepted the position of Director of Professional Education on the staff of the Foundation in 1944. In the same year, the first national office of the APA was established in New York City and the first executive director was hired. Both these actions were made possible by a grant from the Foundation. Also in 1944, a permanent headquarters and staff for the APA enabled the organization to create the House of Delegates to serve as a policy-making body. Other grants from the Foundation provided scholarships to recruit and retain physical therapy students and faculty, funds to hire a consultant to recruit and assign PTs for emergency work relating to polio, and financial support for training in techniques fostered by Sister Elizabeth Kenny for individuals with polio (early application of moist heat to permit mobilization and prevent contractures).

POST-WORLD WAR II PERIOD

The U.S. Army recognized the need to retain PTs in an organized unit to provide service to military personnel. As a result, the Women's Medical Specialist Corps was established in 1947. It consisted of PTs, occupational therapists, and dietitians. A PT, Emma Vogel, became the first chief of the Corps and was accorded the rank of colonel.[11] In 1955, the Corps became the Army Medical Specialist Corps to allow men and women to serve with commissions in the military.[14]

A major breakthrough in the treatment of polio occurred during this period with the introduction of gamma globulin and the Salk vaccine. Finally, the disease could be controlled. PTs played prominent roles during field trials of these medications, which began in 1951.

Name clarification continued as the term *physiatrist* became recognized as the title given to physicians who practiced physical medicine. **Physical therapists** (PTs) could now practice *physical therapy*. This role clarification was reflected in the new name for the national organization, the American Physical Therapy Association, in 1947 and a new title for the journal, *Physical Therapy*, in 1962. It was also demonstrated in the title of the new Essentials, which extensively revised the original document of 1936. The new title, Essentials of an Acceptable School of Physical Therapy, no longer referred to *technicians*. This document was adopted by the AMA in 1955 and was used to approve new and existing educational programs for over 20 years. The new Essentials established minimum curricular standards, including a program length of 12 months.

(NOTE: As the need and interest in unique areas of practice, education, and research continued to develop over the decades, new entities within the APTA were created. These are identified in appropriate time periods that follow, but described in more detail in Chapter 4.)

1960s THROUGH 1980s

The three-decade period of the 1960s through the 1980s was characterized by growth and recognition in education, practice, and research. Societal issues of this period included an aging population, health promotion, and disease prevention. Federal legislation funded health care for a variety of populations, which increased the demand for physical therapy. The profession responded with several actions.

First, the APTA adopted policy statements in the 1960s to clarify the preparation and use of PTAs and aides. These positions were necessary to meet the growing demand for services.

The headquarters of the APTA was relocated to Washington, DC, in 1971 to increase political involvement. Executive operations were further strengthened when two adjacent office buildings were purchased in nearby Alexandria, Virginia, in 1983.

New education programs were developed in an attempt to keep pace with the demand; curricular evolution was inherent as health care in general expanded. This period opened with an APTA policy in 1960 declaring the baccalaureate degree to be the minimum educational requirement for a PT. By the late 1970s, it became clear that a postbaccalaureate degree would be necessary to master the knowledge and skills required for competent practice. Consequently, a critical policy adopted by the APTA in 1979 (amended in 1980) stated that new and existing programs in physical therapy must award a postbaccalaureate degree by December 31, 1990. This requirement had a major impact on curricular development.

This period also saw an evolution in the historical link between the AMA and the APTA (formerly APA) regarding approval (accreditation) of educational programs. The APTA became more actively involved in the accreditation process. In 1974 it adopted the Essentials of an Accredited Educational Program for the Physical Therapist, which represented a dramatic departure from the prescriptions in the 1955 Essentials.[13] In 1977, the Commission on Accreditation in Education (a body separate from, but administratively supported by, the APTA) became recognized by the U.S. Office of Education and Council on Postsecondary Education as an accrediting agency. Standards for Accreditation of Physical Therapy Educational Programs was adopted by the APTA in 1979. In 1983, after contesting the value of the AMA in the accreditation process, the Commission on Accreditation in Education became the sole agency for accrediting education programs for PTs and PTAs. This recognition marked the maturity of the profession.

Increased demand for services and educational requirements resulted in advances in practice opportunities. The profession lobbied aggressively at the state level for direct access: the right to conduct patient examinations and interventions without a physician's referral. The patient was the ultimate beneficiary: health care costs were reduced (no required physician visit), and physical therapy could begin sooner. In 1957, Nebraska became the first state to have direct access. The second state to enact legislation for direct access was California in 1968. Legislation proliferated through the 1980s, and by the end of the decade, direct access was legal in 24 states.

Advances in practice fostered new opportunities to demonstrate excellence. The American Board of Physical Therapy Specialties was created by the APTA in 1978. This provided a mechanism for PTs to become certified and recognized as clinical specialists in certain practice areas.

The need for research to substantiate physical therapy interventions became essential. This was particularly true as insurance providers began to challenge the cost of health care. The Foundation for Physical Therapy was initiated in 1979 to promote and support research in physical therapy.

1990s

During the 1990s, skyrocketing costs of health care resulted in significant cost control measures in the private and government sectors. New methods of financing and reimbursing health care, created by the proliferation of managed care and the Balanced Budget Act of 1997, had a direct impact on the delivery of health care services, including physical therapy. Costs were controlled by limitation of the type, number, and reimbursement amounts for services. The circumstances of PTs and PTAs deteriorated as job availability and salaries plateaued and then declined in some facilities. This unfavorable situation was compounded by the continued proliferation of education programs. One study predicted a surplus of PTs by the end of the decade.[16] Unemployment suddenly became a real issue.

Practice issues had a domino effect on education. With a tight job market, applications to PT and PTA education programs dropped. In fact, many of the programs for PTAs closed voluntarily because of limited enrollment. Eventually, the APTA established a position recommending against the development of new education programs.

The shift to postbaccalaureate education gave rise to several national conferences, which resulted in documents that described the values and preferences in PT and PTA education programs. A Normative Model of Physical Therapist Professional Level Education: Version 2004 was originally developed in 1994-95 to provide guidance to these programs.[17] Similar activities for PTA education programs resulted in a parallel document for these programs first published in 1999 and revised in 2007.[18]

Although the need for clinical research had been known for decades, the controls imposed by third-party payers were a direct call for research that would justify physical therapy services. First published in 1995, the *Guide to Physical Therapist Practice* provided a comprehensive and detailed description of physical therapy services, but research was needed to substantiate these services. A Clinical Research Agenda for Physical Therapy was established to identify areas where research was needed and feasible. Programs offered by the Foundation for Physical Therapy to fund research were expanded. The developing concept of **evidence-based practice** (practice based on proof) was promoted through the new Hooked on Evidence program.[19] (See Chapter 2 for additional description of evidence-based practice.) This provided a user-friendly database of current literature pertinent to the practice of physical therapy. APTA members were able to review journal articles and submit a critical analysis to the database for use by clinicians. New accreditation criteria for PT education programs increased the expectation regarding faculty scholarship. These new opportunities and expectations created by external and internal forces combined to promote further research activities in the profession.

Through the course of this period, the APTA took a strong leadership role in addressing the issues. Extensive lobbying and rallying of public sentiment resulted in legislation that protected patients' rights in managed care organizations and lifted a major funding cap in the Medicare program for physical therapy services. Several task forces were established to consider the role and governance rights of PTAs. Final reports were instrumental in new policies and positions that clarified their clinical role, education level, continuing education opportunities, recognition of advance proficiencies, and governance rights. In 1998 a separate deliberative body for PTAs, the Representative Body of the National Assembly, was approved. The decade closed with a bright outlook for improvements in the future.

TWENTY-FIRST CENTURY

The twenty-first century opened with an evolutionary action by the APTA House of Delegates when, in the year 2000, it adopted the APTA **Vision Statement for Physical Therapy 2020** (Box 1-5; see Box 7-1 for the shortened version, the Vision Sentence).[20] Commonly cited as **Vision 2020**, it has become a beacon for the profession and has provided a distinct direction for current and future action. Its six key components address the areas of practice, education, and research: (1) autonomous practice, (2) direct access, (3) practitioner of choice, (4) Doctor of Physical Therapy (DPT), (5) evidence-based practice, and (6) professionalism. It soon became the source for follow-up action by the Board of Directors and House of Delegates to further define these elements and establish goals and actions to achieve them. Some examples of these actions follow.

In 2003, the APTA Board of Directors issued a position listing and describing the elements of **autonomous practice**. This was subsequently updated and adopted by the House of Delegates (Box 1-6).[21] This position indicates that PTs have the capability to exercise professional judgment to practice under direct access within their scope of practice and refer patients and clients to other health care professionals when necessary. These attributes reiterate the importance of autonomy of judgment as one of the highest, if not the highest, characteristic of a profession.

In the same year the Board of Directors approved another document related to the Vision Statement, "Professionalism in Physical Therapy: Core Values," developed by a consensus conference method (Table 1-1).[22] The purpose of identifying and describing these **core values** was to assist the transition to a doctoring profession by articulating what a PT practitioner would do in her or his daily

BOX 1-5

American Physical Therapy Association (APTA) Vision Statement for Physical Therapy 2020

- Physical therapy, by 2020, will be provided by physical therapists who are doctors of physical therapy and who may be board-certified specialists. Consumers will have direct access to physical therapists in all environments for patient/client management, prevention, and wellness services. Physical therapists will be practitioners of choice in patients'/clients' health networks and will hold all privileges of autonomous practice. Physical therapists may be assisted by physical therapist assistants who are educated and licensed to provide physical therapist–directed and –supervised components of interventions.
- Guided by integrity, lifelong learning, and a commitment to comprehensive and accessible health programs for all people, physical therapists and physical therapist assistants will render evidence-based services throughout the continuum of care and improve quality of life for the society. They will provide culturally sensitive care distinguished by trust, respect, and an appreciation for individual differences.
- While fully availing themselves of new technologies, as well as basic and clinical research, physical therapists will continue to provide direct patient/client care. They will maintain active responsibility for the growth of the physical therapy profession and the health of the people it serves.

From American Physical Therapy Association (APTA): *APTA Vision Sentence for Physical Therapy 2020 and APTA Vision Statement for Physical Therapy 2020*, HOD P06-00-24-35, House of Delegates Policies, Positions, and Guidelines, Alexandria, VA, 2009, APTA.

BOX 1-6

Autonomous Physical Therapist Practice

Physical therapists have the responsibility to practice autonomously in all settings, practice environments, and employment relationships.
Autonomous physical therapist practice is characterized by:
- Independent, self-determined professional judgment within one's scope of practice, consistent with the profession's codes and standards and in the patient's/client's best interest.
- Responsibility and acceptance of risk for all aspects of the physical therapist patient/client management.
- Ability to refer to and collaborate with health care providers and others to enhance the physical therapist patient/client management.
- Recognition of circumstances that necessitate a request for consultation and initiation of such consultation when in the best interest of the patient/client.
- Clinical decision making that is independent of external financial considerations.
- Physical therapist governance and control of physical therapy practice in all settings.

From American Physical Therapy Association (APTA): *Autonomous physical therapist practice: definitions and privileges*, BOD P03-03-12-28, Board of Directors Standards, Positions, Guidelines, Policies, and Procedures, Alexandria, VA, 2009, APTA.

Table 1-1
Core Values of Professionalism in Physical Therapy

Core Value	Definition
Accountability	Accountability is active acceptance of the responsibility for the diverse roles, obligations, and actions of the physical therapist, including self-regulation and other behaviors that positively influence patient/client outcomes, the profession, and health needs of society
Altruism	Altruism is the primary regard for or devotion to the interest of patients/clients, thus assuming the fiduciary responsibility of placing the needs of the patient/client ahead of the physical therapist's self-interest
Compassion/ caring	Compassion is the desire to identify with or sense something of another's experience; a precursor of caring Caring is the concern, empathy, and consideration for the needs and values of others
Excellence	Excellence is physical therapy practice that consistently uses current knowledge and theory while understanding personal limits, integrates judgment and the patient/client perspective, embraces advancement, challenges mediocrity, and works toward development of new knowledge
Integrity	Integrity is steadfast adherence to high ethical principles or professional standards
Professional duty	Professional duty is the commitment to meeting one's obligations to provide effective physical therapy services to individual patients/clients, to serve the profession, and to positively influence the health of society
Social responsibility	Social responsibility is the promotion of a mutual trust between the profession and the large public that necessitates responding to societal needs for health and wellness

From *Professionalism in physical therapy: core values.* BOD P05-04-02-03. American Physical Therapy Association.[21]

practice to demonstrate professional behavior. This document has focused greater attention on professional behaviors and how to teach and emulate them.

Continued lobbying efforts were successful in advancing direct access legislation. Evidence became available to demonstrate the fiscal and human benefits of this practice delivery model. One study concluded the total paid claims for physician-referred physical therapy were 2.2 times higher than paid claims to PTs practicing in direct access states.[23] Direct access finally became legal in all 50 states and the District of Columbia in 2014.[24]

Perhaps the most dramatic impact generated by Vision 2020 was in PT education programs. No one predicted the rapid pace of transition to the DPT degree created by the opening sentence. The first class of PTs with the designation "DPT" graduated in 1996 from Creighton University in Omaha, Nebraska, but by 2010 nearly all professional-level PT education programs were at the doctoral level. One of the reasons for this rapid transition was that most of the existing PT education programs already far exceeded the minimal curricular requirements for the master's degree, which was the common degree awarded. Another was that this was a professional doctorate (e.g., MD, JD), which requires advanced education and practice in the profession, unlike the academic doctorate (e.g., PhD, EdD), which requires extensive research to generate new knowledge.

As the doctoral degree rapidly became the entrance degree for graduates into the profession, these new professionals began to seek advanced education and training to maintain their sense of a "doctoring" profession. The American Board of Physical Therapy Residency and Fellowship Education was created by the Board of Directors to review and accredit postprofessional residency and fellowship programs in physical therapy.[25] These have become increasingly popular as new graduates seek to continue their education and training as they enter the profession. With the growth and development of education for PTs, leaders in physical therapy education decided it was imperative to establish a stronger voice and role. The American Council of Academic Physical Therapy (ACAPT) was created as a council under the Board of Directors of the APTA in 2010 to promote the highest standards of excellence in physical therapist education, including clinical and postprofessional education, and subsequently became a component of the APTA by action of the House of Delegates in 2013.[26]

This period also experienced further analysis and evolution of organizational structure of the APTA as it affected the PTA. In 2005, after an extensive review of the limited effectiveness of the Representative Body of the National Assembly, the APTA House of Delegates replaced it with the PTA Caucus, which had its first meeting in 2006. This entity consisted of representatives from all the chapters of the APTA and provided nonvoting delegates to the House of Delegates. Other mechanisms for direct input from the PTA community to the Board of Directors, such as the Advisory Panel of Physical Therapist Assistants, were also approved. These and other related changes that pertain to PTAs, such as consideration of the baccalaureate degree, are further described in Chapter 3.

Research was further promoted when the Hooked on Evidence program was open to nonmembers of the APTA. This was limited to article searches. Additional resources for article searches were established in the Open Door program, which subsequently became known as Article Search.[27] This program permits APTA members to search several prominent databases in the medical literature and access thousands of publications.

As this period continued, leaders within the profession began to question whether the expectations of Vision 2020 were either met or should be updated. After considerable work by a designated task force and discussion by the House of Delegates, the latter body adopted a new Vision Statement for the Physical Therapy Profession in 2013 (Box 1-7).[28] A companion document, Guiding Principles to Achieve the Vision,[29] was also adopted and described how the profession and society would appear once the vision was achieved. The principles addressed Identity, Quality, Collaboration, Value, Innovation, Consumer-centricity, Access/Equity, and Advocacy. The *Guide to Physical*

BOX 1-7

Vision Statement for Physical Therapy
Transforming society by optimizing movement to improve the human experience.

Vision Statement for Physical Therapy and Guiding Principles to Achieve the Vision. Reprinted from http://www.apta.org, with permission of the American Physical Therapy Association, Copyright © 2015 American Physical Therapy Association.

Therapist Practice was revised and updated to become a more internal document. The document was originally directed to policy makers to inform them about the description of physical therapy. Other resources now provide this information; therefore, the current version is directed to PTs and PTAs.

Although the first decade of the new century opened with a limited job market for PTs and PTAs, the outlook changed dramatically for the better. Employment projections for these two groups over the period from 2012 to 2022 are excellent: 36% for PTs and 41% for PTAs.[30] This presents an excellent future for the profession.

Issues continue to impact the profession and are under review and consideration by the APTA. These include permanent removal of the Medicare cap on reimbursement for outpatient rehabilitation services (combines physical therapy and speech-language pathology), whether there should be service extenders besides PTAs, the possibility of moving the degree requirement for the PTA to the baccalaureate level, and the identification and implementation of best practice in clinical education. The profession continues to "move forward" (APTA's branding campaign) as the needs of society evolve.

SUMMARY

Physical therapy is a profession that enjoys a proud heritage. From the reconstruction aides of World War I to the autonomous practitioners of today, PTs continue to provide services to reduce pain, improve function, and maintain health. As a preamble to the remainder of the text, this chapter provided a definition of physical therapy and the qualities that characterize it as a profession, particularly autonomy of judgment. The history of the profession was traced from its origins in World War I. The influence of poliomyelitis and world wars, relationships with the AMA, development of the APTA, and recognition as a profession were described. In the decades after World War II, growth and development were paramount features of the profession until managed care and other forces for cost control in health care took hold in the 1990s. The millennium ended with a tight job market that had an unfavorable impact on education programs. The twenty-first century opened with Vision 2020, which set new goals and instigated follow-up action. The job market improved, and this helped lead to the rapid establishment of DPT and residency programs. Research was further promoted by the Hooked on Evidence program and higher expectations of faculty. The rights of PTAs within the profession continued to evolve. A new Vision Statement and Guiding Principles focused on the needs of society and how physical therapy can improve that experience. The profession was on the move to achieve the principles of the new Vision Statement.

REFERENCES

1. Hislop HJ: The not-so-impossible dream, *Phys Ther* 55:1069–1080, 1975.
2. Guidelines: Physical Therapist Scope of Practice. BOD G02-14-18-12. American Physical Therapy Association. http://www.apta.org/uploadedFiles/APTAorg/About_Us/Policies/Practice/ScopePractice.pdf#search=%22model%20definition%20of%20physical%20therapy%. Accessed September 23, 2014.
3. Guide to Physical Therapist Practice 3.0. American Physical Therapy Association. http://guidetoptpractice.apta.org/. Accessed September 23, 2014.
4. Provision of Physical Therapy Interventions and Related Tasks. HOD P06-00-17-28. American Physical Therapy Association. http://www.apta.org/uploadedFiles/APTAorg/About_Us/Policies/Practice/ProvisionInterventions.pdf#search=%22provision%20of%20physical%20therapy%20interventions%20related%20tasks%22. Accessed September 24, 2014.
5. Physical Therapy as a Health Profession. HOD P06-99-19-23. American Physical Therapy Association. http://www.apta.org/uploadedFiles/APTAorg/About_Us/Policies/Practice/PhysicalTherapyHealthProfession.pdf#search=%22position%20on%20physical%20therapy%20as%20a%20health%20profession%22. Accessed September 24, 2014.
6. Swisher LL, Page CG: *Professionalism in physical therapy: history, practice, & development,* St. Louis, 2005, Elsevier.
7. Moore WE: *The professions: roles and rules,* New York, 1970, Russell Sage Foundation.
8. Standards and Required Elements for Accreditation of Physical Therapist Education Programs. http://www.capteonline.org/uploadedFiles/CAPTEorg/About_CAPTE/Resources/Accreditation_Handbook/CAPTE_PTStandardsEvidence.pdf. Commission on Accreditation in Physical Therapy Education. Accessed May 18, 2015.
9. Standards and Required Elements for Accreditation of Physical Therapist Assistant Education Programs. http://www.capteonline.org/uploadedFiles/CAPTEorg/About_CAPTE/Resources/Accreditation_Handbook/CAPTE_PTAStandardsEvidence.pdf. Commission on Accreditation in Physical Therapy Education. Accessed May 18, 2015.
10. Granger FB: The development of physiotherapy, *Phys Ther* 56:13–14, 1976.
11. Davies EJ: The beginning of "modern physiotherapy."*Phys Ther* 56:15–21, 1976.
12. Davies EJ: Infantile paralysis, *Phys Ther* 56:42–49, 1976.
13. Pinkston D: Evolution of the practice of physical therapy in the United States. In Scully RM, Barnes ML, editors: *Phys Ther*, Philadelphia, 1989, Lippincott.
14. Beard G: Foundations for growth: a review of the first forty years in terms of education, practice, and research, *Phys Ther Rev* 41:843–861, 1961.
15. Hazenhyer IM: A history of the American Physiotherapy Association, *Physiother Rev* 26(1):3–14, 1946.
16. Vector Research, Inc: *Executive summary, workforce study,* Alexandria, VA, 1997, American Physical Therapy Association.
17. A normative model of physical therapist professional education: version 2004, Alexandria, VA, 2004, American Physical Therapy Association.
18. A normative model of physical therapist assistant education: version 2007, Alexandria, VA, 2007, American Physical Therapy Association.
19. Hooked on Evidence. http://www.hookedonevidence.org/search.cfm?CFID=93323612&CFTOKEN=221c98542241d946-A9FC5E37-B9F3-68D9-B4DFEF392405E119. Accessed September 24, 2014.
20. *Vision 2020.* American Physical Therapy Association. http://www.apta.org/Vision2020/. Accessed September 24, 2014.
21. Autonomous Physical Therapist Practice. HOD P06-06-18-12. American Physical Therapy Association. http://www.apta.org/uploadedFiles/APTAorg/About_Us/Policies/Practice/AutonomousPTPractice.pdf#search=%22autonomous%20practice%22. Accessed September 24, 2014.
22. Professionalism in Physical Therapy: Core Values. BOD P05-04-02-03. American Physical Therapy Association. http://www.apta.org/uploadedFiles/APTAorg/About_Us/Policies/BOD/Judicial/ProfessionalisminPT.pdf. Accessed September 24, 2014.
23. Mitchell JM, de Lissovoy G: A comparison of resource use and cost in direct access versus physician episodes of physical therapy, *Phys Ther* 77:10–18, 1997.
24. New Michigan Law Means All 51 Jurisdictions Allow Direct Access to PTs. http://www.apta.org/PTinMotion/NewsNow/2014/7/1/MichiganDirectAccess/. Accessed September 24, 2014.

25. American Board of Physical Therapy Residency and Fellowship Education. http://www.abptrfe .org/Home.aspx. Accessed September 24, 2014.

26. ACAPT. http://acapt.org/. Accessed September 24, 2014.

27. Article search. http://www.ptnow.org/ArticleSearch/Default.aspx. Accessed September 27, 2014.

28. Vision Statement for Physical Therapy. http://www.apta.org/Vision/. Accessed September 24, 2014.

29. Guiding Principles to Achieve the Vision. http://www.apta.org/Vision/. Accessed September 24, 2014.

30. Occupational Outlook Handbook. United States Department of Labor. Bureau of Labor Statistics. http://data.bls.gov/search/query/results?cx=013738036195919377644%3A6ih0hfrgl50& q=physical+therapy+inurl%3Abls.gov%2Fooh%2F. Accessed September 24, 2014.

ADDITIONAL RESOURCES

American Physical Therapy Association: *Healing the generations: a history of physical therapy and the American Physical Therapy Association,* Lyme, CT, 1995, Greenwich Publishing Group. Comprehensive and detailed description of the history and evolution of the profession and practice of physical therapy in the United States.

Hazenhyer IM: A history of the American Physical Therapy Association: 2. Formative years, 1926-1930, *Physiother Rev* 26(2):66–74, 1946. Describes the pertinent issues confronting the profession during this period, including the first published curriculum and a review of educational programs, controversy over technicians versus professionals, legislation to regulate practice, and growth of the journal.

Hazenhyer IM: A history of the American Physical Therapy Association: 3. Coming of age, 1931-1938, *Physiother Rev* 26(3):122–129, 1946. Continues description of issues in previous article as they evolved during this pre–World War II period.

Hazenhyer IM: A history of the American Physical Therapy Association: 4. Maturity, 1939-1946, *Physiother Rev* 26(4):174–184, 1946. In this final article in the series, the author describes issues involving membership rights, chapter organizations, further curricular changes, impact of the National Foundation for Infantile Paralysis, activities in military service, and the journal.

www.apta.org. Website of the American Physical Therapy Association. Excellent resource for current information and documents pertinent to the profession.

REVIEW QUESTIONS

1. How does the APTA's *definition* of physical therapy differ from its *philosophical statement*?

2. Explain the differences between the practice and the profession of physical therapy, and identify the documents that describe each.

3. Define *profession*, and apply its five characteristics to physical therapy. Is physical therapy a profession?

4. How did polio and World Wars I and II affect the origin and evolution of physical therapy in the United States?

5. Describe how the relationship between the AMA and what was eventually to become the APTA changed from the 1920s through the 1980s.

6. What impact has Vision 2020 had on the profession of physical therapy? How does the new Vision Statement differ from Vision 2020?

7. How has the education of physical therapists evolved since the turn of the century?

All *physical therapists, regardless of title or position, function in multiple capacities, shifting from one to another as the situation demands. For example, the clinician serves as a teacher, a supervisor, a negotiator, a clinician researcher, an advocate, and a business administrator. Physical therapists in other positions not only share those functions but may assume additional ones as well.*
Geneva R. Johnson

2 Roles and Characteristics of Physical Therapists

Michael A. Pagliarulo

Screening
Secondary care
SOAP note
Standards of Practice for Physical Therapy
Systems review
Tertiary care
Tests and measures
Work hardening/conditioning

LEARNING OBJECTIVES

After reading this chapter, the reader will be able to:

1. Describe the roles of the physical therapist in primary, secondary, and tertiary care.

2. Describe the roles of the physical therapist in prevention and health promotion.
3. Describe the components of the patient/client management model.
4. Describe general features of tests and measures and interventions used in physical therapy.
5. Describe other professional roles of the physical therapist in the areas of consultation, education, critical inquiry, and administration.
6. List and describe the demographic characteristics of physical therapists.

In the past two decades, the demand for physical therapists (PTs) and physical therapist assistants (PTAs) and the recognition and reimbursement for services they provide have evolved dramatically. This transformation has resulted from several trends and outside influences, including the aging population, federal legislation entitling children in public schools to health care, a burgeoning interest in personal fitness, and actions taken by insurance companies and the government to contain the rising cost of health care. PTs and PTAs have had to adapt to these rapid and extensive changes, which at times have been frustrating to comprehend and accommodate. A Putnam Investments advertisement aptly summarizes these sentiments: "You think you understand the situation, but what you don't understand is that the situation just changed."[1]

The profession of physical therapy has succeeded and will continue to succeed. We have followed several of the ground rules proposed by Price Pritchett, including becoming quick-change artists, accepting ambiguity, and holding ourselves accountable for our individual actions.[1] To provide a framework for understanding the profession in the context of change, this chapter examines the diverse and shifting roles of PTs, the breadth of services provided, and the variety of employment settings where these services exist. Recent demographic data and information on employment activities and conditions are presented. More specific descriptions of the clinical functions performed by PTs and PTAs in the delivery of services are presented in Part 2 of this text. This chapter focuses on the roles and characteristics of the PT; those for the PTA are covered in Chapter 3.

ROLES IN THE PROVISION OF PHYSICAL THERAPY

The primary role of a PT involves direct patient care. Although PTs engage in many other activities and in some cases no longer participate in clinical practice, patient care remains the predominant employment activity. For this reason, the **Standards of Practice for Physical Therapy** is perhaps the foremost core document approved by the House of Delegates of the American Physical Therapy Association (APTA) and serves as a foundation to the delivery of physical therapy. As noted in the preamble to the document, "These standards are the profession's statement of conditions and performances that are essential for provision of high-quality professional service to society, and provide a foundation for the assessment of physical therapist practice."[2] The sections of the Standards are as follows:

I. Ethical/Legal Considerations.
II. Administration of the Physical Therapy Service.
III. Patient/Client Management.
IV. Education.
V. Research.
VI. Community Responsibility.

Each section provides performance statements for excellence in clinical practice. Note that these areas include those that contribute to high-quality patient care, such as administration of the service and application of research findings.

A second document fundamental to the description of patient care, is the *Guide to Physical Therapist Practice 3.0 (the Guide).*[3] This was revised in 2014 to focus more on the interests of physical therapists and physical therapist assistants, rather than outside parties, such as policy makers, as it did in its original form. It serves as a reference for most of the material that follows in this chapter.

CONCEPTS THAT INFORM PHYSICAL THERAPIST PRACTICE

The *Guide* lists and describes four concepts that are essential to the practice of physical therapy.[3] The first is the International Classification of Functioning, Disability and Health (ICF) and the Biopsychosocial Model. The ICF is a standardized method to classify health used by the World Health Organization. By its very nature, it focuses on *a*bility rather than *dis*ability. It includes both a description of the components of functioning as well as the environment, which could alter the degree of performance (see Figure 12-3 and Table 12-1). The Biopsychosocial model adds the concept of biological, psychological, and social domains, which likewise impact the degree of performance.

Evidence-based practice is the second concept fundamental to the practice of physical therapy. In this approach to health care the therapist combines (1) the best available evidence, (2) clinical expertise of the provider, and (3) the values and circumstances of the patient/client. This ensures that the therapist uses well-documented and supported contemporary practice within the context of the patient/client. Several tools are available to access published literature and other relative information, such as clinical practice guidelines, through PTNow.[4] This electronic resource through APTA was designed and implemented for the convenience and needs of PTs and PTAs in the clinical environment.

The third basic concept in the delivery of physical therapy is Professional Values and Guiding Documents. Professional Values were identified and described following the adoption of Vision 2020 to clearly delineate practice expectations in the area of professionalism (see Table 1-1 for a description of these core values). The *Code of Ethics for the Physical Therapist* also provides practice expectations based upon values through eight principles (see Box 5-2 for the *Code of Ethics*). Another guiding document is the *Standards of Practice for Physical Therapists,* which address not only clinical practice, but the overall service delivery environment as described earlier in this chapter.

Quality Assessment is the final generic concept regarding physical therapist practice. This measures the effectiveness of the service and considers the structure, processes, and outcomes. These measures are done systematically and continuously.

PRIMARY, SECONDARY, AND TERTIARY CARE

Individuals who seek health care, such as physical therapy, may move through multiple levels of providers as they enter the system and may eventually reach a specialist. The first level of care, **primary care**, is defined as the level of health care delivered by a member of the health care system who is responsible for the majority of the health needs of the individual.[3] This level of care usually, but not always, is provided by the first health care provider in contact with the recipient. Family and community members may also provide care at this level. **Secondary care** is provided by clinicians on a referral basis—that is, after the individual has received care at the primary level. In **tertiary care** the service is provided by specialists, commonly in facilities that focus on particular health conditions. These services may also be provided on a referral basis.

PTs are engaged in practice at all three levels of care. Physical therapy is most often delivered by referral as secondary or tertiary care. Tertiary care may be provided in a highly specialized unit, such as a burn care center. The entry point for an individual seeking physical therapy services, however, is shifting to primary care. This is described as **direct access**. As Burch states, the phrase *direct access* is preferred to *practice without referral,* which implies no regard or interest in the critical services provided by practitioners in other disciplines.[5] Direct access is now legal for physical therapists in all 50 states and the District of Columbia. Individuals may obtain physical therapy services without having to obtain a referral from another health care provider. In this role, the PT serves as a gatekeeper for further health care services.

TEAM APPROACH

Regardless of the level of care provided, the PT works in collaboration with other health care professionals, including physicians, nurses, occupational therapists, dentists, social workers, speech-language pathologists, and orthotists/prosthetists. As people seek the services of other health care professionals, PTs collaborate with such practitioners as podiatrists, chiropractors, massage therapists, acupuncturists, and osteopaths. In addition, the therapist may communicate with other individuals, such as educators and insurers, for the ultimate benefit of the patient/client.

This collaborative approach has not only been promoted in practice, but in education as well under the umbrella term of **interprofessionalism**. The APTA supports this approach through action taken by the House of Delegates when it endorsed the four Interprofessional Education Collaborative (IPEC) Core Competency.[6] These competencies address values, roles, communication, and teamwork in both education and practice.

PREVENTION AND HEALTH PROMOTION

Fortunately, the general public has become more aware of healthy lifestyle habits and is engaging in activities and behavior that promote healthy living. By preventing or limiting dysfunction, individuals have more positive work and recreation experiences. In addition, the need for and cost of health care are reduced.

PTs, by virtue of their extensive education in normal body structure and function, are well qualified to provide services that prevent or limit dysfunction. These services may be categorized as **screening** or prevention activities.[3] In screening, the PT determines whether further services are needed from a PT or other health care professional. A common example is posture analysis of schoolchildren to determine whether scoliosis may be present. In **prevention** activities the PT provides services designed to prevent, limit, or reduce pain and dysfunction. These prevention activities are classified as primary (avoids the dysfunction), secondary (decreases the duration), or tertiary (limits the degree of disability). Business and health care industries have been cooperating to provide programs that will prevent injury and disease and thereby reduce health care costs while increasing productivity. PTs are directly involved in health promotion and wellness activities, both as consultants for establishment of programs and as providers of health care on site or in a health-related facility. The PT may conduct a **functional capacity evaluation,** which consists of an analysis of the ability to perform in the work environment, activities of daily living, or leisure activities.[7] The therapist may then design a **work hardening/conditioning** program. This is a treatment program designed to improve the individual's motor, skeletal, and cardiopulmonary systems as they relate to specific tasks. The goal is to return the individual to work.

PATIENT/CLIENT MANAGEMENT MODEL

The *Guide*[3] has been instrumental in defining and describing what PTs do as clinicians. These activities have been summarized in the patient/client management model (Figure 2-1). This model reflects the process of gathering information, analyzing the findings, designing a plan of care, and implementing that plan to result in optimal outcomes for the patient/client. Each phase of the model is described below.

EXAMINATION

The first component of the patient/client management model, **examination**, is the process of gathering information about the past and current status of the patient/client. It begins with a **history** to describe the past and current nature of the condition or health status of the patient/client. The type of information gathered is comprehensive and includes not only medical and surgical history, but several other areas, such as social and employment histories, functional status, status of major body systems, and living environment. Sources for this information include the patient/client, caregivers, other health professionals, and medical records. A **systems review** is then conducted to obtain general

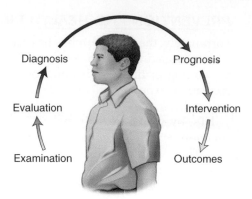

Figure 2-1 ■ The patient/client management model describes the sequence of events by which physical therapists perform the process of examination and intervention for individuals who receive care. (Modified from *Guide to Physical Therapist Practice 3.0.* American Physical Therapy Association. http://guidetoptpractice.apta.org/. Accessed September 29, 2014.)

information about the anatomic and physiologic status of the musculoskeletal, neuromuscular, cardiovascular/pulmonary, and integumentary systems, as well as the communication and cognitive abilities of the patient/client. In the final component of the examination, **tests and measures**, the therapist selects and performs specific procedures to quantify the physical and functional status of the patient/client. A list of these tests and measures as presented in the *Guide* appears in Table 2-1, and some examples are shown in Figure 2-2, *A-E.* Note that these activities involve observation, manual techniques, simple and complex equipment, and environmental analysis.

Along this process of data gathering, the therapist decides whether to: (1) retain the patient/client, (2) refer to other health care providers, (3) consult with other health care providers for advice, or (4) co-manage the patient/client with other providers. If the decision is not to refer to other providers, then the therapists proceed to the other phases of the patient/client management model.

EVALUATION

The **evaluation** is a clinical judgment based upon the findings from the history, systems review, and tests and measures. This step is integrally linked to establishing a diagnosis, prognosis, and plan of care. Throughout the episode of care, evaluation continues to determine whether any adjustments are necessary to these determinations.

DIAGNOSIS

Evaluation is essential to establish a **diagnosis**, the next component of the model. The diagnosis is a categorization of the findings from the examination through a defined process. Unlike a medical diagnosis determined by a physician, the PT

Table 2-1
Tests and Measures Used in a Physical Therapy Examination

Test or Measure	Description
Aerobic Capacity/Endurance	Ability to use the body's O_2 uptake and delivery system
Anthropometric Characteristics	Body dimensions and fat composition
Assistive Technology	Equipment used to improve function
Balance	Ability to maintain the body in equilibrium
Circulation (Arterial, Venous, Lymphatic)	Analysis of blood and lymph movement to determine adequacy of cardiovascular pump, circulation, oxygen delivery, and lymphatic drainage
Community, Social, and Civic Life	Ability to engage in social activity outside of the home
Cranial and Peripheral Nerve Integrity	Assessment of sensory and motor functions of cranial and peripheral nerves
Education Life	Abilities in schools and other education settings
Environmental Factors	Facilitators or barriers in person's physical, social, and attitudinal environment
Gait	Manner in which a person walks
Integumentary Integrity	Health of the skin
Joint Integrity and Mobility	Assessment of joint structure and passive movement
Mental Functions	Global (such as consciousness) and specific (such as memory) functions of the brain
Mobility (Including Locomotion)	Ability to change body positions or location
Motor Function	Control of voluntary movement
Muscle Performance (Including Strength, Power, Endurance, and Length)	Capacity of a muscle or group of muscles to generate force
Neuromotor Development and Sensory Processing	Evolution of movement skills and integration of information from the environment
Pain	Analysis of cause, intensity, quality, and frequency of pain
Posture	Analysis of body alignment and positioning
Range of Motion	Amount of active and passive movement at a joint
Reflex Integrity	Analysis of the neural pathway of the reflex to determine the performance of the neuromuscular system
Self-care and Domestic Life	Analysis of activities necessary for independent living at home

Continued

Table 2-1
Tests and Measures Used in a Physical Therapy Examination—cont'd

Test or Measure	Description
Sensory Integrity	Assessment of peripheral and central sensory processing, including awareness of movement, position, and object recognition
Skeletal Integrity	Analysis of the bony structures of the body
Ventilation and Respiration	Assessment of movement of air into and out of the lungs and exchange of gases to perform activities of daily living and exercises
Work Life	Analyses to determine whether the patient/client can assume or resume a role in work settings

Data from *Guide to Physical Therapist Practice 3.0,* American Physical Therapy Association. http://guidetoptpractice.apta.org/. Accessed September 29, 2014.

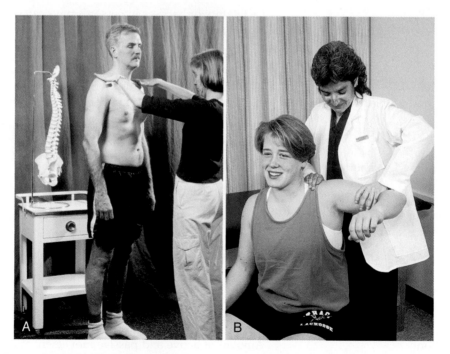

Figure 2-2 ■ Some components of the physical therapy examination that follow a history of the condition. **A**, Observation to determine the overall status of the condition. **B**, Manual muscle test; requires specific positioning and direction of resistance. **C**, Passive range of motion to determine amount of joint movement. **D**, Tests and measures may include the use of technical equipment. Here the therapist measures the conduction velocity of certain nerves. **E**, Physical therapists can conduct cardiovascular and fitness tests with a stationary bicycle. (Courtesy Dewey Neild.)

Continued

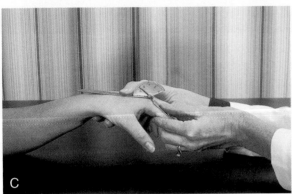

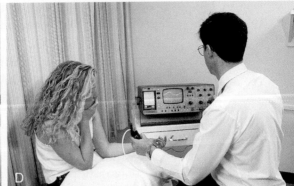

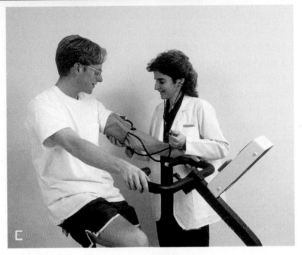

Figure 2-2 ■ Cont'd

establishes a diagnostic label that focuses on the impact that the condition has on function, particularly at the level of the whole person. The diagnosis by the PT is established in accordance with the law promulgated by the appropriate entity and the policy adopted by the House of Delegates of the APTA (Box 2-1).[8] This policy recognizes the professional and autonomous judgment of the PT and stipulates the responsibility for referral to other practitioners when warranted.

PROGNOSIS

Attention now shifts to the future to establish a **prognosis**, or a prediction of the level of improvement in function and time necessary to reach that level. The PT must incorporate the attitude and motivation of the patient/client in order to establish a prognosis that is realistic relevant to the unique characteristics of the individual.

At this point, the PT designs a **plan of care** that consists of the goals, outcomes, and interventions (including the duration and frequency). It is based upon the

BOX 2-1

Diagnosis by Physical Therapists

■ Physical therapists shall establish a diagnosis for each patient/client.

■ Prior to making a patient/client management decision, physical therapists shall utilize the diagnostic process in order to establish a diagnosis for the specific conditions in need of the physical therapist's attention.

■ A diagnosis is a label encompassing a cluster of signs and symptoms commonly associated with a disorder or syndrome or category of impairments in body structures and function, activity limitations, or participation restrictions. It is the decision reached as a result of the diagnostic process, which is the evaluation of information obtained from the patient/client examination. The purpose of the diagnosis is to guide the physical therapist in determining the most appropriate intervention strategy for each patient/client. In the event the diagnostic process does not yield an identifiable cluster, disorder, syndrome, or category, intervention may be directed toward the alleviation of symptoms and remediation of impairments in body structures and function, activity limitations, or participation restrictions.

■ The physical therapist's responsibility in the diagnostic process is to organize and interpret all relevant information collected. The diagnostic process includes obtaining relevant history, performing systems review, and selecting and administering specific tests and measures.

■ When indicated, physical therapists order appropriate tests, including but not limited to imaging and other studies, that are performed and interpreted by other health professionals. Physical therapists may also perform or interpret selected imaging or other studies.

■ In performing the diagnostic process, physical therapists may need to obtain additional information (including diagnostic labels) from other health professionals. In addition, as the diagnostic process continues, physical therapists may identify findings that should be shared with other health professionals, including referral sources, to ensure optimal patient/client care. When the patient/client is referred with a previously established diagnosis, the physical therapist should determine that the clinical findings are consistent with that diagnosis. If the diagnostic process reveals findings that are outside the scope of the physical therapist's knowledge, experience, or expertise, the physical therapist should then refer the patient/client to an appropriate practitioner.

findings of the examination, and the determination of the diagnosis and prognosis. The plan incorporates the input of the patient/client, and may include consultation with others involved with the care of the individual. **Goals** are the intended level of function expected at the conclusion of the episode of care. They must be written in terms that are measureable, oriented to function, and time sensitive. Only after these data-gathering and analysis activities have been completed can interventions begin.

INTERVENTION

Intervention occurs when the PT and PTA conduct procedures with the patient/client to achieve the desired outcomes. An intervention universal to all individuals under the care of the PT is patient or client instruction. This information, education, and training address the condition, current and expected functions, plan of care, and ongoing care. Family members and caregivers may be included in this interaction. The remaining interventions are more classical in that they involve direct therapeutic interaction of the PT or PTA with the patient/client. Categories of interventions are listed alphabetically in Table 2-2. Figure 2-3, *A-F*, illustrates some examples of these interventions, which include manual techniques (high touch) and equipment (high tech). At this point, a PTA would be involved in a substantial component of the care as delegated by the PT. This may include instruction in the community and home settings (Figure 2-4, *A-C*). Further descriptions of procedural interventions can be found in each chapter of Part II of this text.

Table 2-2
List of Intervention Categories Used in Physical Therapy

Intervention	Description
Airway Clearance Techniques	Activities to create or maintain clear airways
Assistive Technology: Prescription, Application, and, as Appropriate, Fabrication or Modification	Selection (or fabrication), fit, and training in the use of devices and equipment to improve function, prevent further impairments, and reduce pain
Biophysical Agents	Use of thermal, acoustic, electrical, or radiant energy, and mechanical equipment to decrease pain and swelling, and improve skin condition, joint movement, and neuromuscular performance
Functional Training in Self-care and in Domestic, Education, Work, Community, Social, and Civic Life	Activities to improve function in home, education, work, and community environments
Integumentary Repair and Protective Techniques	Activities to improve wound healing and scar management
Manual Therapy Techniques	Skilled hand techniques on soft tissues and joints to increase motion and reduce pain
Motor Function Training	Planned physical movements, postures, or activities
Therapeutic Exercise	Planned physical movements or activities to improve physical function and health status

Data from *Guide to Physical Therapist Practice 3.0*. American Physical Therapy Association. http://guidetoptpractice.apta.org/content/1/SEC31.body. Accessed September 29, 2014.

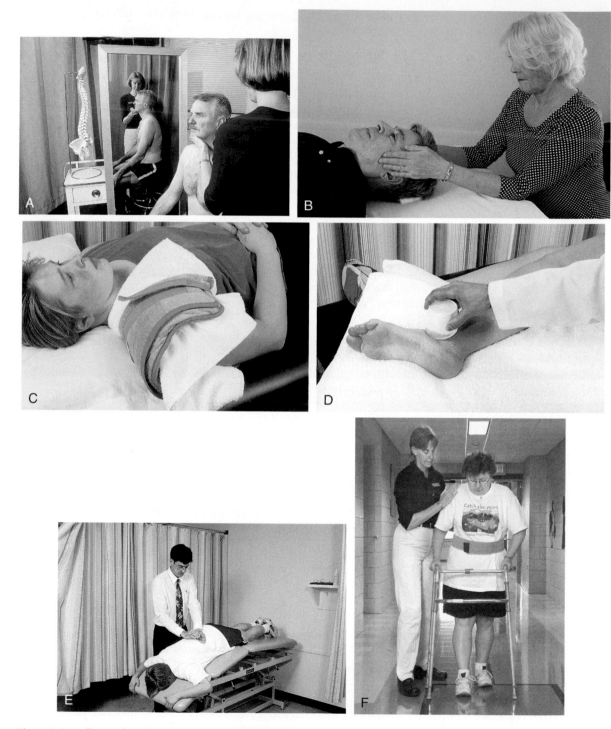

Figure 2-3 ■ Examples of interventions used in physical therapy. **A,** Posture correction with exercises and instruction. **B,** Myofascial release techniques in the temporomandibular joint region. **C,** Hot packs to provide superficial heat. **D,** Ice massage to decrease pain and swelling. **E,** Postural drainage to remove fluid from specific parts of the lungs. **F,** Ambulation training with the use of a walker. (Photo B courtesy Emily Maletz; all others courtesy Dewey Neild.)

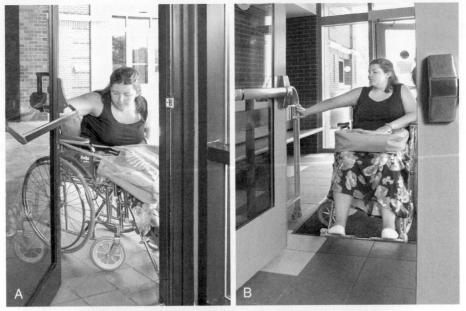

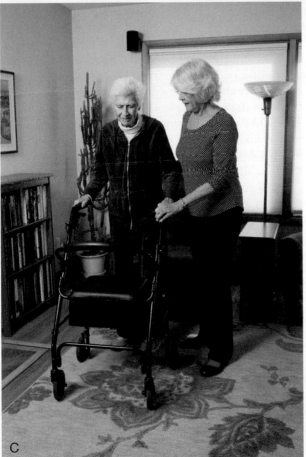

Figure 2-4 ■ Interventions may also involve activities in the community and home environments. **A** and **B**, The patient is instructed in how to negotiate doors without and with automated opening mechanisms. **C**, The patient is instructed in the use of a rolling walker in the home environment. (Photo C courtesy Emily Maletz; all others courtesy Dewey Neild.)

OUTCOMES

Outcomes are the result of the interventions and entire plan of care. Data are collected and analyzed to create reports to improve service.

Throughout the course of the patient/client management model, the PT may periodically conduct reexaminations to determine the effect of the plan of care. If goals and outcomes are not being achieved, the plan, goals, and outcomes may be modified or the patient/client may be referred to other practitioners for services.

COORDINATION, COMMUNICATION, AND DOCUMENTATION

A consistent exchange of information is essential to ensure that all personnel involved in care of the patient/client are well informed about his or her status. Interactions and the status of the patient/client must be documented and communicated with other members of the health care team in order to coordinate the services. Permanent records provide a baseline for future reference. They must be clear, concise, and accurate. Documentation is required by certain federal and state regulations and all insurance carriers. Fortunately, the APTA has constructed a set of guidelines—Physical Therapy Documentation for Patient/ Client Management[9]—to assist PTs in this area.

Written communication can follow many formats. Documentation regarding evaluation and treatment can be written as a narrative. This design allows maximum flexibility, but is unstructured. Standardized forms are frequently used as an efficient method of recording information. They are helpful, but the structure of the form may not apply to the particular patient/client situation.

The **SOAP note** combines the best attributes of the narrative and standardized form. It is taken from the problem-oriented medical record system introduced by Weed in 1969.[10] The SOAP note is structured yet adaptable and is widely used among health care practitioners. The four components are *S* for subjective (what the patient/client, or family member describes), *O* for objective (what the PT observes or measures), *A* for assessment (clinical judgment based on examination; includes goals), and *P* for plan (plan of care). The abbreviations provide an effective and efficient method for outlining and documenting patient information.

Computer technology has influenced documentation in health care and has been incorporated into several commercially available systems to create an **electronic health record.**[11] Some systems simply provide terminals for writing narratives, whereas others use handheld units to record information. This approach to documentation has become common in health care and provides an efficient means to access longitudinal information on the patient/client. It has been shown to reduce waste, errors, and unnecessary variation and utilization in practice, thereby reducing costs of health care. Moreover, payers are converting to this method of data entry and are requiring this for submission of insurance claims by providers.

Ultimately, physical therapy services will be concluded for each **episode of care**, defined as care provided for a specific condition over a set period of time.[2] This occurs when (1) goals or outcomes have been achieved, (2) the individual is no longer able to continue, or (3) the therapist believes that further intervention will not improve the status of the individual. In any case, the PT must plan for the conclusion of services and document reasons, status of the patient/client at that time, and any follow-up care that may be necessary.

OTHER PROFESSIONAL ROLES

CONSULTATION

PTs frequently provide consultation, that is, expert opinion or advice, at the request of the patient/client, another health care provider, an organization, business, school, or government agency. The purpose is to make recommendations concerning the current or proposed physical therapy for the patient/client or for services requested by the entity. Examples of the latter include court testimony, architectural recommendations, and suggestions for health care policies.

EDUCATION

PTs and PTAs are continually providing education to a variety of audiences, because instruction is an inherent part of patient care activity in physical therapy. Patients and sometimes family members are taught exercises or techniques to enhance function. Such instruction requires knowledge and skills that must be conveyed by the PT or PTA.

Instruction also occurs in the clinical facility when students are supervised during internships. Demonstration, supervision, and feedback are important for practicing and perfecting skills.

PTs and PTAs are involved in academic education. They may teach in a formal academic setting or a continuing education program.

CRITICAL INQUIRY

Critical inquiry in physical therapy is essential for the viability of the profession. This is the application of scientific principles to interpret professional literature, conduct research, and assess outcomes and new concepts. PTs and PTAs must be healthy skeptics and constantly ask, "Why?" They must be able to respond when practitioners and those who pay for their services question them about the choice and efficacy of their interventions. Practice must be based on sound evidence that comes from well-designed research (evidence-based practice). Figure 2-5 is an example of a motion analysis lab to conduct research on the movement of body components. Sound practice is an inherent responsibility of every PT and PTA and is based on the selection of appropriate interventions, complete documentation, and outcomes assessment.

ADMINISTRATION

PTs and PTAs may move into a variety of administrative positions. Generally, the promotion ladder in clinical facilities involves more administrative responsibilities at the expense of patient care activities. An individual could also leave the patient care environment and assume an executive position within a health care or related organization. Administrative responsibilities include planning, communicating, delegating, managing, directing, supervising, budgeting, and evaluating. These activities are particularly important when the PT is an owner or partner in an independent practice.

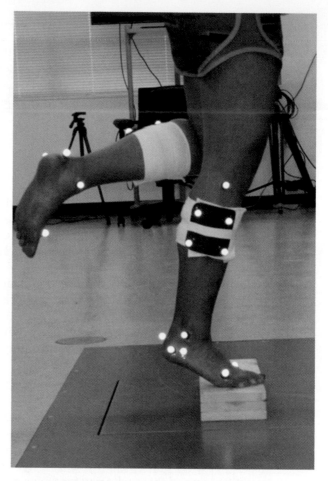

Figure 2-5 ■ Research is essential to demonstrate efficacy of physical therapy interventions.

CHARACTERISTICS OF PHYSICAL THERAPISTS

Demographic information on PTs is presented here; comparable information for PTAs is included in Chapter 3. These data are taken from annual surveys conducted by the APTA based on a sample of members.[12]

DEMOGRAPHICS

GENDER

Women continue to predominate in the profession of physical therapy. In 2013, they accounted for 70% of the PTs who were members of the APTA.

AGE

The mean age of the respondents in 2013 was 44 years. A modest and progressive increase in this figure has been noted (39 years in 2000); however, the members of the profession remain relatively young.

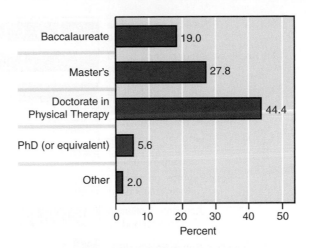

2

Figure 2-6 ■ Highest earned degree achieved by physical therapists who are members of the American Physical Therapy Association. (Data from *Physical Therapist Demographic Information.* http://www.apta.org/WorkforceData/. Accessed September 9, 2014.)

EDUCATION

The highest earned academic degree of PT members is displayed in Figure 2-6. This represents a continual and significant shift toward the Doctor of Physical Therapy (DPT) degree in comparison with past data. For example, in 2005, 30.5% of the respondents in a membership survey held a bachelor's degree, 45.9% held a master's degree, and only 15.2% held the DPT (either entry-level or postprofessional) as the highest earned degree. In 2013, these figures were 19%, 27.8%, and 44.4%, respectively. This reflects the proliferation of DPT degree programs and requirement for programmatic accreditation by December 31, 2015.

EMPLOYMENT FACILITY

A review of Figure 2-7 reveals that the highest percentage of respondents, 33%, are employed in a private office. The distribution of these employment settings has remained essentially unchanged since 2010. Regardless of the type of employment facility, the vast majority of respondents, 81.1%, held full-time positions (salaried, hourly, or self-employed).

SUMMARY

The roles and activities of PTs continue to evolve to meet the changing needs of society and new requirements in the payment systems for services. Despite these changes, diversity and opportunity remain widespread in physical therapy. Direct patient/client care continues to be the primary activity of PTs. Such care involves examination, evaluation, diagnosis, prognosis, intervention, and outcomes as outlined in the patient/client management model. PTs also provide services to prevent pain and dysfunction and promote health. Other roles include consultation, education, critical inquiry, and administration. Regardless of the

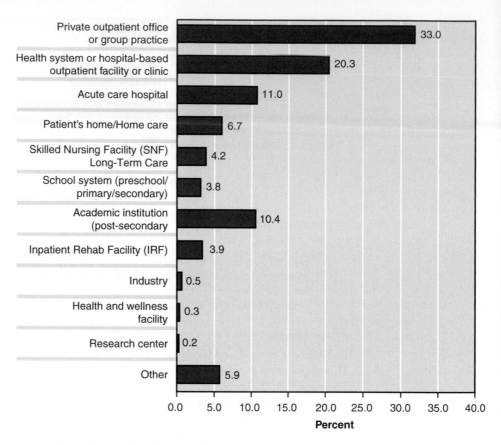

Figure 2-7 ■ Distribution of physical therapists who are members of the American Physical Therapy Association by facility of employment. (Data from *Physical Therapist Demographic Information*. http://www.apta.org/ WorkforceData/. Accessed September 9, 2014.)

area of activity, PTs collaborate with other health care providers as part of an interprofessional team.

In terms of demographics, the majority of PTs continue to be female and relatively young. The DPT degree now predominates as the highest earned degree. The most common employment facility is a private office.

The characteristics described here indicate that the profession continues to evolve and succeed. Such attributes contribute to the popularity of the profession and the enthusiasm of many individuals for pursuing a career as a PT or PTA.

REFERENCES

1. Pritchett P: *The employee handbook of New Work Habits for a radically changing world: 13 ground rules of job success in the information age*, Dallas, 2012, Pritchett & Associates.
2. *Standards of Practice for Physical Therapy*. HOD S06-10-09-06. American Physical Therapy Association. http://www.apta.org/uploadedFiles/APTAorg/About_Us/Policies/Practice/ StandardsPractice.pdf. Accessed September 27, 2014.

2

3. *Guide to Physical Therapist Practice 3.0*. American Physical Therapy Association. http://guidetoptpractice.apta.org/. Accessed September 28, 2014.
4. PTNow. http://www.ptnow.org/Default.aspx. Accessed September 28, 2014.
5. Burch E: Direct access. In Matthews J, editor: *Practice issues in physical therapy*, Thorofare, NJ, 1989, Slack.
6. Endorsement of Interprofessional Education Collaborative core competencies. American Physical Therapy Association. http://www.apta.org/uploadedFiles/APTAorg/About_Us/Policies/Education/EndordementofInterprofessional%20Education.pdf#search=%22interprofessionalism%22. Accessed September 28, 2014.
7. Glossary of workers' compensation terms. American Physical Therapy Association. http://www.apta.org/Payment/WorkersCompensation/Glossary/. Accessed September 29, 2014.
8. Diagnosis by physical therapists. HOD P06-12-10-09. American Physical Therapy Association. http://www.apta.org/uploadedFiles/APTAorg/About_Us/Policies/Practice/Diagnosis.pdf#search=%22diagnosis%2. Accessed September 29, 2014.
9. *Guidelines: Physical Therapy Documentation of Patient/Client Management*. BOD G03-05-16-41. American Physical Therapy Association. http://www.apta.org/uploadedFiles/APTAorg/About_Us/Policies/Practice/DocumentationPatientClientManagement.pdf#search=%22guidelines%20for%20documentation%22. Accessed September 29. 2014.
10. Weed LL: *Medical records, medical education and patient care,* Chicago, 1970, Year Book.
11. Understanding and adopting Electronic Health Records (EHR): Part 1—decision. American Physical Therapy Association. http://www.apta.org/EHR/Guide/Decision/. Accessed September 29, 2014.
12. *Physical Therapist Member Demographic Profile* 2013. American Physical Therapy Association. http://www.apta.org/WorkforceData/. Accessed September 29, 2014.

ADDITIONAL RESOURCES

Dreeben O: *Introduction to physical therapy for physical therapist assistants*, Sudbury, MA, 2011, Jones and Bartlett Learning. Addresses specific areas of work for the PTA. Includes history of the profession and evolution of the PTA.

www.apta.org. Website of the APTA. Excellent resource for current information and documents pertinent to the profession.

REVIEW QUESTIONS

1. Why is the phrase direct access preferred over practice without referral?
2. You go to a PT for treatment of an injury sustained while skiing. Describe what you should expect at the first meeting before intervention begins.
3. Describe the steps in an initial examination.
4. What is included in a plan of care?
5. Discuss how you would decide which documentation format might best suit a PT's needs in any given situation. Show the advantages and disadvantages of each.
6. What is the difference between patient-centered and client-centered consultation?

The development of the physical therapist assistant expanded the quantity and quality of patient care. Getting physical therapy services to people in need was always the underlying goal.... With that goal still in mind today, it continues to be important for the profession to encourage further growth of the physical therapist assistant.

Charles Dorando

3

The Physical Therapist Assistant

John E. Kelly and Pamela D. Ritzline

KEY TERMS

acceptable standard of care
active members
Advisory Panel of Physical Therapist Assistants
Affiliate Assembly
affiliate member
Affiliate Special Interest Group (ASIG)
career ladder
clinical problem solving
direct supervision
general supervision
hand-off communication
National Assembly of Physical Therapist
    Assistants
physical therapist assistant (PTA)
Physical Therapist Assistant Caucus (PTA
    Caucus)
physical therapist assistant members
physical therapist of record
physical therapy aides or technicians
physical therapy interventions
PT/PTA team
PT:PTA ratio
PTA SIGs
recognition of advanced proficiency for the PTA
Representative Body of the National Assembly
    (RBNA)
scope of work
sole extender of the physical therapist
Student Assembly

Values-based behaviors for the physical
    therapist assistant

LEARNING OBJECTIVES

After reading this chapter, the reader will be
able to:

■ Identify historical milestones in the
  development of the role of the physical
  therapist assistant.
■ Distinguish between the roles of the physical
  therapist and the physical therapist assistant
  within the patient/client management model.
■ Describe physical therapist assistant
  educational requirements and models of
  delivery.
■ Discuss legal and ethical factors related to
  delegation of selected interventions and
  direction and supervision of physical
  therapist assistants.
■ Describe the controversy regarding the
  physical therapist assistant in entry-level and
  continuing education, clinical work, and
  American Physical Therapy Association
  membership.
■ Explain how the American Physical Therapy
  Association provides for representation and
  influences the clinical work of the physical
  therapist assistant.
■ Discuss how current trends may influence the
  future of the physical therapist assistant.

A growing demand for physical therapy services spurred the creation of the
physical therapist assistant (PTA) in the 1960s. Debate and controversy have
existed in determining the function of the PTA in physical therapist practice since
the inception of this category of health care provider. Future changes in the role
of the PTA in physical therapist practice will be influenced by a number of factors
including expansion of physical therapist practice, the advancement of physical
therapist entry-level education to the doctoral degree, state and federal legislation, demand for physical therapist services, and payment policy.

To aid in understanding the function of the PTA within the PT/PTA team, this
chapter will examine the education, clinical roles, demographics, American Physical Therapy Association (APTA) representation, and trends influencing the future
of PTAs. A historical perspective will provide some insight into the current discussions regarding the scope of work of the PTA. Clinical utilization of PTAs will be
closely examined in light of legal and ethical considerations, APTA positions and

guidelines, and the many factors to consider when physical therapists (PTs) utilize PTAs to perform selected interventions.

DEFINITION

Defining the term *physical therapist assistant* provides a starting point to understanding the role of the PTA. A PTA is a health care provider whose function is to assist the PT in the provision of physical therapy services in compliance with laws and regulations governing the practice of physical therapy (Box 3-1).[1–3]

ORIGIN AND HISTORY

As described in Chapter 1, the polio epidemic and World War II collectively reinforced the need for physical therapy services. Health care legislation, particularly the Hill-Burton Act of 1946 and the Medicare and Medicaid legislation of 1965, led to increased access to physical therapy. This increased access created tremendous demand for physical therapy services that could not be met, and a shortage of PTs resulted.[4] Although some hospitals and physical therapy clinics created structured on-the-job training for nonprofessional staff to help meet the demand,[5,6] the need for formally educated and regulated support personnel quickly became apparent.[7,8]

Before any action on the part of the APTA, several agencies began to investigate the creation of formalized training of support personnel in physical therapy. Some of these agencies included the American Association of Junior Colleges, the U.S. Department of Labor, the U.S. Department of Health, vocational schools, physician groups, hospitals, rehabilitation centers, nursing homes, and state health departments.[9–11] The APTA became concerned about the development of training programs without the benefit of physical therapy leadership and input, and in 1964

BOX 3-1

Definition of the Physical Therapist Assistant

Physical therapist assistants (PTAs) are the only licensed/certified health care providers that deliver physical therapy services under the direction and supervision of physical therapists (PTs) as part of the PT/PTA team. PTAs are responsible for providing, progressing, and, where appropriate, modifying physical therapy interventions to maximize patient/client safety, comfort, and response within the plan of care established by the supervising physical therapist. PTAs are clinical decision makers who use data collection methods to measure the patient's response to the interventions provided. Additionally, PTAs use value-based behaviors in carrying out the plan of care, including communicating with the supervising physical therapist regarding patient status, treatment outcomes, and any other information that may impact the plan of care. PTAs are graduates of Commission on Accreditation in Physical Therapy Education–accredited PTA education programs and must pass the National Physical Therapy Examination—PTA as a minimum requirement for licensure/certification in all jurisdictions. PTAs comply with all legal requirements of jurisdictions regulating the practice of physical therapy and with the American Physical Therapy Association's Standards of Ethical Conduct for the Physical Therapist Assistant.

From American Physical Therapy Association (APTA): *PTA caucus: description of the physical therapist assistant, PTA caucus annual meeting minutes June*, Alexandria, VA, 2014, APTA.

the APTA House of Delegates (HOD) established a task force to investigate the role of support personnel and the criteria for PTA education programs.[11] In 1967, the task force submitted a proposal for the creation of *physical therapy assistants* (the title was later changed to *physical therapist assistants* to clarify the role that PTAs play in the provision of physical therapy interventions to assist PTs).[12]

On July 5, 1967, the APTA HOD adopted the policy statement, "Training and Utilization of the Physical Therapy Assistant,"[13] essentially giving birth to the PTA. This policy statement included a definition of the assistant, the supervisory relationship with the PT, and the functions that PTAs could perform. Furthermore, the statement established the need for accreditation of 2-year associates degree education programs by what is now the Commission on Accreditation in Physical Therapy Education (CAPTE). Finally, the statement included support for mandatory licensure and APTA membership eligibility. Two PTA education programs were created in 1967 as a result of this action, at Miami Dade College in Florida and St. Mary's Junior College (now known as the Minneapolis Campus of St. Catherine University) in Minnesota. Two years later, in 1969, these institutions graduated the first 15 PTAs.[14]

Development of new PTA education programs was prolific; they eventually exceeded the number of PT education programs (Figure 3-1). As more PTA education programs were established, variability in the preparation of PTA students became evident. In 1975, in an effort to improve uniformity of PTA education programs, the APTA HOD approved *The Essentials of an Interim Approved Educational Program for the Physical Therapist Assistant*.[15] Despite these efforts, debate among physical therapy practitioners and educators regarding the appropriate education, utilization, and supervision of PTAs continued throughout the 1980s and 1990s,[16] leading the APTA Department of Education to organize the Coalition on Consensus for Physical Therapist Assistant Education in 1995.[17] This landmark series of

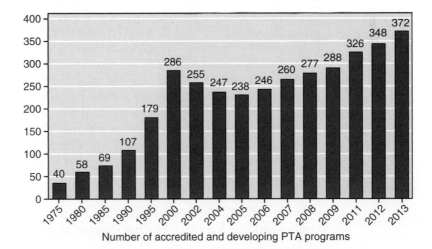

Number of accredited and developing PTA programs

Figure 3-1 ■ Number of physical therapist assistant education programs. (Data from CAPTE 2012-2013 Fact Sheet, Physical Therapist Assistant Programs, June 2013. http://www.capteonline.org/uploadedFiles/CAPTEorg/About_CAPTE/Resources/Aggregate_Program_Data/AggregateProgramData_PTAPrograms.pdf#search=%22factsheet%22. Accessed September 19, 2014.)

conferences eventually led to the development of *A Normative Model of Physical Therapist Assistant Education,* initially approved by the APTA HOD in 1999.[18] This comprehensive document, alongside the CAPTE document *Evaluative Criteria for Accreditation of Education Programs for the Preparation of Physical Therapist Assistants*[19] and the *Guide to Physical Therapist Practice 3.0* (the *Guide*),[20] established increased consistency in the educational preparation and clinical utilization of PTAs.

The physical therapy profession overcame significant obstacles in its growth and development. The Balanced Budget Act of 1997, introduction of the prospective payment system (PPS) under Medicare, and restricted access to physical therapy services resulting from managed care contracts combined to cause a declining job market for PTs and PTAs, as well as for many other health care providers.[21] As a result, the development of new PTA education programs eventually experienced a decline, and some programs were terminated voluntarily. Fortunately, the job market improved in response to continued high demand for physical therapy services and as a result of the expansion of physical therapists' roles.

The role of the PTA continued to be refined through actions of the APTA. In 2000, the position statement *Procedural Interventions Exclusively Performed by Physical Therapists*[22] defined interventions that were beyond the scope of work of the PTA. In 2003, in response to recommendations by a task force to study the role of the PTA, the APTA Board of Directors (BOD) initiated work to define the role of the PTA within the APTA's Vision 2020.[23] In 2007, as part of the revisions to *A Normative Model of Physical Therapist Assistant Education,* a PTA clinical problem-solving algorithm was produced.[18] In 2008, after extensive research, the APTA BOD adopted the document *Minimum Required Skills of Physical Therapist Assistants at Entry-Level*[24]; and in 2009 the APTA BOD issued a resolution reaffirming that the PTA is the **sole extender of the physical therapist**, meaning that the PTA is the "only individual permitted to assist a physical therapist in selected interventions under the direction and supervision of a physical therapist,"[2] that the associates degree is the appropriate degree requirement for the PTA, and that PTAs have "potential for ongoing education after licensure/regulation within the realm of interventions."[25,26]

Further evolution of the PTAs role in physical therapist practice occurred during the 2011 APTA HOD meeting, with the adoption of the position "Physical Therapist accountability and responsibility for the Delivery of Care."[27] This new position statement was effectively silent regarding who may assist the physical therapist in providing **physical therapy interventions.** The position was rescinded at the 2014 HOD meeting, meaning the APTA position supports PTAs as the only individual permitted to assist a PT in providing selected interventions.[28]

EDUCATION AND CURRICULUM

This section reviews the educational level, accreditation requirements, and curriculum for PTA education programs. The purpose of these education programs is described in *A Normative Model of Physical Therapist Assistant Education* (Box 3-2).

ACCREDITATION

As of January 1, 2015, PTAs are licensed or otherwise regulated in all 50 states and the District of Columbia.[29] To complete the licensure examination, a candidate must be a graduate of or graduating from a PTA education program that meets the accreditation standards of CAPTE or is deemed substantially equivalent. CAPTE is the only

3

BOX 3-2

The Purpose of Physical Therapist Assistant Education

The purpose of physical therapist assistant education is to graduate knowledgeable, competent, self-assured, adaptable, and service-oriented patient/client care providers. Physical therapist assistant education prepares the graduate to perform selected components of interventions and data collection and assess the patient's/client's safety and response to the interventions provided under the direction and supervision of the physical therapist in an ethical, legal, safe, and effective manner. Additionally, with other members of the health care delivery team, interact with members of the patient's/client's family and caregivers and work cooperatively with other health care providers. Graduates are prepared to participate with the physical therapist in teaching other health care providers and providing psychosocial support for patients/clients and their families and caregivers with recognition of individual, cultural, and economic differences.

Data from American Physical Therapy Association (APTA): A normative model of physical therapist assistant education: version 2007, Alexandria, VA, 2007, APTA.

accreditation agency recognized by the U.S. Department of Education and the Council for Higher Education Accreditation to accredit PT (professional level) and PTA education programs in the United States. Accreditation staff members are APTA staff hired specifically for CAPTE; however, CAPTE functions independently from APTA, including the accreditation decisions for PT and PTA education programs. Some variability in the structure and design of PTA education programs exists to allow for consistency with the mission and community needs of each university or college; however, CAPTE dictates the minimum requirements. The most recent revisions of the standards for accreditation for PT and PTA education programs adopted by CAPTE were deliberately crafted to parallel similar categories of expectations.[30,31]

DIFFERENTIATION BETWEEN PHYSICAL THERAPIST AND PHYSICAL THERAPIST ASSISTANT EDUCATION

PT professional education programs prepare PT students to perform all aspects of the patient/client management model, including examination, evaluation, diagnosis, prognosis, and intervention.[20] The educational requirements within PTA curricula are designed to prepare PTA students to assist the PT in the delivery of physical therapy interventions and the associated data collection. The curricula for PTA education programs contain many similarities to those for PT education programs, including general and foundational content as well as technical and clinical components. Basic sciences within the general and foundational content include math, chemistry, physics, biology, anatomy and physiology, kinesiology, and pathology, although some variability exists. These courses provide foundational knowledge for further instruction in the application of skilled interventions.

The technical education component of the curriculum is designed to prepare the PTA student to perform physical therapy interventions under the direction and supervision of the PT. These courses include instruction in intervention and associated data collection techniques (Table 3-1).

Table 3-1
Interventions and Associated Data Collection Techniques

Procedural Interventions	Anthropometric Characteristics	Arousal, Attention, and Cognition	Assistive and Adaptive Devices, Orthotics, Prosthetics	Body Mechanics	Environmental, Self-Care, and Home Issues
Therapeutic exercise, aerobic capacity/endurance conditioning/reconditioning	X				
Balance, coordination, and agility training					
Body mechanics and postural stabilization				X	
Flexibility exercises					
Gait and locomotion training			X		X
Neuromotor development training		X			
Relaxation		X			
Strength, power, and endurance training					
Functional training in self-care and home management		X	X	X	X
Manual therapy techniques	X				
Application of devices and equipment	X		X		
Airway clearance techniques					
Integumentary repair and protection techniques	X				
Electrotherapeutic modalities	X	X			
Physical agents	X	X			

Adapted from American Physical Therapy Association (APTA): *A normative model of physical therapist assistant education: version 2007*, Alexandria, VA, 2007, APTA.

Gait, Locomotion, and Balance	Integumentary Integrity	Muscle Performance	Neuromotor Function	Pain	Posture	Range of Motion	Sensory Response	Vital Signs
X								X
X			X		X			
		X			X			
			X	X		X		
X			X					
			X					
			X					X
		X			X			
X			X					
	X			X		X		
	X			X	X		X	
	X							X
	X			X			X	
	X	X	X	X			X	
	X			X		X	X	X

CLINICAL EDUCATION

In addition to the didactic component of the curricula, clinical education is an important component of PTA education programs. CAPTE requires both integrated and terminal clinical experiences.[31] The clinical education requirements include exposing the PTA student to a variety of practice settings and patient/client diagnoses. Clinical education practice settings are similar to those for PT students and may include acute care hospitals, rehabilitation centers, extended-care facilities, outpatient clinics, and school settings. While participating in clinical education, the PTA student may be supervised by a PT or a PTA; however, additional supervision and direction from the supervising PT are necessary when a PTA is the direct clinical instructor.[32]

The APTA provides guidelines,[33,34] clinical assessment tools,[35] and voluntary credentialing for PT and PTA clinical instructors.[36]

BEHAVIORAL CRITERIA

Accreditation criteria emphasize the inclusion of career development and behavioral expectations in addition to the foundational knowledge and technical and clinical skills necessary to become a PTA. These expectations include self-reflection and cultural competence as well as altruism, caring and compassion, continuing competence, duty, integrity, PT/PTA collaboration, responsibility, and social responsibility, which the APTA has deemed **Values-based Behaviors for the PTA.**[37] Graduates of PTA programs are responsible for understanding resource management principles, including the concepts of time management, facility policy and procedures, service delivery models, reimbursement guidelines, regulatory requirements, economic factors, and health care policy, and how these principles affect patient/client care. Additionally, graduates should be able to read and interpret professional literature and implement new concepts in their clinical work.

Communication skills are emphasized throughout the PTA education curriculum. Ongoing communication with patients/clients and family members, including teaching and education, is necessary to ensure effective intervention. Expertise in written, verbal, and nonverbal communication skills is necessary for the PTA program graduate to be proficient in interactions with other health care providers, payers, administrators, and especially the supervising PT.

CLINICAL PROBLEM SOLVING

Clinical problem solving includes the ability to adjust, modify, or discontinue an intervention within the plan of care established by the PT based on clinical indications.[24] A graduate of a PTA program has the skills and knowledge to determine the effectiveness of the intervention; to adjust the intervention in order to improve the patient/client response, or for patient/client safety or comfort; and to collect data documenting the effectiveness of the intervention. Refer to Figure 3-2 for a diagram of the clinical problem-solving process a PTA uses in ensuring patient/client safety and comfort while progressing toward established outcome goals.

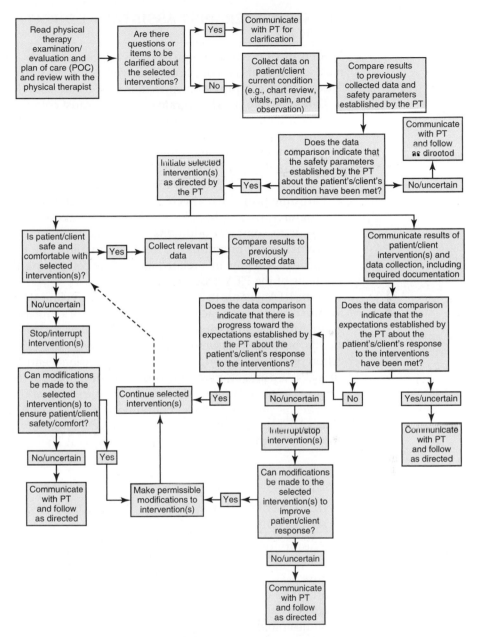

Figure 3-2 ■ The algorithm represents the thought processes occurring during a patient/client interaction or episode of care. The entry point into the algorithm may occur at any point at which the supervising physical therapist delegates selected interventions. The algorithm should not imply a limited opportunity for interaction between the physical therapist and PTA. Communication should be ongoing throughout the episode of care. (From American Physical Therapy Association [APTA]: *A Normative model of physical therapist assistant education: version 2007*, Alexandria, VA, 2007, APTA.)

PHYSICAL THERAPIST ASSISTANT EDUCATION PROGRAM MODELS

Models of PTA education programs vary considerably, based on the perceived needs of students and applicants, as well as the mission of the academic setting. Three commonly provided curricular models are as follows:

■ **One plus one (1 + 1) programs.** Students must complete foundational general education content satisfactorily before being accepted into the PTA program. Once accepted, students complete the technical physical therapy content, including didactic, laboratory, and clinical education segments.

■ **Integrated 2-year programs.** Students accepted into the program complete foundational and physical therapy requirements concurrently.

■ **Part-time programs.** This model may have components of integrated or 1 + 1 programs. Class schedules are designed to allow students to continue working or to complete additional academic requirements (e.g., weekend programs). Some programs are designed to allow the PTA student to pursue a bachelor's degree in a related area while completing the educational requirements of the PTA program.

Some PTAs choose to become PTs, using their clinical knowledge as a head start toward completing the academic requirements of a professional entry-level PT program. Most PT professional education programs do not accept PTA coursework credits, but a limited number of "bridging" programs exist.[38] The purpose of education programs bridging from PTA to professional entry-level PT education is to allow PTAs a unique opportunity to complete the degree requirements and become PTs in a decreased time frame than that required in traditional professional entry-level degree programs, while continuing to work as a PTA. This educational model allows PTAs to receive credit for their PTA coursework and clinical experience and apply it toward an entry-level Doctor of Physical Therapy degree.

THE FUTURE OF PHYSICAL THERAPIST ASSISTANT EDUCATION

The history of increasing numbers of PTA program graduates is a reflection of the ongoing shortage of physical therapy practitioners in the marketplace (Figure 3-3).[39] Although the APTA has determined the associates degree is the appropriate entry-level degree for the PTA,[25] examination of PTA entry-level education is ongoing. Some within the physical therapy profession perceive an undesirable gap in educational levels between the PTA and the PT because the professional entry-level education of the PT has elevated to the doctoral degree. Many barriers exist in increasing the entry-level education of the PTA, including the location of the predominance of PTA education programs in technical and community colleges that would require articulation agreements with four-year institutions in order to confer bachelor's degrees. However, proponents point to the salient qualities of an increased educational level, resulting in PTAs with an increased skill level and, therefore, the best prepared and most qualified individuals to assist PTs in the provision of selected patient/client

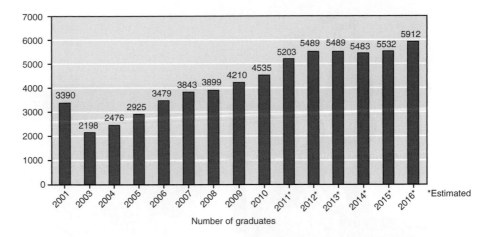

Figure 3-3 ■ Physical therapist assistant program graduates. (Data from CAPTE 2012–2013 Fact Sheet, Physical Therapist Assistant Programs, June 2013. http://www.capteonline.org/uploadedFiles/CAPTEorg/About_ CAPTE/Resources/Aggregate_Program_Data/AggregateProgramData_ PTAPrograms.pdf#search=%22factsheet%22. Accessed September 19, 2014.)

interventions. While discussion is ongoing, any changes that may occur in the entry-level education of PTAs are speculative. Further discussion related to this topic can be found in the Trends section of this chapter.

UTILIZATION The PTA's clinical role lies solely within the intervention component of the patient/client management model (see Figure 2-1). Figure 3-4 provides examples of a PTA performing an intervention (gait training using body weight-supported treadmill training [BWSTT]), and a data collection technique (joint range-of-motion measurement [goniometry]). Even when selected physical therapy interventions are directed to a PTA, the PT remains responsible for the care, documentation, and outcomes related to that intervention. This responsibility highlights the importance of ongoing communication, and direction and supervision throughout the episode of care. Although clinical settings and situations differ greatly, regardless of the setting where the service is provided, the decision to direct selected interventions to a PTA is part of the clinical decision-making process of the evaluating PT.[2]

DELEGATION, DIRECTION, AND SUPERVISION

According to the APTA position statement *Direction and Supervision of the Physical Therapist Assistant*, delegation of selected interventions "requires the education, expertise, and professional judgment of a physical therapist" (Box 3-3).[2] Determining the appropriate utilization of a PTA in a particular clinical setting is essential to ensure safe, legal, ethical, and high-quality patient/client care. Outcomes, efficiency of service delivery, and patient satisfaction can be enhanced by the utilization of a PTA.[40] For this to occur, the supervising PT must carefully

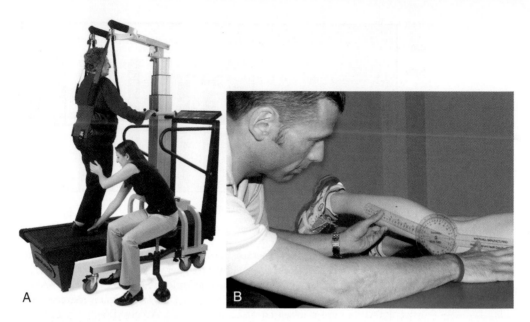

Figure 3-4 ■ **A,** Example of a physical therapist assistant (PTA) performing an intervention (gait training using body weight-supported treadmill training). (Courtesy Mobility Research.); **B,** Example of a PTA performing a data collection technique (joint range-of-motion measurement [goniometry]).

BOX 3-3	*Direction and Supervision of the Physical Therapist Assistant*

Physical therapists have a responsibility to deliver services in ways that protect the public safety and maximize the availability of their services. They do this through direct delivery of services in conjunction with responsible utilization of physical therapist assistants who assist with selected components of intervention. The physical therapist assistant is the only individual permitted to assist a physical therapist in selected interventions under the direction and supervision of a physical therapist.

Direction and supervision are essential in the provision of quality physical therapy services. The degree of direction and supervision necessary for assuring quality physical therapy services is dependent upon many factors, including the education, experiences, and responsibilities of the parties involved, as well as the organizational structure in which the physical therapy services are provided.

Regardless of the setting in which the physical therapy service is provided, the following responsibilities must be borne solely by the physical therapist:
1. Interpretation of referrals when available.
2. Initial examination, evaluation, diagnosis, and prognosis.

BOX 3-3 **Direction and Supervision of the Physical Therapist Assistant—cont'd**

3. Development or modification of a plan of care which is based on the initial examination or reexamination and which includes the physical therapy goals and outcomes.
4. Determination of when the expertise and decision-making capability of the physical therapist requires the physical therapist to personally render physical therapy interventions and when it may be appropriate to utilize the physical therapist assistant. A physical therapist shall determine the most appropriate utilization of the physical therapist assistant that provides for the delivery of service that is safe, effective, and efficient.
5. Reexamination of the patient/client in light of their goals, and revision of the plan of care when indicated.
6. Establishment of the discharge plan and documentation of discharge summary/status.
7. Oversight of all documentation for services rendered to each patient/client.

The physical therapist remains responsible for the physical therapy services provided when the physical therapist's plan of care involves the physical therapist assistant to assist with selected interventions. Regardless of the setting in which the service is provided, the determination to utilize physical therapist assistants for selected interventions requires the education, expertise, and professional judgment of a physical therapist as described by the *Standards of Practice, Guide to Professional Conduct,* and *Code of Ethics.*

In determining the appropriate extent of assistance from the physical therapist assistant (PTA), the physical therapist considers:

- The PTA's education, training, experience, and skill level
- Patient/client criticality, acuity, stability, and complexity.
- The predictability of the consequences.
- The setting in which the care is being delivered.
- Federal and state statutes.
- Liability and risk management concerns.
- The mission of physical therapy services for the setting.
- The needed frequency of reexamination.

Physical Therapist Assistant
Definition
The physical therapist assistant is a technically educated health care provider who assists the physical therapist in the provision of physical therapy. The physical therapist assistant is a graduate of a physical therapist assistant associate degree program accredited by the Commission on Accreditation in Physical Therapy Education (CAPTE).

Utilization
The physical therapist is directly responsible for the actions of the physical therapist assistant related to patient/client management. The physical

Continued

| BOX 3-3 | *Direction and Supervision of the Physical Therapist Assistant—cont'd* |

therapist assistant may perform selected physical therapy interventions under the direction and at least general supervision of the physical therapist. In general supervision, the physical therapist is not required to be on-site for direction and supervision but must be available at least by telecommunications. The ability of the physical therapist assistant to perform the selected interventions as directed shall be assessed on an ongoing basis by the supervising physical therapist. The physical therapist assistant makes modifications to selected interventions either to progress the patient/client as directed by the physical therapist or to ensure patient/client safety and comfort.

The physical therapist assistant must work under the direction and at least general supervision of the physical therapist. In all practice settings, the performance of selected interventions by the physical therapist assistant must be consistent with safe and legal physical therapist practice and shall be predicated on the following factors: complexity and acuity of the patient's/client's needs; proximity and accessibility to the physical therapist; supervision available in the event of emergencies or critical events; and type of setting in which the service is provided.

When supervising the physical therapist assistant in any off-site setting, the following requirements must be observed:

1. A physical therapist must be accessible by telecommunications to the physical therapist assistant at all times while the physical therapist assistant is treating patients/clients.
2. There must be regularly scheduled and documented conferences with the physical therapist assistant regarding patients/clients, the frequency of which is determined by the needs of the patient/client and the needs of the physical therapist assistant.
3. In those situations in which a physical therapist assistant is involved in the care of a patient/client, a supervisory visit by the physical therapist will be made:
   a. Upon the physical therapist assistant's request for a reexamination, when a change in the plan of care is needed, prior to any planned discharge, and in response to a change in the patient's/client's medical status
   b. At least once a month, or at a higher frequency when established by the physical therapist, in accordance with the needs of the patient/client
   c. A supervisory visit should include:
      i. An on-site reexamination of the patient/client
      ii. On-site review of the plan of care with appropriate revision or termination
      iii. Evaluation of need and recommendation for utilization of outside resources

Direction and Supervision of the Physical Therapist Assistant, HOD P06-05-18-26. House of Delegates Standards, Policies, Positions, and Guidelines. Alexandria, VA, American Physical Therapy Association, 2009.

consider the many factors influencing the suitability of delegation of selected interventions and the need for ongoing supervision and direction. These factors are discussed in the following sections.

THE PRACTICE ACT

The state practice act is the legal statute intended to "protect public health, safety and welfare, and provide for state administrative control, supervision, licensure, and regulation of the practice of physical therapy."[41] Many state practice acts establish the maximum **PT:PTA ratio**, type and frequency of communication with the supervising PT, frequency of patient/client reexamination by the PT, and minimum level of supervision. Levels of supervision are defined by the APTA (Box 3-4).[42]

Practice acts differ widely from one jurisdiction to another and must be examined carefully.[29] For example, New Jersey requires PTAs to work under **direct supervision** and that the supervising PT may supervise a maximum of two PTAs.[43] This means the PTA may treat patients only when a supervising PT is on-site at the facility. Texas, on the other hand, requires only **general supervision**, meaning the supervising PT may be off-site as long as the PT is available by phone, does not stipulate a maximum PT:PTA ratio, and allows for PTAs to screen patients for possible referral.[44] This regulation allows the PTA to provide physical therapy interventions off-site and opens many work

BOX 3-4

Levels of Supervision

The American Physical Therapy Association recognizes the following levels of supervision:
1. **General Supervision:** The physical therapist is not required to be on-site for direction and supervision but must be available at least by telecommunications.
2. **Direct Supervision:** The physical therapist is physically present and immediately available for direction and supervision. The physical therapist will have direct contact with the patient/client during each visit that is defined in the *Guide to Physical Therapist Practice* as all encounters with a patient/client in a 24-hour period. Telecommunications does not meet the requirement of direct supervision.
3. **Direct Personal Supervision:** The physical therapist or, where allowable by law, the physical therapist assistant is physically present and immediately available to direct and supervise tasks that are related to patient/client management. The direction and supervision is continuous throughout the time these tasks are performed. Telecommunications does not meet the requirement of direct personal supervision.

Reprinted from Direction and Supervision of the Physical Therapist Assistant, HOD P06-05-18-26. House of Delegates Standards, Policies, Positions, and Guidelines. Alexandria, VA, American Physical Therapy Association, 2009. Reprinted from http://www.apta.org, with permission of the American Physical Therapy Association, Copyright © 2015 American Physical Therapy Association.

opportunities where shortages of PTs exist, including home care and rural clinics. These rules were developed to promote quality service delivery and to protect patient/client safety, in some cases eliminating overutilization of PTAs and ensuring appropriate ongoing direction and supervision. Reading and understanding your state practice act is an important part of working within the PT/PTA team.

State practice acts also contain definitions, entry-level education and continuing education requirements, examination and licensure standards, and professional misconduct disciplinary procedures.[29] The Federation of State Boards of Physical Therapy (FSBPT) developed a model practice act that can be used by states as they update their rules to increase uniformity across jurisdictions.[41] See Chapter 5 for detailed information on this subject.

FACILITY POLICY

To ensure high-quality provision of physical therapy services, as well as to comply with state practice acts, many facilities develop specific procedures for managing PTA delegation issues. For example, some facilities may require cosigning PTA treatment notes or may use specific forms to document ongoing communication. Clinical staffing patterns, especially when coordinating schedules around sick days, vacations, and weekend coverage, dictate the establishment of **hand-off communication** procedures and a **physical therapist of record**. These concepts are critical to decrease errors related to poor communication and to establish primary responsibility for patient/client management. The PT of record is accountable for the coordination, continuation, and progression of the plan of care.[45] Through establishment of a facility procedure to clearly identify the PT of record and the process of hand-off communication, confusion regarding the responsibility for patient/client management is reduced. Refer to Box 3-5 for an example of a hospital policy addressing delegation and supervision issues.

BOX 3-5 *Example of Hospital Policy to Ensure Appropriate Direction and Supervision*

Hospital Policy: Physical Therapist/Physical Therapist Assistant Team
I. Purpose
a. To establish the procedures to ensure adherence to legal practice standards, including all federal and state regulations related to the relationship of the physical therapist to the physical therapist assistant in the delivery of patient care. The physical therapist assistant is the only individual permitted to assist a physical therapist in selected interventions under the direction and supervision of a physical therapist.

BOX 3-5   *Example of Hospital Policy to Ensure Appropriate Direction and Supervision—cont'd*

b. To establish the procedures to reduce errors and improve communication regarding patient care in order to maintain quality patient care.

II. Policy statements

a. Physical Therapist Assistants will work in a team with a Physical Therapist, who will have knowledge and responsibility for the patients to which he/she has assigned to the care of the PTA. In general, the PT performing the initial evaluation will be responsible for the ongoing care of the patient assigned to the PTA. If for some reason, due to staffing conditions, the evaluating PT is not available for direction and supervision of the PTA, another partner therapist will be assigned to assume responsibility for those patients.

III. Procedure

a. Inpatient Physical Therapy
   i. PT/PTA teams will be aligned for each acute care team within Rehabilitation Services. Realignment may occur as needed at the beginning of each new rotation period or as staff changes occur.
   ii. A PT in each PT/PTA team will become the PT of record for this team and will cover assigned floor(s) within the bigger team.
   iii. Each PT/PTA team will have a brief daily stand-up meeting at a determined place and time to discuss the current patients.
   iv. New evaluations completed on the weekend will be coded by the evaluating PT, indicating either "PT should see" or "PTA can see" for Monday. The Triage Coordinator will be responsible to assign the patients accordingly.
   v. The newly assigned PT will do a brief chart review and check in on the patient within 24 hours to assume the PT of Record role for each patient evaluated by a different PT.
   vi. The PTA may see the new patient assigned to him/her before the new PT of Record sees the patient, because the patient was previously evaluated and the plan of care is established and because the daily communication process is in place. The PTA will contact the PT of Record if he/she determines direction is needed after reviewing the patient chart or after attempting to see the patient.
   vii. For days off during the week (Monday through Friday), patients will be assigned to the appropriate PT of Record. If the PT of Record for any team is off, the Team Leader or Triage Coordinator may become the PT of Record for that team.
   viii. A physical therapist working on the weekend will be assigned the PT of Record role on Saturday and Sunday. The "Therapist in

Continued

BOX 3-5

Example of Hospital Policy to Ensure Appropriate Direction and Supervision—cont'd

charge" may also be consulted by a PTA, and/or the PT/PTA team working may discuss complex patients during the day. A patient may be deferred back to the original PT of Record for Monday.

    ix. When patients are transferred to different floors, communication should occur between the current PT/PTA team and the new PT of Record. This communication should include whether the new PT of Record should take the patient or if the PTA for the team can take the patient. The new PT of Record will do a brief chart review or reevaluation as needed.

    x. At rotations (two times per year), the current PT/PTA team will discuss the patients with the new PT/PTA team.

b. Outpatient Physical Therapy

    i. The PT of Record will be identified on the front of the chart on a sticker.

    ii. Most of the time the PT of Record will be the evaluating PT.

    iii. The PT of Record will be a consistent PT at that facility, not a "fill-in" (e.g., supplemental coverage for a PTO).

    iv. The PTA will utilize and contact the PT of Record for questions regarding patient care.

    v. If the evaluating PT is not the ongoing PT of Record:

        1. In Adult areas, the patient must be scheduled with a PT (who then becomes the PT of Record) prior to assigning to a PTA.

        2. In Pediatric areas, the PTA will consult with the evaluating PT and/or newly assigned PT of Record regarding assigned patients.

    vi. If a patient transfers facilities after initial evaluation, then the patient must be scheduled with a PT (who then becomes the PT of Record) prior to assigning to a PTA.

    vii. The PT/PTA teams will have coinciding schedules to allow face-to-face conversation regarding patient care on a daily basis.

    viii. PTA in a clinic without the Primary Therapist (i.e., PTO day)

        1. A "partner" PT will be designated and on call for the PTA to contact regarding patient care.

        2. The Manager and Team Leaders will set up schedules for partner PTs coinciding with PTO schedule.

        3. The Manager and Team Leaders will be utilized as the partner PT in the case of unexpected absences.

c. For All PT/PTA Teams

    i. The PT of Record will reevaluate Inpatients assigned to PTAs every 14 days.

    ii. The PT of Record will reevaluate Outpatients the earlier of every thirty (30) days or every fifteen (15) physical therapy visits.

[Note: PTO = Paid time off.]

PAYER REIMBURSEMENT POLICIES

Depending on the funding source, additional requirements may need to be met when selected interventions are delegated to a PTA. For example, Medicare, the federally administered system of health insurance available to persons age 65 years or older, has specific requirements for supervision based on the type of setting where the care is provided (Table 3-2).[46] Some private insurance plans limit reimbursement for physical therapy interventions provided by a PTA. This alarming trend, known as tiered payment, whereby reimbursement rates are lower when interventions are provided by a PTA will be discussed in the Trends section of the chapter.

PHYSICAL THERAPIST ASSISTANT COMPETENCE

Delegation and supervision should be predicated on the experience, skill level, and continuing competence demonstrated by the PTA. A PTA with 10 years of experience and continuing education, and competence will have skills well beyond entry level.[25] For the PT, this skill level will allow increased confidence when making delegation decisions and a decreased need for direction and supervision. The supervising PT must understand the skill level of the PTA when making delegation decisions. Incumbent on the PTA is the responsibility to request a PT reexamination or consultation, when appropriate, to ensure ongoing supervision in the event of the following:

■ A change in patient/client status.
■ An unsafe or unexpected response to an intervention.
■ A lack of expected progress in response to an intervention.
■ A request to advance the patient/client beyond the established plan of care.
■ A need for clarification regarding the plan of care.
■ Inappropriate delegation of interventions that are beyond the PTA's skill level.[2]

RISK MANAGEMENT

The supervising PT remains responsible for physical therapy services when directing selected interventions to a PTA, and this concept has been adopted by the courts. Therefore, it is very rare for a PTA (or other support personnel)

Table 3-2
Medicare Supervision Requirements

Medicare Therapy Provider Setting	PTA Supervision Level	Supervisory Requirement
Outpatient Hospital, Nursing Facility, CORFs, ORFs, HHAs	General	PT presence not required on premises; PT must be available by phone
PT in Private Practice	Direct	PT present in the office suite
Physician Office	Direct	PT present in the office suite

CORFs = Comprehensive Outpatient Rehabilitation Facilities; ORFs = Outpatient Rehabilitation Facilities; HHAs = Home Health Agencies.
Modified from Centers for Medicare and Medicaid Services: *Medicare benefit policy transmittal 88*, Publication 100-02, Baltimore, 2008, Department of Health and Human Services.

to be solely named in a professional liability claim.[47] Failure to appropriately supervise a treatment or procedure is the most frequent allegation in liability claims against physical therapy practitioners when PTAs or other support personnel are involved in providing patient care.[48] Besides the risk of liability, inappropriate direction and supervision decisions also can carry the risk of license revocation, fines, and/or denial of payment for services by third-party payers.[49] Although APTA positions may be more stringent than many state practice acts, a court of law may consider APTA documents to be the **acceptable standard of care** when selected interventions are directed to a PTA.

PHYSICAL THERAPY AIDES

In addition to directing care to a PTA, a PT may select other support personnel such as a physical therapy aide to assist with tasks related to patient care. **Physical therapy aides or technicians** are unlicensed support personnel who complete tasks associated with the operation of a physical therapy service as assigned by the supervising PT or PTA, where permitted by law. Some examples of these tasks include transporting patients to the treatment areas, assisting patients on and off equipment, cleaning equipment, and stocking supplies.

State practice acts differ significantly regarding the regulation of aides, causing confusion regarding their role. The APTA position *Provision of Physical Therapy Interventions and Related Tasks,* identifies the roles of aides for consistency within the profession.[50] Although aides and other nonphysical therapy practitioners are sometimes employed by physical therapy clinics, it is important to note the HOD position that includes "the patient/client management element of interventions should be represented and reimbursed as physical therapy only when performed by a physical therapist or physical therapist assistant performing selected interventions under the direction and supervision of a physical therapist."[51]

CLINICAL CONSIDERATIONS

Patient/client condition and the practice setting are additional considerations when determining appropriate utilization of a PTA. According to the APTA position statement *Direction and Supervision of the Physical Therapist Assistant* "patient/client criticality, acuity, stability, and complexity, the predictability of the consequences, and the setting in which the care is being delivered" must be considered when determining the extent of delegation and the need for direction and supervision (see Box 3-3).[2] Consider the example of a busy outpatient orthopaedic clinic. Physical therapy clinics with patients/clients who have less complicated issues, who are progressing quickly, and who have on-site supervision may facilitate greater utilization of PTAs. The close proximity or availability of the supervising PT as well as the predictability of the situation ease the PT's burden of supervision. In contrast are physical therapy services provided off-site, such as in home health care settings, involving patients/clients with complex medical issues, or with frequently changing PT/PTA teams. These circumstances may present decreased opportunity to utilize a PTA or increase the need for and frequency of PT reassessment of the patient/client.

SCOPE OF WORK

In addition to the previously presented factors, the APTA has deemed two selected interventions beyond the **scope of work** of a PTA. These interventions are selective sharp debridement, which is a component of wound care, and spinal and peripheral joint mobilizations, which are components of manual therapy. This position is controversial because of several factors:

1. Before the year 2000, these interventions were widely included in the curricula of PTA programs, CAPTE requirements, and licensure examinations; therefore, many PTAs in the workforce were trained in these interventions and contend they have the skills to perform them clinically.
2. Patients need these interventions to achieve their goals in physical therapy; however, shortages in the number of licensed PTs, especially in rural settings, compromises best practice when their care is being directed to PTAs who are restricted from providing these interventions.
3. The 2011 FSBPT clinical practice analysis showed that 43% of entry-level PTAs were performing peripheral joint mobilization and 28% were performing spinal joint mobilization.[52]
4. Most state practice acts do not restrict PTAs from performing these interventions.

Although differences exist in the practice and regulatory environments, the APTA position states these interventions "require the skills of evaluation, examination, diagnosis, and prognosis which fall solely within the scope of practice of the physical therapist."[22]

Figure 3-5 presents a conceptual model that illustrates the multiple factors that must be considered by the PT when making decisions about direction of selected interventions to a PTA and the level of supervision required.

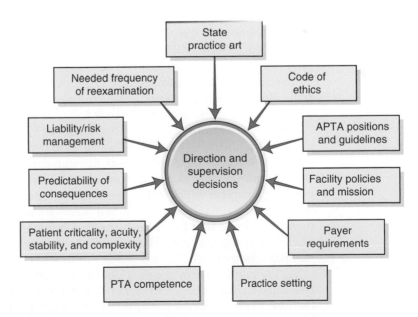

Figure 3-5 ■ Factors influencing direction and supervision. Conceptual model to illustrate the factors the physical therapist must consider when making decisions regarding direction of selected interventions and appropriate levels of supervision.

THE PHYSICAL THERAPIST/PHYSICAL THERAPIST ASSISTANT TEAM

Teamwork between the supervising PT and the PTA is the key to successful outcomes regardless of the clinical setting or interventions directed to the PTA. The **PT/PTA team** must include ongoing effective communication to be successful. Regularly scheduled structured meetings as well as opportunities for impromptu discussion are essential. Patient/client management can be enhanced through use of direction of selected interventions to a PTA when the PT/PTA team is "characterized by trust, mutual respect, adaptability, cooperation, and an appreciation of individual and cultural differences."[53]

The APTA has developed two resources to help PTs and PTAs understand the multiple steps involved in direction and supervision decisions. Refer to Figures 3-6 and 3-7 for algorithms helpful in guiding PT/PTA teams.

CONTINUED COMPETENCE

Another role of the APTA is to advance the practice of physical therapy to meet the future needs of society. Critical to the advancement of the profession is continuing advancement of clinical skills. The APTA provides opportunity and supports PTA participation in continuing education beyond entry-level skills.[54] Previously, some controversy existed regarding PTAs attending continuing education courses alongside their PT counterparts. This controversy was the result of some PTs questioning the ability of PTAs to attain advanced skills once provided by only the PT and because of the content of many continuing education courses in the areas of examination, evaluation, diagnosis, and prognosis. Although these areas of the patient/client management model are outside of the scope of work of the PTA, PTAs benefit from understanding the process the supervising PTs must use in establishing a plan of care. Both PTs and PTAs are obligated to utilize only the information from continuing education courses that is within their scope of practice or work.

To remain clinically competent, PTAs must seek ways to improve their clinical skills after graduation. Many jurisdictions require Continuing Education Units (CEUs) to maintain licensure. Even if CEUs are not required for licensure, the PTA is bound by the *Standards of Ethical Conduct for the Physical Therapist Assistant* to be lifelong learners (see Box 5-2). Standard 6 states, "Physical therapist assistants shall enhance their competence through the lifelong acquisition and refinement of knowledge, skills, and abilities."[55] Setting career development goals regarding clinical work and specialization and advancement will facilitate increased knowledge attainment and lifelong learning in the areas of physical therapy practice that best match the PTA's interests. Ongoing self-assessment of clinical competence can help the PTA identify practice areas to address to maintain competence.[56]

APTA members may access a tool for evaluating potential clinical opportunities, titled *Considerations for Practice Opportunities and Professional Development*.[57] Because PTA utilization varies across jurisdictions, practice settings, and management structures, this tool can help objectify the pros and cons associated with choosing a particular career opportunity. In addition, in 2008, the APTA BOD established a task force to determine appropriate career pathways for the PTA.[25] In response, the task force created the Advanced Proficiency Pathway

PTA Direction Algorithm

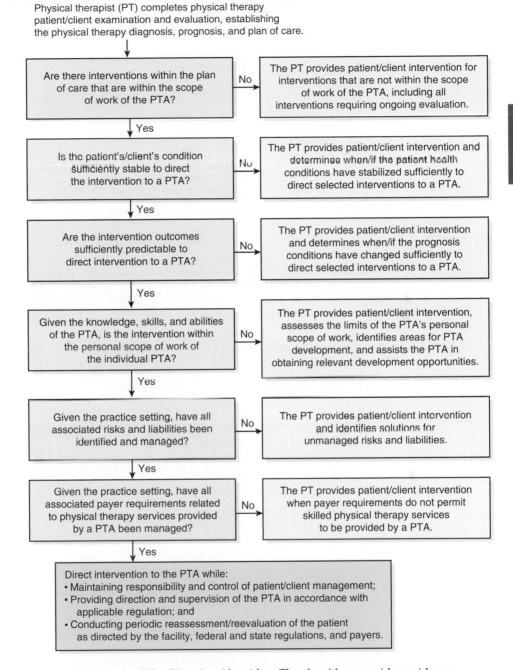

Physical therapist (PT) completes physical therapy patient/client examination and evaluation, establishing the physical therapy diagnosis, prognosis, and plan of care.

Are there interventions within the plan of care that are within the scope of work of the PTA?

No → The PT provides patient/client intervention for interventions that are not within the scope of work of the PTA, including all interventions requiring ongoing evaluation.

Yes ↓

Is the patient's/client's condition sufficiently stable to direct the intervention to a PTA?

No → The PT provides patient/client intervention and determines when/if the patient health conditions have stabilized sufficiently to direct selected interventions to a PTA.

Yes ↓

Are the intervention outcomes sufficiently predictable to direct intervention to a PTA?

No → The PT provides patient/client intervention and determines when/if the prognosis conditions have changed sufficiently to direct selected interventions to a PTA.

Yes ↓

Given the knowledge, skills, and abilities of the PTA, is the intervention within the personal scope of work of the individual PTA?

No → The PT provides patient/client intervention, assesses the limits of the PTA's personal scope of work, identifies areas for PTA development, and assists the PTA in obtaining relevant development opportunities.

Yes ↓

Given the practice setting, have all associated risks and liabilities been identified and managed?

No → The PT provides patient/client intervention and identifies solutions for unmanaged risks and liabilities.

Yes ↓

Given the practice setting, have all associated payer requirements related to physical therapy services provided by a PTA been managed?

No → The PT provides patient/client intervention when payer requirements do not permit skilled physical therapy services to be provided by a PTA.

Yes ↓

Direct intervention to the PTA while:
• Maintaining responsibility and control of patient/client management;
• Providing direction and supervision of the PTA in accordance with applicable regulation; and
• Conducting periodic reassessment/reevaluation of the patient as directed by the facility, federal and state regulations, and payers.

Figure 3-6 ■ PTA Direction Algorithm. The algorithm provides guidance for PT/PTA teams regarding decisions to direct selected interventions. (From APTA, Crosier J. PTA Direction and Supervision Algorithms: Step-by-step problem-solving diagrams to guide PTs and PTAs. *PT in Motion.* 2010;2(8):47–50. Reprinted from http://www.apta.org, with permission of the American Physical Therapy Association, Copyright © 2015 American Physical Therapy Association.)

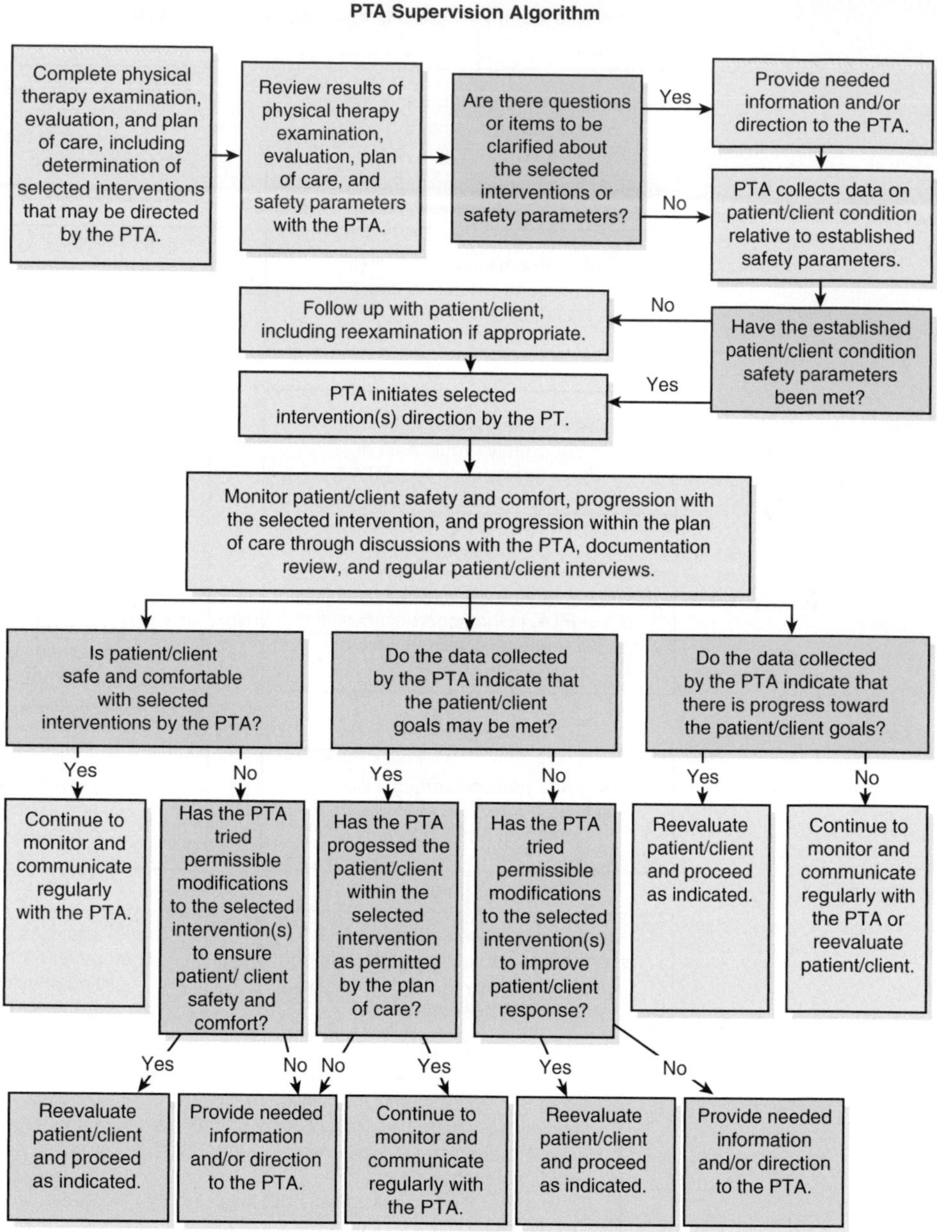

PTA Supervision Algorithm

Figure 3-7 ■ PTA Supervision Algorithm. The algorithm reflects current APTA policies and positions and provides guidance in the appropriate supervision of the PTA. (From Crosier J., PTA Direction and Supervision Algorithms: Step-by-step problem-solving diagrams to guide PTs and PTAs. *PT in Motion*. 2010;2(8):47–50. Reprinted from http://www.apta. org, with permission of the American Physical Therapy Association, Copyright © 2015 American Physical Therapy Association.)

Program.[58] The Advanced Proficiency Pathways are postgraduation curricula specifically designed to increase the PTA's knowledge and skill in a specific physical therapy clinical practice area, and consists of:

■ Core educational courses.
■ Clinical practice area specific courses.
■ Knowledge examinations.
■ Mentored clinical experiences with skill checks.

Clinical practice areas include Acute Care, Cardiopulmonary, Geriatric, Oncology, Pediatrics, and Wound Management.

3

CHARAC-TERISTICS OF PHYSICAL THERAPIST ASSISTANTS

Demographic characteristics and employment information regarding physical therapist assistants are presented in this section. Comparable information for physical therapists is included in Chapter 2.

DEMOGRAPHICS

The demographic information in this section was obtained from 2013 APTA membership data.[59] Although data are specific to PTAs who are APTA members, the information likely is representative of the workforce.

Gender. Women accounted for 75% of PTA members, compared to 70% of PT members.

Age. Forty-four percent of PTA members reported being under the age of 40, compared with 54% in 2005. This shift may be indicative of the high number of non-traditional students enrolled in PTA education programs.

Race. Eighty-seven percent of PTA members report being white. All other races combined account for just 13% of PTA members.

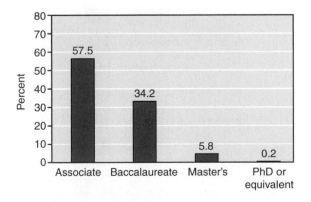

Figure 3-8 ■ Highest earned academic degree achieved by physical therapist assistants who are members of the American Physical Therapy Association (APTA). (Data from American Physical Therapy Association [APTA]: Year End Membership Database: *PTA demographics: highest earned degree,* Alexandria, VA, 2014, APTA.)

Education. The associate degree was the highest academic degree earned by 57.5% of PTA members (Figure 3-8), which reflects the degree requirement. A bachelor's degree was held by 34.2% of PTA members, and 5.8% held a master's degree. The number of PTAs with education beyond the required associates degree has increased by 9% compared to 2005. Data do not reflect the number of PTAs who became physical therapists and therefore received an advanced degree.

EMPLOYMENT FACILITY

Employment patterns for PTAs are similar to those of PTs. Private practice accounts for approximately one-third of employed PTAs (Figure 3-9). The most significant difference between PT and PTA employment patterns is in the skilled nursing facility (SNF)/long-term care setting, where 21% of PTA members report employment compared to only 5% of PTs. This difference may represent higher PT:PTA ratios than in many other clinical settings. Refer to the case studies at the end of this chapter for a discussion about direction and supervision considerations in the face of challenging staffing patterns.

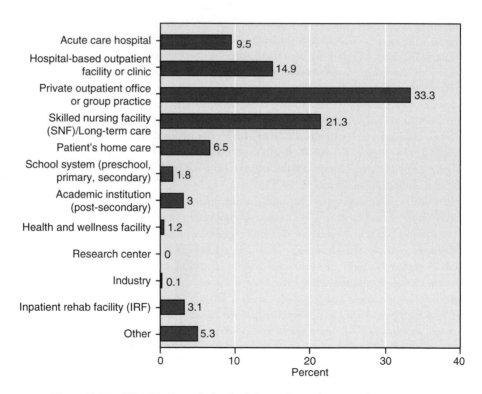

Figure 3-9 ■ Distribution of physical therapist assistants who are members of the American Physical Therapy Association (APTA) by facility of employment. (Data from American Physical Therapy Association [APTA]: Year End Membership Database: *PTA demographics: type of facility in which PTA members work,* Alexandria, VA, 2014, APTA.)

CAREER DEVELOPMENT

The demand for physical therapy services is projected to continue to grow; therefore, the job market for PTAs is expected to be favorable. The U.S. Bureau of Labor Statistics predicts that PTA employment numbers will grow by 41% over the 10-year period ending 2022.[60] Coupled with the large variety of clinical settings, PTAs have many employment options and will likely enjoy a secure future. In addition to multiple clinical setting options, PTAs have increasing opportunities for career advancement. Some clinical settings include a **career ladder** for PTAs. Career ladders stipulate post-entry-level qualifications and work experience. Additional responsibilities and/or expertise in specialized clinical procedures are rewarded with department or facility recognition and increased compensation. Career ladders may provide opportunities to advance into leadership roles.[61] Other opportunities for career advancement as a PTA may include (but are not limited to) the following:

- Becoming a clinical instructor for PTA students.
- Providing clinical in-services.
- Serving as a graduate assistant.
- Marketing physical therapy services.
- Assisting in research.
- Serving in an APTA leadership role.
- Coordinating staffing patterns.
- Working in program development.
- Becoming an administrator.
- Teaching.
- Serving as a member of a state licensure board.

AMERICAN PHYSICAL THERAPY ASSOCIATION MEMBERSHIP AND REPRESENTATION

In 1967, the APTA HOD voted to adopt standards for the creation of PTA education programs. No one at the time could have predicted the heated debates, turmoil, and controversy that would occur over the years regarding PTA membership and representation! Beginning with the initial debate over creating a PTA membership category, the structure of PTA representation within APTA has evolved in an effort to provide increased integration and leadership opportunities.

EVOLUTION

The evolution of the PTA representation structure began with the formation of the **Affiliate Special Interest Group (ASIG)** and has included the **Affiliate Assembly**, the **National Assembly of Physical Therapist Assistants**, the **Representative Body of the National Assembly (RBNA)**, and currently, the **Physical Therapist Assistant Caucus (PTA Caucus).** Now known as **physical therapist assistant members**, PTAs initially were known as **affiliate members** when a membership category was created for them in 1973.[62] Affiliate members were granted one half of a vote in APTA elections at the component level and within their chapter's delegation at the HOD. As PTA membership began to grow, the need for a formalized structure of representation became apparent, and in 1983 the ASIG was formed. The ASIG provided a regional structure for representation of PTAs and an elected chairperson who served as a liaison to the APTA BOD.[11]

In 1989 the Affiliate Assembly was created, replacing the ASIG as the representative structure for the PTA. An assembly was a new type of component of the APTA, eventually adding the **Student Assembly** in 1990. The formation of an assembly allowed members of the same classification to meet, confer, and promote the interests of their constituents within the APTA as well as externally. The Affiliate Assembly included officers elected by their peers, who served as liaisons with APTA officers and staff.[62]

In 1992, the APTA HOD adopted a new policy allowing PTAs to hold offices at the component level (chapters and sections).[11] This policy allows a PTA member to hold any office at the component level that is not in direct succession to the office of president. This policy further integrated PTAs into the association by providing leadership opportunities alongside their PT counterparts.[63]

In 1998 the APTA HOD voted to create a new membership category for PTAs, the *physical therapist assistant*. The affiliate member became the physical therapist assistant member, and the **active member** category for PTs became the physical therapist member. A new entity, the National Assembly of Physical Therapist Assistants, or simply the National Assembly, was structured similarly to the HOD. Representation was provided by the RBNA, which included two RBNA delegates to the APTA HOD. The RBNA delegates were permitted to speak, debate, and make motions in the HOD, but they could not vote. The RBNA included national officers, regional directors, and chapter representatives, which provided increased cohesiveness and a more organized system of promotion and protection of PTA members.

The RBNA solely addressed issues related to PTAs and met separately from the HOD.[64] Because this new structure removed the PTA's voting privilege from the HOD, many PTAs became disenfranchised with the new direction the RBNA assumed. Rather than increased integration within the APTA, the RBNA structure separated PTAs from their PT counterparts. An unfortunate result was a dramatic decrease in PTA membership within the APTA (Figure 3-10). In 2015 the APTA HOD voted to amend the bylaws to allow chapters and sections to provide PTAs with a full vote at chapter and section meetings. Previously only provided a 1/2 vote, the change signifies a significant increase in PTA inclusiveness within the APTA.[65]

THE PHYSICAL THERAPIST ASSISTANT CAUCUS

The organizational structure of PTA representation was changed yet again after an in-depth study conducted by a task force formed by the HOD.[66] As a result, the RBNA was dissolved in 2005, and two new bodies were formed to represent the PTA membership: the **Advisory Panel of Physical Therapist Assistants** and the PTA Caucus.[67] The Advisory Panel of Physical Therapist Assistants was later dissolved as a part of governance review along with all advisory panels. The PTA Caucus continued and is the current structure for PTA representation within the APTA.

The PTA Caucus provides representation for the PTA member in APTA governance. The PTA Caucus includes the Chief Delegate, four Delegates, and 51 PTA Caucus Chapter Representatives. The PTA Caucus meets formally each year immediately before the annual meeting of the HOD. During this annual

3

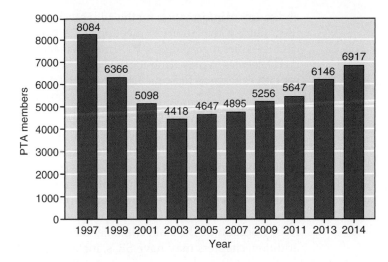

Figure 3-10 ■ Physical therapist assistant (PTA) membership in the American Physical Therapy Association (APTA). (Data from APTA Department of Member Development, Alexandria, VA, 2014.)

meeting, the Chief Delegate and Delegates are elected by the PTA Caucus Chapter Representatives for 3-year terms. The PTA Caucus Chapter Representatives are elected or selected by their chapter (states and District of Columbia). The mission of the PTA Caucus is reflective of the role the PTA plays in the clinical setting, supporting the practice of the PT (Box 3-6).[68]

The role of the PTA Caucus Delegates and the Chief Delegate is to be the voice in the HOD of PTA members. In the HOD, the PTA Caucus Delegates can make and debate motions, which have the potential to become policies and positions of the APTA. They participate in discussions on the floor of the HOD equally with chapter and section delegates, but do not have a vote, which is restricted to chapter delegates. To facilitate ongoing communication regarding issues involving the PTA members they represent, the PTA Caucus Delegates meet regularly throughout the year. The PTA Caucus Chief Delegate attends APTA BOD meetings and interacts with the chief executive officer (CEO), president, board members, and APTA staff.

PTA Caucus Representatives represent the interests of PTA members within their chapter. This involves participation in chapter activities as well as national PTA Caucus activities. Most PTA Caucus Representatives are members of their chapter BOD, where they are the voice of the PTA members they represent, as well

BOX 3-6

The Mission of the Physical Therapist Assistant Caucus

The Physical Therapist Assistant Caucus, serving with integrity and responsiveness, will be the voice of the physical therapist assistant in meeting the vision, goals, and objectives of the American Physical Therapy Association and the profession.

Data from the American Physical Therapy Association (APTA): APTA Physical Therapist Assistant Caucus Procedure Manual, Alexandria, VA, 2009, APTA.

as a source of information for their chapter leadership regarding PTA Caucus activities. During their annual meeting, PTA Caucus Representatives elect officers, discuss issues regarding the PTA members they represent, and assist the PTA Caucus Delegates in preparing for the HOD. During the HOD, the PTA Caucus Representatives serve as liaisons between the PTA Caucus and their chapter delegates.

SPECIAL INTEREST GROUPS

Additional opportunities exist for PTA involvement via participation in special interest groups (SIGs). SIGs are formed as a way for members who "share a special professional interest that cannot be served through existing means to meet and participate in activities related to that special interest within a component's structure."[69] Many of the APTA's specialty practice sections have SIGs that focus on specific areas of physical therapy practice, such as the Stroke SIG within the Neurology Section or the Pain Management SIG within the Orthopaedic Section. In addition, chapters may have SIGs, including student SIGs and **PTA SIGs**, which provide additional ways to connect with colleagues, serve as a conduit for PTA members to be integrated into chapter activities, and provide leadership opportunities, membership recruitment, and retention activities at the grass roots level.

HONORS AND AWARDS

The APTA recognizes PTAs for advanced clinical skills in acute care, aquatic, cardiovascular and pulmonary, education, geriatric, integumentary, musculoskeletal, neuromuscular, and pediatric physical therapy. The standards for receiving **recognition of advanced proficiency for the PTA** are detailed in Box 3-7. Benefits of receiving recognition of advanced proficiency include official recognition from the APTA, designation as an expert within a clinical specialty area, reinforcement of lifelong learning, and merit that may assist with career advancement. PTAs are eligible to receive honors and awards as APTA members, including the F.A. Davis Award for Outstanding PTA Educator, the Mary McMillan Scholarship Award for outstanding student contributions, the Outstanding PTA Award, and the Outstanding PT/PTA Team Award (Box 3-8).[70]

TRENDS

The profession of physical therapy continues to evolve and progress, yet many issues affecting the role of the PTA remain unresolved. As the clinical role of the PT has expanded to include patient/client systems screening, diagnosis of impairments, interpretation of tests and imaging, and consultation with other health professionals, the need for highly educated and technically proficient assistants has become ever more apparent. Expansion into emerging practice areas including wellness and prevention, emergency departments, and women's health ensures continued demand for physical therapy services, which will include utilization of PTAs. Being recognized as the practitioners of choice in the management of musculoskeletal conditions, practicing autonomously, and having direct access will allow additional opportunities for PTs and the PTAs they supervise.

PTA education programs are increasing in number to meet the demand for physical therapy services. With this increase in the number of education programs, and with advancement to the doctor of physical therapy as the professional-level degree for PTs, many questions are raised regarding the

BOX 3-7 ■ *Criteria for APTA's Recognition of Advanced Proficiency for the PTA*

Physical Therapist Assistants who meet the following minimum requirements are eligible for recognition:
1. Current member of APTA.
2. Five years of work experience that must include a minimum of 2000 hours total and at least 500 hours in the past year in 1 of the following categories of work: Acute Care, Aquatic, Cardiovascular and Pulmonary, Education, Geriatrics, Integumentary, Musculoskeletal, Neuromuscular, Oncology, Pediatrics.
3. Completion of at least 60 contact hours (6 CEUs) of continuing education in physical therapy within the last 5 years that includes a minimum of 45 contact hours in the selected area of proficiency. Continuing education must be related to physical therapy and within the scope of work of the PTA as defined by APTA positions, standards, guidelines, policies, and procedures and the *Guide to Physical Therapist Practice.* Continuing education may include topics that are both clinical and nonclinical.
4. Consistent, above-average job performance within the PT/PTA team, verified through a letter of reference from a supervising physical therapist.
5. Evidence of involvement in at least three activities that demonstrate the applicant's leadership abilities and contributions to the community. At least two of these activities must be related to physical therapy or health care.

Adapted from Recognition of Advanced Proficiency for the Physical Therapist assistant, BOD Y09-09-10-11, Board of Directors Policies, Positions, and Guidelines, Alexandria, VA, American Physical Therapy Association, 2009.

clinical role and appropriate educational level for PTAs. The APTA continues to investigate the appropriate entry-level education requirement for PTAs; however, the future of PTA education remains unknown.[25,26]

In attempts to determine the appropriate entry-level education requirement for the PTA in the future, the central question should be, "What level of education best prepares the PTA to assist the PT in providing high-quality, evidence-based patient/client care?" Although increasing the entry-level education requirements in PTA curricula would involve monumental changes to the current educational model and overcoming significant obstacles, the advancement of the entry-level professional education requirement for PTs from the baccalaureate degree to the doctorate of physical therapy faced similar challenges.[71] Possible advantages in increasing the entry-level requirement to the baccalaureate include the following:
■ A stronger scientific foundation on which to build.
■ Increased technical and manual skills.
■ Improved professionalism.
■ Enhanced ability to analyze and apply evidence to clinical work.
■ A possible increase in scope of work.

BOX 3-8	APTA's *Outstanding* PT/PTA Team Award

Purpose

To recognize outstanding clinical practice interaction between physical therapists and physical therapist assistants who are a part of a highly functional PT/PTA Team.

Eligibility

1. Each physical therapist or physical therapist assistant nominee must have been engaged in providing clinical services for at least 5 years.
2. Been licensed or regulated if required by the jurisdiction where the individual is working.
3. The composition of the team may include one or more physical therapists and one or more physical therapist assistants.

Physical therapist and physical therapist assistant teams must have:

4. Worked together (existed) in a clinical practice of any setting for at least 3 years.
5. Positively affected the quality of physical therapy care provided to patients/ clients in their practice setting as a result of their ability to work as a team.
6. Contributed to the enhancement of the overall delivery of physical therapy services in their practice setting as a result of their teamwork.
7. A formal (written) or informal (communicated) team protocol that includes team structure, method of communication, determination of assignments to patients/clients, and method of supervision related to patient/client needs.

Criteria for Selection

The PT/PTA team relationship:

1. Is characterized by trust, mutual respect, adaptability, cooperation, and an appreciation of individual and cultural differences.
2. Involves direction, supervision, and effective communication.
3. Has been enhanced through mentoring, continuing education, and professional development.
4. Has had an effect on the delivery of high quality physical therapy services to patients/clients within their practice setting.

Adapted from Policy and Procedures for the Outstanding Physical Therapist/Physical Therapist Assistant Team Award, BOD Y06-08-02-02, Board of Directors Policies, Positions, and Guidelines, Alexandria, VA, American Physical Therapy Association, 2009.

- Deflection of encroachment on physical therapy practice.
- Bolstering of the drive for direct access in all jurisdictions.
- Decreased restriction of reimbursement for PTA-delivered interventions.
- Attraction of highly qualified students.
- Easing of the "bridge" to PT education.

Disadvantages in increasing the degree requirements may include the following:

- A possible increase in inappropriate utilization of unlicensed support personnel.

■ A potential expectation for increased compensation by baccalaureate-prepared PTAs, although this may not be the case, and was not the case for PTs when degree requirements were advanced.

■ Increased time and expense of a bachelor's degree, which may affect the applicant pool.

■ The possibility that PTA programs located within community colleges may be forced to close or develop articulation agreements with a 4-year institution.

The future of the PTA in the delivery of physical therapy services is being carefully examined by the APTA.[1,71] As the APTA leads the way to clearly define the "roles and responsibilities of the PT and PTA in ensuring effective communication, professional relationships, competent service delivery, assessment of ongoing clinical competence, and skill development,"[25] unwarranted variation in the practice arena exists in the clinical utilization of PTAs.[72,73] Use of clinical practice guidelines developed by APTA related to PT/PTA teams can be useful in reducing this variability.[74] In addition, ensuring that PT students are educated in the appropriate utilization of PTAs is essential to ensure that high-quality outcomes are achieved while selected interventions are directed to PTAs.

Although the clinical role of the PTA remains strictly within the intervention component of the patient/client management model, development of post-entry-level education and specialization will allow for further expansion of the clinical roles PTAs may play in the future. Acquiring specialized clinical techniques, applying newly developed equipment, using technology, and becoming involved in research are some ways PTAs may advance their skills beyond entry-level. PTAs who acquire advanced clinical skills beyond entry level allow their supervising PT greater capacity in quality management of patient/client care.

While the current climate is positive for the PTA, some disturbing trends must be overcome for the PTA to flourish. The current trend of some public and private insurers denying payment or paying at a reduced rate for physical therapy interventions when provided by the PTA is especially troubling. The APTA, alongside other stakeholders within the physical therapy profession, must demonstrate the cost-effective, high-quality service that PTAs provide. Information provided to insurers must include positive clinical outcome data, as well as new practice guidelines specifying direction and supervision standards. A need exists for high-quality clinical research, stressing outcomes, efficiency, and patient/client satisfaction under the PT/PTA team model to justify reimbursement for services provided by PTAs.

As the "baby boomer" generation ages, the demand for physical therapy services is predicted to increase dramatically.[60] Uncertainty exists, though, in part because of recent health care legislation impacting physical therapy practice, and therefore PTAs, including the Medicare therapy cap and sustainable growth rate, the Affordable Care Act of 2010, pay-for-performance legislation, and Veterans Administration (VA) health care reform.[75] Legislation must address fair payment for services, direct access and referral for profit arrangements, all of which are potential hurdles in the future of the profession of physical therapy and of the PTA.[76]

How the PTA membership category of the APTA evolves will have an effect on the future role of the PTA within the profession of physical therapy. Evolution will undoubtedly occur, if history serves as a model for the future. The APTA provided increased integration of the PTA into governance activities, but progress must continue. The PTA Caucus, in its short existence, has influenced a growth in membership, recognition, and value of membership. The APTA and the PTA Caucus must continue to work collaboratively to nurture the relationship with potential PTA members, and with each other. Once they become members, PTAs are able to take advantage of the benefits, services, and professional relationships they will form from APTA involvement to further develop the role of the PTA in the delivery of physical therapy services.

SUMMARY

Since the graduation of the first PTAs in 1969 to the recent APTA investigation of the feasibility of a transition to an entry-level baccalaureate, the PTA has proven to be a cost-effective and high-quality provider of physical therapy interventions. Currently the associates degree is appropriate for preparing the PTA; however, the clinical skills demanded of PTAs necessitate close examination of their educational preparation to ensure that they remain the most qualified persons to meet the needs of the physical therapy profession in the future. The APTA will continue to be the authority in guiding PTA education programs, accreditors, professional licensing agencies, state boards of physical therapy, and clinicians in creating a clear definition of the role of the PTA in the future.

PTAs presently have the opportunity to be recognized by the APTA for advanced proficiency in 10 clinical specialty areas. Advanced Proficiency Pathways provide an opportunity for development of post-graduate specialization. Career ladders use this recognition in some clinics to provide advancement opportunities. After an evolution of membership categories and statuses, the PTA Caucus provides an effective structure for PTA representation within the APTA. PTA leadership has the opportunity for collaboration with their PT counterparts in helping to determine the policies and positions of the APTA. Although state practice acts vary greatly, PTAs are licensed or otherwise regulated in all 50 states and the District of Columbia. Many factors, including legislation, reimbursement, economic trends, and an aging population, influence the demand for physical therapy services, but the future of the profession and of the PTA is promising.

To produce high-quality outcomes efficiently, the PT/PTA team must be one of mutual respect, collaboration, and ongoing communication. Within the PT/PTA team, careful consideration of a multitude of factors affecting patient care is vital to practice and work legally, ethically, and effectively. The controversy concerning the role of the PTA will diminish as the profession of physical therapy continues to mature and develop. As PTs and PTAs work collaboratively in the clinic, so must the PT and PTA leadership within the APTA to achieve the vision for the profession of physical therapy.

CASE STUDIES

The following case studies illustrate examples of the roles and variety of practice settings for PTAs and their supervising PTs. Case Study One is an example of an effective PT/PTA team using communication, mutual respect, and ethical practice patterns to provide high-quality care in a demanding clinical setting. Case Studies Two through Four illustrate practical applications of the many factors that must be considered when making direction and supervision decisions and include reflection questions for consideration.

<table>
<tr>
<td>

CASE STUDY ONE

</td>
<td>

Brody, a PT with 9 years' experience in a variety of settings, is responsible for patient care at two small physical therapy clinics. The clinics are in a state that allows general (off-site) supervision of PTAs. Each setting employs one PTA, who is responsible for providing selected interventions within the clinic. Brody carries a cellular phone and is available for consultation continuously. Shae, a PTA with 4 years' experience, works at the first clinic, which is a rural hospital setting. Shae has participated in continuing education courses several times a year since graduating as a PTA, even though CEUs are not required to maintain licensure in her state. She averages 8 to 12 patient/client treatments per day. Piper, a PTA employed at the second clinic, has 14 years of clinical experience and was a recipient of the APTA's Recognition of Advanced Proficiency for the Physical Therapist Assistant in geriatrics. This clinic serves older adults living in the retirement village, as well as inpatients at the attached ECF. Brody's office is at the ECF, where he is available for examinations, evaluations, patient/client treatment, and on-site supervision.

</td>
</tr>
</table>

After completing an examination and evaluation at the ECF, Brody meets with Piper to review the plan of care he established for the new patient, and her ongoing patient caseload. Piper discusses treatment techniques, patient response, and progress toward established goals. She requests adding stair training to the plan of care for a patient who is supposed to be discharged home in 4 days and has three steps to enter her front door. After their meeting, Brody performs joint mobilization for a patient with adhesive capsulitis of the shoulder (frozen shoulder) before going to the hospital. Piper remains busy throughout the day, treating a variety of patients/clients. Late in the day, while working with Mrs. Gaddis, an 89-year-old woman who recently was discharged to her home in the retirement village after hip replacement surgery, Piper noticed the patient's calf on her involved lower extremity was edematous, red, and painful to the touch. Because this was a new clinical presentation, and because these signs are suspicious for a deep vein thrombosis (DVT), Piper decided to stop the intervention and contact Brody on his cell phone. Brody instructed Piper to contact the physician on call, who was making rounds in the ECF.

Meanwhile, at the hospital, Shae has been performing wound care on Mr. Helton, a 38-year-old man with a lower extremity ulcer. Shae provides pulsed-lavage cleansing to the wound in the physical therapy department, which involves the use of pressurized saline solution to remove loosely attached cellular debris and surface pathogens contained in wound exudate. Brody has arrived from the ECF and has been reviewing two new referrals received for physical therapy evaluations. When Shae inspects the wound bed, she notices adherent necrotic tissue is preventing the wound bed from healing and she asks Brody to examine the wound. After examining the wound, Brody decides to remove the necrotic tissue using sharp debridement. Brody then contacts the referring physician to suggest adding a topical agent that assists in the regeneration of healthy tissue.

As Brody proceeds to the neurologic floor to complete one of the new evaluations, Shae provides wound care interventions to two more patients per their established plans of care. After completing the evaluation, Brody and Shae briefly meet in the nurse's station to discuss treatment options and goals for the new patient who is recovering from a cerebrovascular accident (CVA). Shae suggests using body weight supported treadmill training (BWSTT) with the patient, as she is having difficulty with standing and walking as the result of hemiparesis (weakness on one side of the body).

Shae continues with her busy day, providing physical therapy interventions throughout various hospital areas and with a variety of patient/client types and diagnoses. After lunch Shae receives a call in the physical therapy gym from Paige, the hospital social worker. Paige informs Shae that Mr. Wasson, a 56-year-old man with a surgically repaired femur fracture, is being discharged by his orthopedist that afternoon, as long as Mr. Wasson is able to safely ambulate and maintain his non-weight-bearing (NWB) status. Shae had treated Mr. Wasson only one time after the physical therapy evaluation the day before, and the patient had required minimal assistance for walking short distances with his crutches. After discussing the situation with Brody, Shae asks the physical therapy aide to transport Mr. Wasson to the department for additional gait training. After Mr. Wasson experiences continued struggles using crutches, Shae instructs him in the use of a standard walker. Mr. Wasson is able to maintain his NWB status with the walker, and Shae decides this is the best option. Before leaving the physical therapy department, Mr. Wasson demonstrates his patellar joint mobilizations and gait pattern using the walker for Brody, who has just arrived. Brody completes the discharge summary with input from Shae, and Mr. Wasson is able to go home that afternoon.

CASE STUDY TWO	You are a new graduate PTA working in an outpatient pediatric clinic. Your supervising PT, Owen, is scheduled to work the same hours as you, to perform evaluations and reassessments, and to provide on-site supervision and patient/client treatments in the same gym. One morning as Ella, your first patient, arrives, you are informed by Stephanie, the occupational therapist, that Owen will not be coming to work because of illness.

Discuss the legal and ethical dilemma presented in Case Study Two. Under what conditions would you provide treatment to Ella? What conditions would prevent you from providing treatment in this situation? What policies or procedures should the clinic adopt to deal with this type of situation in the future?

CASE STUDY THREE	You are a PT with 5 years of experience, and a board-certified neurologic clinical specialist (NCS). Although you have advanced clinical skills, you have never supervised a PTA. You have taken a position in an inpatient acute rehabilitation hospital on the stroke team, where you will be supervising André, a PTA with 17 years' experience. One Monday morning you notice André gait-training a patient in the gym who had been evaluated over the weekend by James, a part-time PT. On reviewing the chart, you notice that the plan of care does not include gait training because the patient was too weak to stand up during the evaluation. When you ask André

3

about this, he states, "The nurse said she helped her into the bathroom this morning, and told me it was okay to start her gait training today."

Discuss the legal and ethical dilemma presented in Case Study Three. Who is considered the "physical therapist of record" in this situation? How would you address the missing communication component in ensuring all factors are considered when directing selected interventions to a PTA?

CASE STUDY FOUR	You are a PTA with 6 years of experience working with pediatric patients in an inpatient rehabilitation hospital, and a certified athletic trainer experienced in working with young athletes. You have decided to take a position working with adults in their homes so that you can have more flexibility in your schedule. After receiving an orientation to the paperwork and meeting Yvette, your supervising PT, you are given a stack of charts to review before beginning to provide treatments. While reviewing the chart for Mr. Westerfield, a 76-year-old man recovering from a trimalleolar (ankle) fracture, you notice that his plan of care includes performing joint mobilization of the subtalar and talocrural joints of the ankle. Although you are familiar with normal and pathologic arthrokinematics (accessory joint movement) of these joints, you have not been instructed in performance of these techniques. In addition, you are aware that although your state practice act is silent regarding joint mobilization, an APTA position statement indicates that this technique is "exclusively performed by the physical therapist."

Discuss the legal and ethical dilemma presented in Case Study Four. How would you communicate with Yvette regarding Mr. Westerfield's plan of care? How might your inability to perform this technique adversely affect patient outcomes in this situation?

REFERENCES

1. American Physical Therapy Association (APTA): *Distinction between the physical therapist and the physical therapist assistant in physical therapy, HOD P06-01-18-19. House of Delegates Standards, Policies, Positions, and Guidelines,* Alexandria, VA, 2009, APTA.
2. American Physical Therapy Association (APTA): *Direction and supervision of the Physical Therapist Assistant, HOD P06-05-18-26. House of Delegates Standards, Policies, Positions, and Guidelines,* Alexandria, VA, 2009, APTA.
3. American Physical Therapy Association (APTA): *PTA caucus: description of the physical therapist assistant, PTA caucus annual meeting minutes June,* Alexandria, VA, 2014, APTA.
4. Worthingham CA: Nonprofessional personnel in physical therapy: the dilemma of the profession, *Phys Ther* 45:112–115, 1965.
5. Fowles B: On-the-job training, *Phys Ther* 45:124–126, 1965.
6. Robins V: The challenge of the profession, *Phys Ther* 45:116–118, 1965.
7. Killen MB: Supportive personnel in physical therapy, *Phys Ther* 47:483–490, 1967.
8. McDaniel L: Formal training for assistants to physical therapists, *Phys Ther* 42:562–565, 1962.
9. Blood H, Blood H, Blood H: Report of the ad hoc committee to study the utilization and training of nonprofessional assistants, *Phys Ther* 47(11, Part 2):31–39, 1967.
10. Hislop H: Man power versus mind power, *Phys Ther* 43:711, 1963.
11. Woods EN: PTAs: their history and development, *PT Mag Phys Ther* 1(4):34–39, 1993.
12. White B: Physical therapy assistants: Implications for the future, *Phys Ther* 50:674–679, 1970.
13. American Physical Therapy Association (APTA): *Training and utilization of the physical therapy assistant, policy statement adopted by the House of Delegates, 1967:* Alexandria, VA, 1967, APTA. www.eric.ed.gov/PDFS/ED026493.pdf. Accessed September 26, 2014.
14. Carpenter-Davis C: Physical therapist assistant education over the decades, *J Phys Ther Educ* 17(3):80–85, 2003.

15. Essentials of an Interim Approved Educational Program for the Physical Therapist Assistant: *American Physical Therapy Association, House of Delegates Minutes, June 16, 18-19, 1975,* Alexandria, VA, 1975, APTA.
16. Bashi HL, Domholdt E: Use of support personnel for physical therapy treatment, *Phys Ther* 73:421–429, 1993.
17. American Physical Therapy Association (APTA): *Coalitions for consensus: a shared vision for Physical Therapist Assistant Education,* Alexandria, VA, 1997, APTA.
18. American Physical Therapy Association (APTA): *A normative model of physical therapist assistant education: version 2007,* Alexandria, VA, 2007, APTA.
19. *Evaluative criteria for accreditation of education programs for the preparation of physical therapist assistants, 2013:* Commission of Accreditation in Physical Therapy Education. http://www.capteonline.org/uploadedFiles/CAPTEorg/About_CAPTE/Resources/Accreditation_Handbook/EvaluativeCriteria_PTA.pdf. Accessed April 26, 2014.
20. American Physical Therapy Association (APTA): *Guide to physical therapist practice 3.0, 2014:* Alexandria, VA, 2014, APTA. http://guidetoptpractice.apta.org/. Accessed April 26, 2014.
21. Enchelmayer KB, Hamby EF, Martindale C: The impact of the balanced budget act of 1997 on the physical therapy profession, *Health Care Manag* 19:58–69, 2001.
22. American Physical Therapy Association (APTA): *Procedural interventions exclusively performed by physical therapists, HOD P06-00-30-36. House of Delegates standards, policies, positions, and guidelines,* Alexandria, VA, 2012, APTA.
23. American Physical Therapy Association (APTA): *Board of Directors Meeting Minutes, March 2003,* Alexandria, VA, 2003, APTA.
24. American Physical Therapy Association (APTA): *Minimum required skills of physical therapist assistants at entry-level BOD G11-08-09-18. Board of Directors Policies, Positions, and Guidelines,* Alexandria, VA, 2012, APTA.
25. American Physical Therapy Association (APTA): *Physical therapist assistant in practice and education mega issue discussion resolution. Board of Directors Meeting Minutes, March 2009,* Alexandria, VA, 2009, APTA.
26. Ward S: A valuable resource: recent actions confirm the important role of the PTA in the practice of physical therapy and in APTA, *PT Mag Phys Ther* 17(5):14–16, 2009.
27. American Physical Therapy Association (APTA): *RC 3-11: physical therapist responsibility and accountability for the delivery of care. House of Delegates Minutes, June 2011,* Alexandria, VA, 2011, APTA.
28. American Physical Therapy Association (APTA): *RC 22-14: rescind: physical therapist responsibility and accountability for the delivery of care. House of Delegates Minutes, June 2014,* Alexandria, VA, 2014, APTA.
29. Jurisdictional Licensure Reference Guide. Alexandria, VA, Federation of State Boards of Physical Therapy. https://www.fsbpt.org/FreeResources/RegulatoryResources/LicensureReferenceGuide.aspx. Accessed September 26, 2014.
30. Standards and required elements for accreditation of physical therapist assistant education programs. Commission of Accreditation in Physical Therapy Education. http://www.capteonline.org/uploadedFiles/CAPTEorg/About_CAPTE/Resources/Accreditation_Handbook/CAPTE_PTAStandardsEvidence.pdf. Accessed May 19, 2015.
31. Standards and required elements for accreditation of physical therapist education programs. Commission on Accreditation in Physical Therapy Education. http://www.capteonline.org/uploadedFiles/CAPTEorg/About_CAPTE/Resources/Accreditation_Handbook/CAPTE_PTStandardsEvidence.pdf. Accessed May 19, 2015.
32. American Physical Therapy Association (APTA): *Supervision of student physical therapist assistants, HOD P06-11-09-17. House of Delegates Standards, Policies, Positions, and Guidelines,* Alexandria, VA, 2012, APTA.
33. American Physical Therapy Association (APTA): *Guidelines: clinical education sites, HOD G06-93-27-52. House of Delegates Standards, Policies, Positions, and Guidelines,* Alexandria, VA, 2012, APTA.
34. American Physical Therapy Association (APTA): *Guidelines: clinical instructors, BOD G03-06-21-55. Board of Directors Policies, Positions, and Guidelines,* Alexandria, VA, 2012, APTA.

35. American Physical Therapy Association (APTA): *Clinical performance instruments, 2014:* Alexandria, VA, 2014, APTA. http://www.apta.org/Educators/Assessments/. Accessed September 26, 2014.

36. American Physical Therapy Association (APTA): Clinical Instructor Education and Credentialing Program. Alexandria, VA, APTA. http://www.apta.org/CCIP/. Accessed September 26, 2014.

37. American Physical Therapy Association (APTA): *Values-base behaviors for the PTA, 2011:* Alexandria, VA, 2011, APTA. http://www.apta.org/uploadedFiles/APTAorg/PTAs/Careers/Values/ValuesBasedBehaviorsforPTA.pdf. Accessed November 18, 2014.

38. American Physical Therapy Association (APTA): Education programs bridging from PTA to PT. Alexandria, VA, APTA. http://www.capteonline.org/Programs/Bridge/. Accessed September 26, 2014.

39. American Physical Therapy Association (APTA): *2012-2013 fact sheet: physical therapist assistant education programs,* Alexandria, VA, 2014, APTA. http://www.capteonline.org/uploadedFiles/CAPTEorg/About_CAPTE/Resources/Aggregate_Program_Data/AggregateProgramData_PTAPrograms.pdf#search=%22fact%22. Accessed September 26, 2014.

40. Saunders L: A systematic approach to delegation in out-patient physiotherapy, *Physiotherapy* 83 (11):582–589, 1997.

41. The Model Practice Act for Physical Therapy: A tool for public protection and legislative change, ed 5. Alexandria, VA, the Federation of State Boards of Physical Therapy. https://www.fsbpt.org/FreeResources/RegulatoryResources/ModelPracticeAct.aspx. Accessed September 26, 2014.

42. American Physical Therapy Association (APTA): *Levels of supervision, HOD P06-00-15-26. House of Delegates Standards, Policies, Positions, and Guidelines,* Alexandria, VA, 2012, APTA.

43. New Jersey Administrative Code, Title 13: law and public safety, chapter 39A: state board of physical therapy. http://www.njconsumeraffairs.gov/chapters/Chapter%2039A%20State%20Board%20of%20Physical%20Therapy.pdf. Accessed September 26, 2014.

44. Texas Board of Physical Therapy Examiners: rules, June 2014. http://ptot.texas.gov/idl/9A3B2FEE-52C0-8DC6-2A09-265FCE7DED3F. Accessed September 26, 2014.

45. American Physical Therapy Association (APTA): *Physical therapist of record and "Hand Off" communication, HOD P06-08-16-16. House of Delegates Standards, Policies, Positions, and Guidelines,* Alexandria, VA, 2012, APTA.

46. Publication 100-02 Medicare Benefit Policy Transmittal 88, Centers for Medicare and Medicaid Services, 2008: Baltimore, MD, 2008, Department of Health and Human Services. https://www.cms.gov/Regulations-and-Guidance/Guidance/Transmittals/downloads/r88bp.pdf. Accessed September 26, 2014.

47. Nicholson SK: Managing risk. In Nicholson SK, editor: *The physical therapist's business practice and legal guide,* Sudbury, MA, 2008, Jones & Bartlett Learning, pp 289–297.

48. Physical therapist professional liability claims study, 2006: Chicago, IL, 2006, CNA Financial Corp. https://www.cna.com/vcm_content/CNA/internet/Static%20File%20for%20Download/Risk%20Control/Medical%20Services/Physical_Therapy_Claims_Study.pdf. Accessed September 26, 2014.

49. Welk P: Risk management considerations for physical therapy service delegation, *PT Mag Phys Ther* 16(11):18–21, 2008.

50. American Physical Therapy Association (APTA): *Provision of physical therapy interventions and related tasks, HOD P06-00-17-28. House of Delegates Standards, Policies, Positions, and Guidelines,* Alexandria, VA, 2012, APTA.

51. American Physical Therapy Association (APTA): *Reimbursement for physical therapy services, HOD 06-01-12-15. House of Delegates Standards, Policies, Positions, and Guidelines,* Alexandria, VA, 2012, APTA.

52. Federation of State Boards of Physical Therapy (FSBPT): *Analysis of practice for the physical therapy profession: entry-level physical therapist assistants,* Alexandria, VA, 2011, FSBPT.

53. American Physical Therapy Association (APTA): *Policy and procedures for the outstanding physical therapist/physical therapist assistant team award, BOD Y08-14-04-07. Board of Directors Policies, Positions, and Guidelines,* Alexandria, VA, 2014, APTA.

54. American Physical Therapy Association (APTA): *Professional development, lifelong learning, and continued competence in physical therapy, HOD P05-07-14-14. House of Delegates Standards, Policies, Positions, and Guidelines,* Alexandria, VA, 2012, APTA.
55. American Physical Therapy Association (APTA): *Standards of ethical conduct for the physical therapist assistant HOD S06-09-20-18. House of Delegates Standards, Policies, Positions, and Guidelines,* Alexandria, VA, 2012, APTA.
56. Curtis KA, DeCelle Newman P: *The PTA handbook: keys to success in school and career for the Physical Therapist Assistant,* ed 2, Thorofare, NJ, 2014, SLACK, pp. 253–267.
57. Considerations for practice opportunities and professional development. Alexandria, VA, American Physical Therapy Association Department of Education. http://www.apta.org/CareerManagement/ConsiderationsforOpportunities/. Accessed September 26, 2014.
58. American Physical Therapy Association (APTA): *PTA Advanced Proficiency Pathways (APP).* August, 2014. http://www.apta.org/APP/. Accessed September 26, 2014.
59. Physical Therapist Member Demographic Profile 2013. Alexandria, VA, American Physical Therapy Association. Available at http://www.apta.org/WorkforceData/. Accessed May 23, 2014.
60. Bureau of Labor Statistics, U.S. Department of Labor, *Occupational Outlook Handbook, 2014-15 Edition,* Physical Therapist Assistants and Aides. http://www.bls.gov/ooh/healthcare/physical-therapist-assistants-and-aides.htm. Accessed May 23, 2014.
61. Desilets MPTA: Viewpoint: climbing the ladder: constructing a clinical career path for PTAs, *PT Mag Phys Ther* 16(11):46–49, 2008.
62. American Physical Therapy Association (APTA): RC 10-73: *Affiliate Membership, House of Delegates Minutes. June 27, 1973,* Alexandria, VA, 1973, APTA.
63. American Physical Therapy Association (APTA): *Bylaw amendment: rights and privileges of members, article iv, section 2-3-b. House of Delegates Minutes, June 13-15, 1992,* Alexandria, VA, 1992, APTA.
64. American Physical Therapy Association (APTA): RC 1-98: *National Assembly of Physical Therapist Assistants, House of Delegates Minutes, June 5, 1998,* Alexandria, VA, 2015, APTA.
65. American Physical Therapy Association (APTA): RC 3-15: *Amend: Bylaws of the American Physical Therapy Association to Grant Components the Option of Amending their Bylaws to Provide a Full Vote for Physical Therapist Assistant Members. House of Delegates Minutes, June 2015,* Alexandria, VA, 2015, APTA.
66. American Physical Therapy Association (APTA): *The Future Role of the Physical Therapist Assistant-Replacement Packet II, House of Delegates Minutes, June 18-20, 2001,* Alexandria, VA, 2001, APTA.
67. American Physical Therapy Association (APTA): *Amendment to the bylaws of the APTA, House of Delegates Minutes, June 6-8, 2005,* Alexandria, VA, 2005, APTA.
68. American Physical Therapy Association (APTA): *Physical therapist assistant Caucus procedure manual,* Alexandria, VA, 2014, APTA.
69. American Physical Therapy Association (APTA): *Guidelines; formation and structure of component special interest groups, BOD G03-99-30-95. House of Delegates Standards, Policies, Positions, and Guidelines,* Alexandria, VA, 2012, APTA.
70. American Physical Therapy Association (APTA): *Policy and Procedures for the Outstanding Physical therapist/Physical Therapist Assistant Team Award, BOD Y06-08-02-02. Board of Directors Policies, Positions, and Guidelines,* Alexandria, VA, 2012, APTA.
71. American Physical Therapy Association (APTA): RC20-12: *Feasibility study for transitioning to an entry-level Baccalaureate physical therapist assistant degree. House of Delegates Minutes, June 2012,* Alexandria, VA, 2012, APTA.
72. Resnik L, Feng Z, Hart DL: State regulation and the delivery of physical therapy services, *Health* 41:1296–1316, 2006.
73. Resnik L, Liu D, Mor V, Hart D: Predictors of physical therapy clinic performance in the treatment of patients with low back pain syndromes, *Phys Ther* 88:989–1004, 2008.
74. American Physical Therapy Association (APTA): PT/PTA Teamwork: Models in Delivering Patient Care. June, 2013. http://www.apta.org/SupervisionTeamwork/Models/. Accessed September 26, 2014.
75. *Report to Congress: Increasing the Value of Medicare: Toward Better Value in Purchasing Outpatient Therapy Services,* Washington, DC, 2006, Medicare Payment Advisory Commission. http://67.59.137.244/publications%5Ccongressional_reports%5CJun06_Ch06.pdf. Accessed September 26, 2014.
76. American Physical Therapy Association (APTA): Understanding Health Care Reform. Alexandria, VA, APTA. http://www.apta.org/HealthCareReform/. Accessed September 26, 2014.

ADDITIONAL RESOURCES

Clynch H: *The role of the physical therapist assistant: regulations and responsibilities*, Philadelphia, PA, 2012, F. A. Davis. Comprehensive text on PTA history, education, practice and regulation.

Bradford B: PTAs today: The history makers, celebrating 40 years of PTAs: A four part series, PT in Motion 1(1):60–63, 2009:1(2):56–59, 2009; 1(3):44–46, 2009; 2(1):52-57, 2010. A four-part series describing the origin, history, and perspectives on the future of the PTA.

Solberg J: The Entry-Level Baccalaureate: pro, *PT in Motion* 5(11):38–42, 2014.

Dougherty J: The Entry-Level Baccalaureate: Con, *PT in Motion* 5(12):64–70, 2014. Together these two articles discuss the pros and cons of advancing the entry-level degree requirement of the PTA to the Bachelor's degree.

Dreeben O: *Physical therapy clinical handbook for PTAs*, ed 2, Sudbury, MA, 2012, Jones and Bartlett. A comprehensive reference regarding the PT/PTA relationship, clinical documentation, and provision of interventions.

Information for Physical Therapist Assistants. http://www.apta.org/PTA/. This section of the APTA website contains all of the PTA-specific information and documents that APTA has developed for PTA members. Members are able to access information on education, career planning and development, leadership opportunities, scholarship opportunities, and more.

"PTAs Today." In: PT in Motion (formerly PT: Magazine of Physical Therapy). The professional issues magazine of the American Physical Therapy Association (APTA). "PTAs Today" is a regular feature, authored by PTAs, that provides a human interest look at issues concerning PTA members.

The Federation of State Boards of Physical Therapy. www.fsbpt.org. Website contains links to practice acts in all jurisdictions, information about the National Physical Therapy Examinations for physical therapists and physical therapist assistants, and the model practice act.

REVIEW QUESTIONS

1. Name and describe the current structure within the APTA to provide representation for PTA members.
2. Identify the factors that must be considered by a physical therapist when making direction and supervision decisions following an evaluation.
3. Describe current trends in the health care environment and/or physical therapy practice that may provide further opportunity or limitations for PTA clinical work.
4. Discuss the arguments for and against increasing the level of PTA education to the bachelor's degree.
5. List the requirements for and benefits of obtaining the APTA's Advanced Proficiency for the Physical Therapist Assistant.
6. Explain clinical problem solving. Why is it an essential skill for the PTA to master?
7. Define "unwarranted variation" in practice as it relates to PTA utilization. Discuss steps that can decrease variation in clinical utilization of PTAs.

If you want to increase knowledge in your field, expand networking possibilities, or jump-start your job hunt, a professional association membership is an option worth exploring.[1]

Marybeth Gunner Pulliam

4

American Physical Therapy Association

Michael A. Pagliarulo

Federation of State Boards of Physical Therapy
    (FSBPT)
Foundation for Physical Therapy
House of Delegates (HOD)
NEXT Conference and Exposition
Physical Therapy Political Action Committee
    (PT-PAC)
section
special interest group (SIG)
World Confederation for Physical Therapy
    (WCPT)

LEARNING OBJECTIVES

After reading this chapter, the reader will be
able to:

- Describe the structure and function of the
  American Physical Therapy Association.
- Distinguish between sections and
  assemblies within the Association.
- Identify and describe organizations that are
  related to the Association.
- Describe the benefits of belonging to the
  Association.

The definition of physical therapy presented in Chapter 1 demonstrates that
this discipline is a profession because it possesses all the qualities or criteria of
a profession. One of these criteria is a representative organization. This chapter
focuses on the **American Physical Therapy Association (APTA)**, which is a
national organization that represents the physical therapy profession. The organization's mission, structure, and benefits are described here. A historical
account of the Association was presented in Chapter 1. Affiliated and related
organizations representing physical therapy interests are included at the end
of this chapter.

VISION, MISSION, AND GOALS

The APTA is a national member-driven organization that represents the profession of physical therapy (Figure 4-1). It is composed of more than 90,000 physical
therapists (PTs), physical therapist assistants (PTAs), and students throughout
the United States and abroad. Membership is strictly voluntary.

A strategic plan of a typical organization commonly opens with a vision, a
mission, and goals before proceeding to objectives and action plans. The Vision
Statement of the APTA, "Transforming society by optimizing movement to
improve the human experience," was described in Chapter 1. Mission and goals
are described here.

In 1993 the House of Delegates (HOD) of the APTA adopted a mission statement and related position to fulfill the mission. The mission statement[2] (Box 4-1)
and fulfillment position[3] (Box 4-2) demonstrate the profession's interest in serving the public and its members through practice, education, and research.

Goals for the APTA are proposed by the Board of Directors (BOD). They are
then reviewed and approved by the HOD. The goals as of this writing were
approved by the HOD in June 2005 and are presented in Box 4-3.[4] These goals
direct the activities and funding priorities for the APTA and reiterate the ground-
ing in education, research, and practice. They are anchored to the Vision 2020
Statement and further promote activities to attain this vision. Now that the
Vision Statement has been updated, the Goals will no doubt reflect this in the
future (see Chapter 1 for further description of Vision 2020 and the Vision Statement for Physical Therapy).

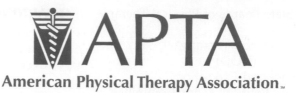

Figure 4-1 ■ Logo for the American Physical Therapy Association. (Courtesy American Physical Therapy Association.)

BOX 4-1	Mission of the American Physical Therapy Association

The mission of the American Physical Therapy Association (APTA), the principal membership organization representing and promoting the profession of physical therapy, is to further the profession's role in the prevention, diagnosis, and treatment of movement dysfunctions and the enhancement of the physical health and functional abilities of members of the public.

BOX 4-2	Mission Statement Fulfillment

To fulfill the American Physical Therapy Association's (APTA's) Mission, to meet the needs and interests of its members, and to promote physical therapy as a vital professional career, the Association shall:

■ Promote physical therapy care and services through the establishment, maintenance, and promotion of ethical principles and quality standards for practice, education, and research.

■ Influence policy in the public and private sectors.

■ Enable physical therapy practitioners to improve their skills, knowledge, and operations in the interest of furthering the profession.

■ Develop and improve the art and science of physical therapy, including practice, education, and research.

■ Facilitate a common understanding and appreciation for the diversity of the profession, the membership, and the communities we serve.

■ Maintain a stable and diverse financial base from which to fund the programs, services, and operations that support this mission.

BOX 4-3

Goals That Represent the Priorities of the American Physical Therapy Association

Goal I: Physical therapists are universally recognized and promoted as the practitioners of choice for persons with conditions that affect movement and function.

Goal II: Physical therapists are universally recognized and promoted as providers of fitness, health promotion, wellness, and risk-reduction programs to enhance quality of life for persons across the life span.

Goal III: Academic and clinical education prepares doctors of physical therapy who are autonomous practitioners.

Goal IV: Physical therapists are autonomous practitioners to whom patients/clients have unrestricted direct access as an entry point into the health care delivery system and who are paid for all elements of patient/client management in all practice environments.

Goal V: Research advances the science of physical therapy and furthers the evidence-based practice of the physical therapist.

Goal VI: Physical therapists and physical therapist assistants are committed to meeting the health needs of patients/clients and society through ethical behavior, continued competence, collegial relationships with other health care practitioners, and advocacy for the profession.

Goal VII: Communication throughout the American Physical Therapy Association (APTA) enhances participation of and responsiveness to members and promotes and instills the value of belonging to the APTA.

Goal VIII: APTA standards, policies, positions, guidelines and the *Guide to Physical Therapist Practice, Normative Model of Physical Therapist Education, Evaluative Criteria for Accreditation of Education Programs for the Preparation of Physical Therapists, Normative Model of Physical Therapist Assistant Education, Evaluative Criteria for Accreditation of Education Program for the Preparation of Physical Therapist Assistants,* and *Professionalism in Physical Therapy: Core Values* are recognized and used as the foundation for physical therapist practice, research, and education environments.

These goals are based upon APTA Vision Statement for Physical Therapy 2020 (Vision 2020), developed by the Association in 2000. The goals encompass the Association's major priorities as it moves toward realization of the ideals set forth in Vision 2020. The Board is committed to these goals as the foundation from which to lead the Association. The Association's awareness of cultural diversity, its commitment to expanding minority representation and participation in physical therapy, and its commitment to equal opportunity for all members permeate these goals. These goals are not ranked and do not represent any priority order.

4

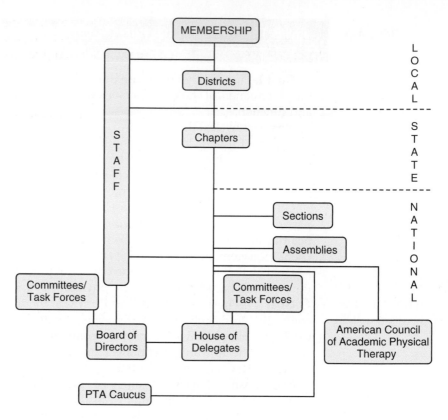

Figure 4-2 ■ Three levels of organization within the American Physical Therapy Association. Note how the membership drives this organization. Staff members provide support at all levels, including membership, local, state, and national. Washington, DC, is also a chapter.

ORGANIZA-TIONAL STRUCTURE

The organizational structure of the APTA is depicted in Figure 4-2. This structure provides a three-tiered approach—districts at the local level, chapters at the state level, and several units at the national level—to serve the membership, which is the heart and soul of the organization. Chapters at the state level, and sections, assemblies, and the newly formed American Council of Academic Physical Therapy at the national level are the **components** of the APTA. The BOD and HOD, with their respective committees and task forces, the Physical Therapist Assistant Caucus, and staff complete the general plan of this organization. Each level is described in this section, beginning with the primary unit, the membership.

MEMBERSHIP

As stated earlier, membership in the APTA is voluntary; however, it is estimated that approximately two-thirds of licensed PTs in the United States are members. This extensive membership provides strength and diversity to the organization.

The primary membership categories of the APTA are physical therapist, physical therapist assistant, and their respective student categories.[5] Other categories include life, retired, honorary (not a member in any other category and has made outstanding contributions to the APTA or health of the public), and Catherine Worthingham Fellow of the APTA (physical therapist member for at least 15 years who has made notable contributions to the profession; may use the initials *FAPTA*). Requirements for membership include graduation from (or enrollment in) an education program approved by (or seeking candidacy from) a recognized accrediting agency. In addition, the applicant must sign a pledge indicating compliance with the *Code of Ethics* (physical therapist and related categories) or *Standards of Ethical Conduct for the Physical Therapist Assistant* (physical therapist assistant and related categories) and pay dues.

Service to the membership has always been one of the main purposes of the APTA. Members have had a sense of pride and commitment to the organization. In fact, during the formative years of the profession, membership in this organization was considered the standard for competence. This proud heritage remains today; however, membership is not required to demonstrate competence.

DISTRICTS

As noted in Figure 4-2, a **district** is the most local organizational unit in the structure of APTA. Districts do not exist in all jurisdictions, such as small states. Membership is automatic where they do exist and may be based on the location of residence or employment as provided in the bylaws of APTA.

Districts are more common in locations with high population densities or large geographic areas and frequently consist of one or more counties. This arrangement provides a mechanism for convenient meetings and participation. It also provides a basis for representation in a body that conducts business at the next level of organization, the chapter.

CHAPTERS

In accordance with the standing rules of APTA, a **chapter** "must coincide with or be confined within the legally constituted boundaries of a state, territory, or commonwealth of the United States or the District of Columbia."[6] In 2015, APTA consisted of 51 chapters—one for each state and the District of Columbia. Membership in a chapter is automatic and based on location of residence, employment, education, or greatest active participation (in the last case, only in an immediately adjacent chapter). In contrast to districts, which are not permitted to assess dues, each chapter requires dues from PT and PTA members and, in a few cases, student members.

Chapters are an important component of APTA. They provide a mechanism for participation at a state level and proportionate representation at the national level (see later discussion of the HOD). Chapters also provide an important voice for members at the state level of government. This capacity is essential to maintain statewide legislation and regulations appropriate to the profession and practice of physical therapy.

SECTIONS

A **section** is organized at the national level exclusively. In accordance with the bylaws of APTA, sections provide an opportunity for members with similar areas of interest to "meet, confer, and promote the interests of the respective sections."[5] Membership in one or more of the 18 sections listed in Table 4-1 is

Table 4-1
Sections of the American Physical Therapy Association

Section	Area(s) of Interest	Publication(s)
Acute Care	Physical therapy practitioners working with patients with acute care needs across the life span	*Acute Care Perspectives*
Aquatic Physical Therapy	Advance the practice of aquatic physical therapy	*Journal of Aquatic Physical Therapy, Waterlines*
Cardiovascular and Pulmonary	Development, application, and advancement of cardiovascular and pulmonary physical therapy practice, education, and research	*Cardiopulmonary Physical Therapy Journal*
Clinical Electrophysiology and Wound Management	Electrotherapy and physical agents, electrophysiologic evaluation, physical agents, and wound management SIGs: Electrophysiology, Electrotherapy, and Wound Management	*Clinical Electrophysiology and Wound Management*
Education	Developing new practitioners, academic educators, educational leaders, and administrators SIGs: Academic Faculty, PTA Educators, and Clinical Educators	*Journal of Physical Therapy Education*
Federal Physical Therapy	High-quality physical therapy within federal medical services	e-Newsletter
Geriatrics	Clinical excellence of PTs and PTAs working with older adults SIGs: Balance and Falls, Health Promotion and Wellness, and Osteoporosis	*Journal of Geriatric Physical Therapy*
Hand Rehabilitation	Hand and upper extremity rehabilitation	*Hand Prints*
Health Policy and Administration	Leadership development, health policy and administration SIG: Global Health and Technology in Physical Therapy	*The HPA Resource, HPA Journal*
Home Health	Practice in home health care and other "out-of-hospital" settings	*Quarterly Report*
Neurology	Evidence-based practice, education, and research in neurologic physical therapy SIGs: Brain Injury, Degenerative Diseases, Spinal Cord Injury, Stroke, Balance and Falls, and Vestibular Rehabilitation	*Journal of Neurologic Physical Therapy*

Continued

Table 4-1
Sections of the American Physical Therapy Association—cont'd

Section	Area(s) of Interest	Publication(s)
Oncology	Physical therapy for individuals diagnosed with cancer or HIV or AIDS SIGs: HIV/AIDS, Palliative and Hospice Care, and Lymphedema	*Rehabilitation Oncology*
Orthopaedic	Management of patients with musculoskeletal disorders SIGs: Occupational Health, Foot and Ankle, Performing Arts, Pain Management, Imaging, and Animal Rehabilitation	*Journal of Orthopaedic and Sports Physical Therapy, Orthopaedic Physical Therapy Practice*
Pediatrics	Highest quality of life for all children, people with developmental disabilities, and their families SIGs: Adolescents and Adults with Developmental Disabilities, Academic and Clinical Educators, Early Intervention, Hospital-based Physical Therapy, Neonatology, Pediatric Sports-Fitness, and School-based Physical Therapy	*Pediatric Physical Therapy*
Private Practice	Growth, economic viability, and business success of PT-owned physical therapy services	*Impact*
Research	Fosters and enhances physical therapy-related research SIG: Qualitative Research	*Section on Research* Newsletter
Sports Physical Therapy	Athletic injury management, including acute care, treatment and rehabilitation, prevention, and education	*Journal of Orthopaedic and Sports Physical Therapy, North American Journal of Sports Physical Therapy*
Women's Health	Women's health across the life span	*Journal of the Section on Women's Health, Highlights in Women's Health*

Data from APTA Sections. http://www.apta.org/Sections/. Accessed October 7, 2014.

voluntary; however, only a member of APTA can join a section. Students are permitted and encouraged to join.

In addition to the publications listed in Table 4-1, section members share information at an annual **Combined Sections Meeting (CSM)** in early February. This meeting provides a mechanism for educational and business sessions, and extensive product demonstrations in an exhibit hall. Registrants can attend educational sessions of any section regardless of membership in that section. This has become the most popular national education meeting of the APTA and commonly attracts over 10,000 registrants.

A specialty area within a section may form a **Special Interest Group (SIG)**. Bylaws authorize SIGs within chapters, sections, and assemblies, but they are most common in sections. This capability provides an opportunity for members in one of these components to further organize into smaller areas of common interest. For example, the Orthopaedic Section has six SIGs: Occupational Health Physical Therapy, Foot & Ankle, Performing Arts, Pain Management, Imaging, and Animal Rehabilitation. Participation in any SIG is voluntary.

ASSEMBLIES

An **assembly** is similar to a section in that it provides a mechanism for members with common interests to meet, confer, and promote their objectives. The differences are that assemblies are composed of members of the same class (category) and may exist at the state and national levels. One exception to the class limitation applies to student and student physical therapist assistant members, who may combine into one assembly. In fact, the Student Assembly is the only assembly that currently exists at the national level. This provides an important vehicle for communication and a voice for students.

AMERICAN COUNCIL OF ACADEMIC PHYSICAL THERAPY

The **American Council of Academic Physical Therapy (ACAPT)** became a component of the APTA by action of the HOD in 2013. This entity has an interesting brief history. Its origin is from the now defunct Academic Administrators SIG within the Education Section and was composed of the program directors of PT and PTA education programs. These members believed that their influence over physical *therapy* education (inclusive of PT and PTA programs) should be more significant than a SIG within a section. A council was formed and approved by the BOD in 2010, and the council subsequently became a component in 2013. The purpose of ACAPT is "to advance the enterprise of academic physical therapy by promoting the highest standards of excellence."[7] Its focus is on physical *therapist* (PT) education including clinical and postprofessional education.

PHYSICAL THERAPIST ASSISTANT CAUCUS

The PTA Caucus was created by the HOD in 2005 to serve as a representative body of PTAs. It consists of representatives from each of the chapters and the District of Columbia, as well as five delegates who sit at the HOD. The Caucus meets once a year immediately preceding the HOD meeting to provide a mechanism for representation and discussion of issues and perspectives pertinent to PTAs and presentation to the HOD. See Chapter 3 for further details of the origin and operation of this unit.

BOARD OF DIRECTORS

Six officers of the APTA and nine directors constitute the **Board of Directors**. The officers are the President, Vice President, Secretary, Treasurer, Speaker of the HOD, and Vice Speaker of the HOD. The fundamental duties of the BOD are to carry out the mandates and policies established by the HOD, as well as to manage the affairs of the APTA.

The BOD and HOD must work closely together for effective operation of APTA. Whereas the HOD establishes the policies and positions of APTA, the BOD, elected by the HOD, communicates these issues to internal and external personnel or agencies. This communication of issues is an important representative function of the BOD. The BOD may create ad hoc committees and task forces to carry out its business. These units will also have specific charges and time lines. In addition, the BOD may establish advisory groups and councils to respond to unique service needs of the APTA.

HOUSE OF DELEGATES

The **House of Delegates** is the highest policymaking body of the APTA. It has the authority to establish the policies and directives of the APTA and elect members of the BOD and Nominating Committee. Its general powers, noted in Box 4-4,[5] are derived from the bylaws of the APTA.

The HOD is composed of voting delegates from all chapters and nonvoting delegates (who may speak and make motions) from each section, the PTA Caucus, the Student Assembly, and the BOD. Representation is proportionate; however, the complex formula for determining the size of the HOD ensures that the total number of delegates will always be slightly more than 400. In addition, each chapter is entitled to at least two delegates; each section, one delegate; the PTA Caucus, five delegates; and the Student Assembly, two delegates.

BOX 4-4

General Powers of the House of Delegates

The House of Delegates has authority to determine directives and policies of the Association, to elect the Board of Directors and the Nominating Committee; and to:
A. Amend and repeal these bylaws;
B. Amend, suspend, or rescind the standing rules;
C. Adopt ethical principles and standards to govern the conduct of members of the Association in their roles as physical therapists or physical therapist assistants; and
D. Modify or reverse a decision of the Board of Directors.
All of the general powers of the House of Delegates are subject to the Board of Directors' fiduciary duty to manage the affairs of the Association.

From American Physical Therapy Association (APTA): APTA core documents and bylaws, Alexandria, VA, 2009, APTA. Available at: www.apta.org/AM/Template.cfm?Section=PoliciesandBylaws&Template=/TaggedPage/TaggedPageDisplay.cfm&TPLID=248&ContentID=74026. Accessed September 13, 2010.

In accordance with the bylaws, the annual session (business meeting) of the APTA is the HOD meeting. This session spans 3 days and is held each June immediately preceding the **NEXT Conference and Exposition.** The NEXT Conference continues for another 2 to 3 days and includes an extensive program of educational sessions, exhibits, and activities, such as honors and awards.

Ad hoc committees and task forces, in addition to standing committees, may be created by the HOD to address issues that it deems important. When these groups are created, definite charges and time lines are stipulated in the motion that created the unit.

STAFF

The organizational chart in Figure 4-2 indicates that APTA staff serves the organization at multiple levels. During any business hour, a member (or nonmember) can call the APTA headquarters in Alexandria, Virginia, at its toll-free number, 800-999-APTA (2782), and speak to any of its more than 180 staff members. Staff may also be contacted through links from the APTA website (www.apta.org). This direct benefit is important to access information and services. Staff members also provide support for activities of the chapters, sections, and assemblies and for operation of the HOD, BOD, PTA Caucus, and all national-level committees and task forces.

Key staff members also provide important representative functions to outside agencies, similar to the duties of the BOD. This role is particularly true for the chief executive officer and senior vice presidents. These individuals are responsible for the following units: Financial and Business Affairs, Public Affairs, Member Affairs, and Professional Affairs.

RELATED ORGANIZATIONS

In addition to the components identified in Figure 4-2, several other organizations have a mission and set of goals that complement those of APTA. Some of these agencies function independently of APTA, whereas for others, the link is more than philosophical. In all cases, the relationship is mutually beneficial. These organizations are briefly described in the following sections and labeled in Figure 4-3.

AMERICAN BOARD OF PHYSICAL THERAPY RESIDENCY AND FELLOWSHIP EDUCATION

The **American Board of Physical Therapy Residency and Fellowship Education (ABPTRFE)** is the agency that accredits postprofessional residency and fellowship training programs in physical therapy.[8] This is an extensive process that requires first recognition as a developing program and application for candidate status before eventual accreditation. Residency programs must be at least 1500 hours in length and provide advanced knowledge and skills either in patient/client management or in a nonclinical area that serves as career development. Current content areas for residency programs are cardiovascular and pulmonary, clinical electrophysiology, geriatrics, neurology, orthopaedics, pediatrics, sports, women's health, and wound care management. Fellowship programs are at least 1000 hours in length and have a similar focus as the residency programs, except that they are more specific in the area of practice or career development. Current content areas for fellowship programs are critical care, educational leadership, hand therapy, movement science, neonatology, orthopaedic manual physical therapy, spine, sports division 1, and upper extremity athlete.

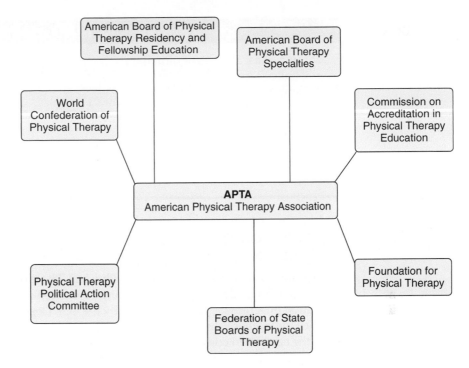

Figure 4-3 ■ Organizations related to the American Physical Therapy Association.

AMERICAN BOARD OF PHYSICAL THERAPY SPECIALTIES

The **American Board of Physical Therapy Specialties (ABPTS)** was created by the HOD in 1978 to provide a formal mechanism to recognize PTs with advanced knowledge, skills, and experience in a special area of practice.[9] A specialization program was established to achieve board certification and enhance the quality of care in the specialty area. Participation in the program is voluntary; however, PTs shall not present themselves as "board-certified clinical specialists" unless they have successfully completed the certification process.

Each specialty area must be approved by the HOD, but criteria for each area are established by the ABPTS. Eight specialty areas have been approved and are listed in Box 4-5.

The first three specialists were recognized in 1985 in the area of cardiopulmonary physical therapy. More than 16,000 clinical specialists have been certified. To be recognized as a "board-certified clinical specialist," a PT must pass a written examination and present the following qualifications: licensure to practice physical therapy in one of the chapters of APTA, Puerto Rico, or the Virgin Islands, and evidence of at least 2000 hours of clinical practice in the specialty area, at least 25% of which must have been done within the 3 years preceding the examination. Certain other requirements and options exist, depending on the specific area of specialization.

BOX 4-5

| Approved Specialty Areas in Physical Therapy |

- Cardiovascular and Pulmonary
- Clinical Electrophysiology
- Geriatrics
- Neurology
- Orthopaedics
- Pediatrics
- Sports
- Women's Health

COMMISSION ON ACCREDITATION IN PHYSICAL THERAPY EDUCATION

The **Commission on Accreditation in Physical Therapy Education (CAPTE)** is responsible for evaluating and accrediting professional (entry-level) PT and PTA education programs.[10] It is recognized by the U.S. Department of Education and Council for Higher Education Accreditation. CAPTE is composed of 31 members from the education community, the physical therapy profession, and the public. It reviews and accredits more than 200 physical therapist and 250 physical therapist assistant education programs. This process begins with applying for and achieving Candidate for Accreditation status for a developing program. Before graduation of the first cohort of students, the program applies to achieve accreditation status. Once achieved, annual reports are required, with full reviews to maintain the status scheduled every 10 years.

The relationship between APTA and CAPTE is integrated, yet they are technically independent. The Accreditation Department within APTA manages the accreditation program; however, CAPTE reviews the data and determines the accreditation status of each education program. Moreover, CAPTE establishes the standards for the accreditation decisions.

FOUNDATION FOR PHYSICAL THERAPY

The **Foundation for Physical Therapy** was established in 1979 by an action of the APTA HOD to promote and provide financial support for research in physical therapy. Its mission is "to fund and publicize physical therapy research that determines the scientific basis and value of services intended to optimize physical functioning by physical therapists, and to develop the next generation of researchers."[11] Because it is an independent entity, its governing body is separate from APTA and consists of clinicians, researchers, and business leaders. The Foundation has awarded more than $14 million in the areas of research grants, scholarships for doctoral degree education, and postdoctoral fellowships. Through these comprehensive programs, the Foundation promotes clinically focused research to improve the practice and cost-effectiveness of physical therapy.

FEDERATION OF STATE BOARDS OF PHYSICAL THERAPY

The **Federation of State Boards of Physical Therapy (FSBPT)** is an independent agency that has been instrumental in coordinating activity among all of the state boards that regulate physical therapy.[12] It exists to protect the public by promoting safe and competent physical therapy practice. Areas of attention include the licensing examination and state practice acts for physical therapy. This organization is particularly helpful for identifying the licensure requirements in each jurisdiction across the nation. Regarding the examinations, FSBPT develops, maintains, and administers the national licensing examination for PTs and PTAs. It has been involved in revising the examination and standardizing passing criteria among the states. Reports on the examination results of program graduates can be helpful to academic programs in identifying curricular strengths and areas that need attention. Concerning state practice acts, FSBPT has created a model practice act for physical therapy to be used in these laws. This model is an attempt to standardize language and legal references to the practice of physical therapy.

PHYSICAL THERAPY POLITICAL ACTION COMMITTEE

The **Physical Therapy Political Action Committee (PT-PAC)** is a fundraising organization to support legislation that addresses the interests of physical therapists at the federal level.[13] This activity is a fundamental necessity in the American political process and assists the profession in addressing the health care needs of society. For the 2012 federal election cycle, $1.85 million was raised and more than $1.37 million was disbursed in contributions to candidates and political party committees. In terms of contributions to political campaigns during that election cycle, PT-PAC was listed as the eighth highest among health care providers' PACs. This is impressive, given the size and financial resources of some of the other leading professions, such as orthopaedic surgeons, dentists, and radiologists.

WORLD CONFEDERATION FOR PHYSICAL THERAPY

Physical therapy is represented on a global level by the **World Confederation for Physical Therapy (WCPT)**.[14] This organization promotes health on a worldwide level by fostering high standards in physical therapy research, education, and practice, and by providing vehicles for the exchange of information and collaboration among related organizations. Member organizations are from 106 nations around the world, including APTA. A WCPT Congress is held every 4 years in a different international location to provide an opportunity for presentations on research and special interests regarding the practice, management, and education in physical therapy.

BENEFITS OF BELONGING

Benefits of belonging to APTA are both intangible and tangible. The intangible benefits relate to the commitment to high-quality service that the organization provides to its members and the public. As the recognized voice for the physical therapy profession in the United States, it is appropriate for PTs, PTAs, and students to join APTA. Through the organizational structure described previously, members are represented in a wide variety of public and governmental areas. Many individuals join simply because they recognize it as their professional responsibility to participate and support the interests of the profession at the national and local levels. No other organization will advocate for the best interests of PTs, PTAs, or the patients and clients whom they serve.

The tangible benefits of belonging to APTA are identified in Table 4-2 and briefly described here. Legislative efforts are provided through lobbying, direct contact with government officials, and a strong infrastructure to represent the members. In this era of rapidly changing health care management and reimbursement, this membership benefit is critical for success of the profession. Information is made available through the APTA website, phone contact with staff, and publications. The website contains a great deal of current and reference information; however, some of it is restricted to members. Continuing education offerings, including annual events, workshops, and home study courses, are available to members at considerable discount from nonmember prices.

Professional development occurs through interaction at the local, state, and national levels, which is available through district, chapter, section, caucus, and assembly events. Practice and research activities include promoting clinical

Table 4-2
Benefits of Belonging to the American Physical Therapy Association

Benefit	Examples
Legislative efforts	Lobbying for Medicare direct access Legislation on concussion management
Information	Publications: *Physical Therapy* *PT in Motion* Access to journal articles and clinical practice guidelines via PTNow Staff assistance on issues affecting practice, education, and research
Continuing education	NEXT Conference and Exhibition Combined Sections Meeting National Student Conclave Workshops and home study courses
Professional development	Networking and education through districts, chapters, sections, PTA Caucus, and Student Assembly
Research	Promotes research funding and activities by supporting the efforts of the Foundation for Physical Therapy
Discounts	Group rates for insurance and credit card programs Reduced conference registration rates

competency through guidelines and policies, advising government agencies and insurance companies of practice standards, and defending the need for research funding to appropriate sources. Insurance and other financial benefits include low-cost group programs and reduced conference registration rates.

Special incentives are provided for student membership. Fees for membership and participation in activities are generally 10–25% of the cost for a physical therapist member. In addition, the Career Starter Dues program eases the transition from student to physical therapist or physical therapist assistant membership. On graduation, student members automatically convert to the respective physical therapist or physical therapist assistant membership category for the remainder of the membership period. For the next year of membership, dues are 50% of those for the respective category. This also includes a free registration to the NEXT Conference and Exhibition.

SUMMARY

This chapter described the purposes, infrastructure, benefits, and organizations related to APTA. Purposes of APTA include serving the public and its members to enhance the profession and practice of physical therapy. Its governing bodies are organized into three levels: local (districts), state (chapters), and national (HOD and BOD). Opportunities for participation in areas of special interest exist in sections and assemblies. Staff members are readily available to support the organization at all levels and interact with external agencies. Other related organizations in the United States and across the globe further promote physical therapy, and APTA participates in these organizations through either direct membership or interaction. Benefits of belonging include outcomes that are intangible (professional commitment) and tangible (legislative efforts, information, continuing education, professional development, practice and research support, and low-cost insurance). Through its purpose, organization, and activities, APTA provides widespread opportunities and strong representation for the profession and practice of physical therapy.

REFERENCES

1. Pulliam M: Discover the benefits of joining a professional organization. Excelsior College Career Corner, # 14 in a series. http://www.excelsior.edu/c/document_library/get_file?uuid=4e4751b8-4675-4fce-91d1-5573a84203c9&groupId=37019. Accessed October 6, 2014.
2. *Mission statement of APTA,* HOD P06-93-05-05. American Physical Therapy Association. http://www.apta.org/uploadedFiles/APTAorg/About_Us/Policies/Goals_Missions/MissionStatementAPTA.pdf. Accessed October 6, 2014.
3. *Mission statement fulfillment,* HOD P06-93-06-07. American Physical Therapy Association. http://www.apta.org/uploadedFiles/APTAorg/About_Us/Policies/Goals_Missions/MissionStatementFulfillment.pdf. Accessed October 6, 2014.
4. *Goals that represent the priorities of the APTA,* HOD P06-05-15-24. American Physical Therapy Association. http://www.apta.org/uploadedFiles/APTAorg/About_Us/Policies/Goals_Missions/GoalsRepresentPrioritiesAPTA.pdf#search=%22goals%22. Accessed October 6, 2014.
5. Bylaws of the American Physical Therapy Association. American Physical Therapy Association. http://www.apta.org/uploadedFiles/APTAorg/About_Us/Policies/General/Bylaws.pdf. Accessed October 6, 2014.
6. *Standing Rules of the American Physical Therapy Association.* American Physical Therapy Association. http://www.apta.org/uploadedFiles/APTAorg/About_Us/Policies/General/Bylaws.pdf. Accessed October 6, 2014.
7. American Council of Academic Physical Therapy. http://acapt.org/. Accessed October 7, 2015.

8. American Board of Physical Therapy Residency and Fellowship Education. http://www.abptrfe.org/Home.aspx. Accessed October 8, 2014.
9. American Board of Physical Therapy Specialties. http://www.abpts.org/home.aspx. Accessed October 8, 2014.
10. Commission on Accreditation in Physical Therapy Education. http://www.capteonline.org/home.aspx. Accessed October 8, 2014.
11. Foundation for Physical Therapy. APTA. http://foundation4pt.org/. Accessed October 8, 2014.
12. Federal of State Boards of Physical Therapy. https://www.fsbpt.org/index.asp. Accessed October 8, 2014.
13. Physical Therapy Political Action Committee. http://www.ptpac.org/. Accessed October 8, 2014.
14. World Confederation of Physical Therapy. http://www.wcpt.org/. Accessed October 8, 2014.

REVIEW QUESTIONS

1. Select at least three components of the APTA mission statement and apply them to Figure 4-2 by indicating at what level of APTA each goal should be most logically tackled. (There may be more than one answer.)
2. Apply the goals listed in Box 4-3 to the various levels of APTA's organizational structure (see Figure 4-2) and compare them with your applications in question 1 and with the definitions of the various APTA components given in this chapter.
3. What is the difference among an assembly, a section, and a SIG? How do they differ in function and membership?
4. Visit the website of one of the organizations associated with the APTA to discern differences in scope and function. What advantage does it offer over membership in APTA alone?

No civilization…would ever have been possible without a framework of stability, to provide the wherein for the flux of change. Foremost among the stabilizing factors, more enduring than customs, manners, and traditions, are the legal systems that regulate our life in the world and our daily affairs with each other.

Hannah Arendt

5

Laws, Regulations, and Policies

Laurie A. Walsh

KEY TERMS

Affordable Care Act (ACA)
Americans with Disabilities Act (ADA)
Certification
Civil law
Code of Ethics for the Physical Therapist
Common law
Contract
Criminal law
Essential Health Benefits (EHB)
Federalism
Health Insurance Marketplace
Health Insurance Portability and
    Accountability Act (HIPAA)
Law
Licensure
Malpractice
Negligence
Policy
Practice act
Professional misconduct
Registration
Regulation
Risk management
Standards of Ethical Conduct for the
    Physical Therapist Assistant
Statute
Tort
Vicarious liability

LEARNING OBJECTIVES

After reading this chapter, the reader will be able to:

- Distinguish among laws, regulations, and policies and how they are made.
- Understand basic concepts regarding how various laws, regulations, and policies affect physical therapy practice.
- Identify resources that physical therapists and physical therapist assistants may use to find out more about laws, regulations, and policies that affect physical therapy practice.
- Identify ways in which individuals and groups can effect change in the regulation of physical therapy practice.
- Understand basic principles involved in the various ways that physical therapists and physical therapist assistants can be held legally liable for the care they provide and the consequences of liability.

The laws, regulations, and policies affecting the practice of physical therapy exist, fundamentally, to protect the public by (1) trying to ensure that providers are competent and (2) where services are paid for by government programs, trying to ensure that taxpayer dollars are being spent appropriately. Laws, regulations, and public policies serve to create, in legal terms, a scope of practice for physical therapy and to distinguish it from other professions. Government regulation is a double-edged sword for physical therapists (PTs) and physical therapist assistants (PTAs): providers receive rights and protection under regulation, but they must also accept responsibilities and limits imposed by regulation. The policies of private organizations also affect the practice of physical therapy.

A detailed examination of the legal regulation of physical therapy practice is beyond the scope of this chapter, and the reader is referred elsewhere for more detail. As you read this chapter, the following basic principles should be kept in mind:

- Many of the laws, regulations, and policies that affect physical therapy practice vary from state to state and from program to program. This chapter focuses on general principles, so readers should look to individual state laws, program regulations, and the like for specific information.
- Various aspects of practice may be governed by both state and federal law. When they come into conflict, federal law generally prevails.
- Some laws, regulations, and public policies govern what services PTs and PTAs may legally provide, whereas others may address how these services are reimbursed. The fact that reimbursement may be denied does not necessarily mean that the services cannot legally be provided, only that the therapist must look elsewhere for reimbursement.

STATUTES AND REGULATIONS

Law is "a body of rules of action or conduct prescribed by the controlling authority and hav[ing] binding legal force.[1]" *Public* policies are the ways in which governmental bodies act to address issues in society and include statutes, regulations, and executive orders.[2] Public policy may be considered the sum of all of the "law" of a jurisdiction on a particular issue, regardless of which body of government is the source. The law of a jurisdiction, therefore, may be composed of laws created by legislatures (called *statutes*), decrees handed down by courts (common law), regulations created by government agencies, executive orders issued by the governor or president or, as is usually the case, some combination of these actions. *Private* policies are developed by private organizations and cannot be enforced in the same way that laws are. Private policies will be discussed later in this chapter.

The various kinds of law may address offenses against society or private wrongs that one individual commits against another. This section addresses the various components of the law and how they affect the practice of physical therapy. This section also discusses the distinctions between the two major topic areas in the law: criminal and civil law.

STATUTES

Statutes, as noted previously, are a type of law that is "enacted and established by the will of the legislative department of government."[1] Statutes affecting the practice of physical therapy may be passed at the federal level by Congress, or at the state level by the various state legislatures, and then signed into law by the relevant executive. Provisions of federal and state statutes can be enforced through the state and federal court systems.

FEDERAL STATUTES

Federal statutes address those areas that the federal government is constitutionally permitted to regulate, such as federal civil rights, interstate commerce, and taxation. Federal statutes apply consistently to all citizens across state lines and, where they conflict with related state laws, generally supersede state law. All the laws passed by the U.S. Congress are known collectively as the U.S. Code.

A number of federal statutes may affect the provision of physical therapy services, including the following:

- The **Americans with Disabilities Act (ADA)** prohibits discrimination against persons with disabilities and requires that goods and services that are available to the public (including health care) be made accessible to persons with disabilities.[3]
- The Individuals with Disabilities Education Act requires that special education and related services (including physical therapy) be provided at public expense to students with disabilities when needed for students to benefit from an education program (see Chapter 12).[4]
- The Social Security Amendments of 1965 contain, among other provisions, the foundation for (1) the Medicare program, the federally subsidized health insurance program for people aged 65 years and older,[5] and (2) Medicaid, jointly funded by the state and federal governments to provide health care services to the poor. Physical therapy is among the health care services reimbursed under Medicare and Medicaid.[6] The year 2015 will mark the 50th anniversary of these programs and significant changes have been made to both over the years in terms of program eligibility, coverage or treatment, and reimbursement mechanisms.[7,8] At the time the law was enacted, only about half of all elderly Americans had health insurance coverage. The dramatic increase in the number of newly insured Americans significantly increased the demand for therapy services.
- The **Health Insurance Portability and Accountability Act (HIPAA)** requires that, among other things, all health care providers who transmit patient

information electronically adhere to federal guidelines as to the type of patient information they disclose, to whom they may disclose it, and how they store it, in order to protect patient confidentiality.[9]

■ The Patient Protection and Affordable Care Act of 2010, commonly known as the **Affordable Care Act (ACA),** the most significant addition to the federal regulation of health care since the creation of Medicare, was signed into law on March 30, 2010.[10,11] The law was intended, among other things, to significantly reduce the number of uninsured and underinsured nonelderly Americans, reduce the cost of health care services, and improve the quality of service provision. An in-depth analysis of the wide-ranging provisions of this law are beyond the scope of this chapter; however, major provisions of the law will be briefly noted as follows:

  − Employers with 50 or more employees must provide those employees with health insurance that meets federal requirements or else pay a financial penalty. The imposition of those penalties has been postponed, however, until at least 2015.

  − Individuals who do not receive insurance through their employer (or some other government program) and can afford to pay for it, must purchase insurance that meets federal requirements or else pay a financial penalty. Those penalties became effective in 2014. Low-income Americans are eligible for various federal subsidies to make insurance more affordable. As originally enacted, the ACA also required states to reduce the number of uninsured Americans by expanding their Medicaid programs in exchange for substantial federal funding; however, the U.S. Supreme Court declared that provision unconstitutional in 2012. Nonetheless, as of this writing, 26 states and the District of Columbia have expanded their Medicaid programs and several others are still considering it.

  − The ACA requires each state to have an insurance exchange, or **Health Insurance Marketplace**, where small employers and individuals can shop for low-cost health insurance plans that meet federal requirements. These marketplaces must certify that all plans offered meet federal requirements, which includes coverage of the following **Essential Health Benefits (EHB)** ambulatory patient services, emergency services, hospitalization, maternity and newborn care, mental health services, substance abuse services, rehabilitative and habilitative services (including therapies and devices), laboratory services, prevention and wellness services, chronic disease management, and pediatric services.

  − Each state will determine what specifically is covered under the plans, but they must be comparable to what is offered by typical employer-provided plans. Some items are required to be covered, such as certain kinds of preventive care, and plans must cover people with preexisting medical conditions and adult-dependent children up to age 26.

  − Each state must offer plans that vary in terms of expense, but not coverage of services. Some plans will have high premiums, but low deductibles/copays, others will have low premiums, but high deductibles/copays.

  − Each state must develop its own marketplace or allow the federal government to run one for state residents.

- Various other provisions in the ACA also create programs to find and reduce health care fraud, link reimbursement to quality of care measures, and promote better coordinated and more efficient care delivery. Many of these and other provisions in the ACA are similar to programs that already exist in commercial, employer-based insurance plans.
- As with the Medicare and Medicaid programs, one can expect that implementation of the ACA will change over time. As happened with enactment of the Medicare and Medicaid programs, there is considerable political opposition to the ACA. Various lawsuits regarding the constitutionality of certain ACA provisions are working their way through the federal court system as of this writing. The outcomes of federal elections may change the balance of power in Congress sufficiently to amend provisions in the law, though an outright repeal of the law seems unlikely. Additionally, as will be discussed later in this chapter, the federal government must continually develop and revise regulations needed to implement the various provisions in the ACA, just as it would with any law. If the bulk of the law survives, one can expect increasing demand for therapy services as previously uninsured Americans gain coverage. Health care providers, including therapists and therapist assistants, must keep track of the implementation process and communicate with their legislators to ensure that any laws affecting health care provision are implemented in ways that best benefit patients.

The consequences for violating federal laws vary. Violations of the ADA may result in fines or injunctions (e.g., in this case, court orders requiring defendants to make their businesses more accessible to persons with disabilities).[12] As noted above, failure of individuals to purchase health insurance under the ACA, or employers to provide it, will result in financial penalties that increase over time.[11]

At this point, it is appropriate to briefly discuss fraud. Legally, fraud occurs when someone intentionally misleads someone else in order to induce that person to do something that will harm that person.[1] With relation to physical therapy, fraud typically means insurance fraud: intentionally providing the payer with false information in order to obtain reimbursement that the provider is not legally entitled to. Insurance fraud may occur with respect to both government-run (federal and state) and private insurance programs. Fraud within the healthcare system is a serious problem. One estimate places losses due to fraud in the U.S. health care system at approximately $750 billion per year.[13]

A detailed explanation of fraud is beyond the scope of this chapter, but a few points will be noted. Fraudulent billing of federal benefit programs, such as Medicare, is vigorously prosecuted. Regulations require auditing of bills submitted to the Medicare program, both before and after payment is made, to look for billing patterns that may indicate fraud.[14] Where there is evidence of intentional misrepresentation, the government can not only begin proceedings to get the money back, there are also civil and criminal laws that can provide further penalties. Therapists can be permanently barred from participating in government-run insurance programs, and the federal False Claims Act, for example, can impose fines up to three times the value of fraudulently obtained reimbursement. Related criminal fraud statutes can impose additional fines and imprisonment.[14] Unfortunately, from time to time, therapists have been guilty of committing fraud. One recent and extreme example involved a PT who defrauded the Medicare program of millions of dollars by filing false claims. The therapist was ultimately sentenced to 10 years in federal prison and ordered to pay $10 million in restitution.[15]

It is essential, then, that therapists and assistants be knowledgeable of, and in full compliance with, any state and federal laws with respect to fraud. Fraud, waste, and abuse are also addressed in Chapter 6.

STATE STATUTES

While the U.S. Constitution requires that certain areas of law, such as interstate commerce and foreign policy, only be dealt with by the federal government, most areas of law are left to the states to govern or can be governed jointly by state and federal government. This division of political power between the federal and state governments is known as **federalism.**[2] State statutes are enacted by state legislatures in areas that states are constitutionally permitted to regulate, such as education, professional licensing, and insurance. When no superseding federal law exists, each state is entitled to tailor its laws to meet the needs of its citizens. Consequently, laws in these topic areas vary from state to state.

State statutes can affect the practice of physical therapy in a number of ways, such as through regulation of the insurance industry, availability of state health care funding for the poor, and state health department requirements. Regarding physical therapy practice, however, the single most important statute is the state physical therapy practice act. The **practice act** is the legal foundation for the scope and protection of physical therapy practice.[16] Among the areas generally covered by practice acts are the state definition of physical therapy practice, identification of providers who may legally provide physical therapy services, identification of tasks that may be delegated (and to which persons they may be delegated), and supervisory requirements.[17] Physical therapy providers are legally permitted to practice only when they comply with their state's practice act, and it is assumed that they are knowledgeable about the provisions of the practice act in the state in which they are licensed. The practice act is the final word regarding what is legal physical therapy practice in a given state; it supersedes the provisions of other state practice acts and the guidelines of private organizations, such as the American Physical Therapy Association (APTA). The consequences of violating state practice acts are often stated in the act itself or accompanying regulations. In some states, such as New York, the unlawful practice of physical therapy is a crime.[18]

A copy of a state practice act may be obtained in many ways. Most state legislatures and PT licensing boards have official websites with all state laws, including practice acts, available online. State practice acts may also be accessed in a variety of other places on the Internet.[19] (Note: Although much information on the APTA website is currently available to the public, some information is accessible only to APTA members. In addition, the reader should note that websites often change the links to content, so links current at the time of publication may be changed at a later date.)

Although a great deal of overlap is seen among state practice acts, they also have significant differences. Given that physical therapy providers are legally responsible for knowing their own practice acts, providers must educate themselves and cannot assume that what is legal therapy practice in another state is also legal in their own state. One example is direct access to physical therapy services, which permits a patient to receive services without first obtaining a referral from another provider, usually a physician. All 50 states and the District of Columbia permit varying degrees of direct access to treatment.[20] State laws vary, for example, in terms of the amount of experience therapists must have before they can provide services without a referral, or the length of time during which service may be provided before a referral must be obtained. Therapists and assistants must then be clear on the rules and regulations of the state in which they practice.

The manner in which physical therapy providers are regulated also varies from state to state. All 50 states license PTs. A license, however, cannot automatically be transferred from one state to another. If a provider moves to another state, that person must apply for a new license according to that state's requirements and procedures.[16] **Licensure** creates a scope of practice, authorizes the individual to practice in a given state, and legally protects use of the professional title.[21] All states require graduation from an accredited program and a passing score on the National Physical Therapy Examination in order to be licensed, but exact procedures, forms, costs, and other requirements vary from state to state. The reader should contact a specific state licensing board to find out what that particular state requires.[19]

The PTA is also recognized under the practice act of every state and the District of Columbia and must be licensed or certified in the respective jurisdiction.[22] Functionally, **certification**, like licensure, legally protects the title of the PTA. Unlike licensure, however, it does not create a separate scope of practice or a monopoly to provide a particular service.[21] Requirements for licensure or certification of PTAs also vary from state to state.

Registration is the least rigorous form of governmental regulation and requires only that registrants periodically provide the state with updated information on their names, addresses, and qualifications and pay a registration fee.[21] Individuals who are licensed or certified are generally required to register periodically, usually every several years, as well. As with PTs, then, the requirements for PTA practice vary from state to state, and PTAs must check with the licensing board of a particular state to determine requirements.

The reader should not confuse state certification with certification by private organizations. The APTA, for example, has a program to recognize PTAs who have achieved advanced proficiency in particular areas of their clinical work, and another program to certify PTs as specialists (see Chapters 3 and 4). The Neuro-Developmental Treatment Association, among other organizations, also has programs to certify practitioners. These private forms of certification establish that an individual has met the standards of these private organizations in terms of competency in a certain therapeutic approach or specialty area.[21] Unlike state certification, they neither create a legally enforceable professional title nor modify the scope of practice.

With respect to efforts to obtain more consistent physical therapy regulation, there is the Model Practice Act for Physical Therapy (MPA). The MPA is not a statute and does not have the force of law, but it is intended to be "the preeminent standard and most effective tool available for revising and modernizing physical therapy practice acts"—a key resource to be consulted when PTs and PTAs seek to lobby for changes in the practice acts.[23] The MPA was developed by the Federation of State Boards of Physical Therapy, a private organization consisting of members of physical therapy licensing boards from all 50 states and the federal territories. The Federation periodically revises the MPA, most recently in 2011.[23] The Federation is also responsible for developing the national licensing examinations for the PT and PTA. More information about the Federation, including licensing information in all states and the District of Columbia, can be obtained from their website (www.fsbpt.org).

REGULATIONS

Unlike statutes, **regulations** are developed by government agencies, not the legislature. Administrative agencies exist at all levels of government within the executive branch and serve a variety of functions, including the regulation of industries and government benefit programs such as Medicare and Medicaid. Such agencies are created by legislatures through statutes. Agencies are overseen by the legislative branch and are to perform only those duties delegated by the legislature; however, agencies are often given a great deal of discretion in terms of how policy is implemented.[2] Unlike legislators, appointees to agencies generally have specific expertise and experience in the industry or program being regulated.

Having been delegated authority in a specific area by the legislature, agencies have the authority to develop rules and regulations and enforce them within a specific industry or program. Statutes are often broadly worded and can be vague; agencies make the regulations that provide the details needed to implement the provisions of a statute.[2] For example, regulations may support, clarify, or give further definition to terms in the statutes that created the agency, or they may set forth procedures for programs created by statute. A practice act, for example, may require that a PTA be supervised on site by a PT. The legislature may then delegate to an appropriate state agency, such as the state's PT board or education department, the responsibility for developing a regulation defining what constitutes appropriate supervision. Consequently, one must be familiar with *both the statutes and regulations* of a given jurisdiction to have full knowledge of the law governing physical therapy practice.

FEDERAL REGULATIONS

Federal agencies regulate a wide variety of industries and benefit programs. Implementation of a piece of legislation as complex as the ACA, for example, will involve a number of federal agencies, including the Department of Labor, the

Social Security Administration, the Internal Revenue Service, and the Centers for Medicare and Medicaid Services (CMS).[24] CMS is particularly important to the provision of physical therapy services because it is responsible for regulation of the Medicare and Medicaid programs. Although a detailed discussion of these programs and the role of CMS is beyond the scope of this chapter, CMS regulations determine, for example, to what extent therapists may participate as providers within the Medicare program and how much and for what services they will be reimbursed (see Chapter 6).[6]

Radical changes have occurred regarding reimbursement within the various aspects of Medicare since the late 1990s.[6] Many of these changes have been driven by congressional amendments to the Medicare legislation; implementation and enforcement of these changes have generally been left up to CMS. One example has been repeated congressional efforts over the years to place an annual monetary "cap" on the amount of reimbursement available under the Part B section of Medicare (which generally covers outpatient services) for physical therapy services provided in a private practice setting.[6] Once a patient's Medicare physical therapy expenses under Part B reached the cap, regardless of need, no further Part B Medicare reimbursement for physical therapy services would be available for the rest of that year. APTA has struggled on behalf of consumers and the profession to restore adequate levels of reimbursement. In the case of the Medicare cap, APTA successfully lobbied Congress in 2006 for a change in the law, allowing CMS to develop a process to provide for exceptions to the cap for patients who demonstrated a continued need for services.[25] Since that time, ongoing budgetary battles in Congress have at times eliminated the cap exceptions process, only to have successful lobbying efforts result in a push for reinstatement. As of this writing, the Part B Medicare cap stands at $1940 per year (to cover both PT and speech pathology services, with a separate cap for occupational therapy services),[26] and the passage of the Patient Protection and Affordable Care Act and other amendments have continued the cap exceptions process, but only as temporary fixes.[25] Physical therapy advocates, therefore, need to be constantly vigilant regarding this and other efforts to limit physical therapy reimbursement under government programs.

Failure to abide by Medicare regulations will result in denial of reimbursement for services rendered. Federal statutes and regulations also prohibit fraudulent billing—that is, intentionally billing Medicare for services the provider knew, or should have known, could not be billed to Medicare.[6] Consequently, when evidence of fraud is uncovered, fines and criminal prosecution may follow, as noted earlier in this chapter. In the absence of fraud, however, the denial of reimbursement does not mean that services were illegally provided, only that they are not covered by the Medicare program and providers must seek reimbursement elsewhere.

APTA updates members frequently regarding the activities of CMS and other government agencies through publications such as the monthly magazine, *PT in Motion*, and *PT in Motion—News Now*, which is updated daily. Both of these publications can be accessed online on the APTA website, which also includes a Payment tab containing information on a variety of reimbursement issues. The

Advocacy section of the APTA website also maintains current information and links to federal and state government websites. Information specific to CMS may be accessed on its website at www.cms.gov.

STATE REGULATIONS

State agencies also regulate a variety of industries and programs. Among the most important for the practice of physical therapy is the state physical therapy board. The composition and functions of the physical therapy boards are set by each state's legislature through statutes. Although they cannot change the practice acts adopted by the state legislatures, state boards serve many important functions.[17] They may advise the legislature or other government bodies to clarify the scope of practice, as well as provide advice to state-licensed practitioners seeking guidance on practice issues in that state. They also assist in administering the state licensing procedures and are generally at least consulted by prosecutors in professional misconduct cases. More information on the role of a state board can be obtained directly from the licensing board of an individual state and the state practice acts.

Professional conduct is regulated by a state disciplinary agency and is a topic that deserves further discussion. **Professional misconduct** involves actions by licensed professionals that demonstrate an inability to meet professional standards and competently perform the duties of a licensed professional.[27] Actions that constitute professional misconduct are defined in the practice act or accompanying regulations and may include physical or sexual abuse of a patient, patient abandonment (discharge of a patient while services are still needed), improper delegation or supervision of treatment activities, provision of unnecessary treatment, fraud, incompetence, and practicing while intoxicated, among other activities.[27] Complaints of unprofessional conduct are typically prosecuted by the state through administrative bodies set up for that purpose, rather than being prosecuted in courts of law, and are completely separate from criminal prosecutions and civil lawsuits.

A finding that the PT or PTA has committed professional misconduct may result, among other things, in a reprimand, fine, requirement to obtain remedial professional education, probation, suspension or revocation of license, or some combination of these penalties.[27] Final disciplinary actions are often published on state agency websites.

CREATING STATUTES AND REGULATIONS

Considering the profound effects statutes and regulations can have on the practice of physical therapy (and the consequences of violations), therapists and assistants must remain aware of, and be in compliance with, the applicable statutes and regulations. When statutes and regulations unnecessarily limit the provision of services to the public, therapists and assistants must work to educate lawmakers to change them. First, however, given that statutes and regulations are created by different government entities, physical therapy providers must educate themselves as to how statutes and regulations are made in order to have an impact on the final outcome.

HOW STATUTES ARE MADE

Enacting or amending statutes is often a lengthy process involving negotiation and compromise. It varies somewhat from state to state and between the state and federal governments. In general, however, the process involves introducing a proposed statute (or bill) in one house of the legislature, where it will be referred to at least one legislative committee that has been assigned to address all bills pertaining to a certain topic (e.g., Finance, Education, Appropriations).[2] Committees gather additional information on the bill, debating and amending it. If passed, the committee's version of the bill is referred to the entire house (or "floor") for debate. If not, the bill "dies" in committee and will have to be reintroduced in the legislature at the next session. Multiple committees may send various versions of a bill to the floor. Debate regarding the bills will continue on the floor, amendments will continue to be put forth, and eventually one bill may obtain the support of the majority. If passed by one house of the legislature after a floor vote, the bill is then forwarded to the other house to undergo the same process again. If not, the bill will be returned to the various committees. Only when passed by both legislative houses in identical form is a bill forwarded to the executive branch (president or governor) to be signed into law or vetoed. Given the complexity of this process, only a tiny fraction of the bills proposed each year will actually become law. Additionally, Congress and many state legislatures have become very politically polarized in recent years, unable to make compromises and find the middle ground necessary to pass legislation. One analysis of Congressional action in 2014 showed that it passed only 212 substantive laws (as opposed to purely ceremonial laws such as renaming government buildings) out of thousands of bills proposed, making it one of the least productive sessions in U.S. history.[28] Each state has a very different political environment, but most states only pass approximately 15% or less of proposed legislation in a given year, though some may pass 50% or more.[29] Changing laws regarding practice, then, often requires persistence and dedication and may take a number of years.

Although the process of enacting statutes is lengthy and complicated, the many steps involved give interested parties, such as physical therapy providers, ample opportunity to contact their legislators to make sure that the interests of the profession and the public are represented. The process of persuading lawmakers, or lobbying, is essential to ensure the well-being of the public and the health of the profession. The APTA is actively involved at both the state and national levels to ensure that the profession's interests are represented. Therapists and assistants must keep abreast of pending legislation that may affect the practice of physical therapy and become involved in lobbying efforts, such as contacting their legislators at various points in the process.[6]

As noted earlier, APTA keeps members updated on current legislative issues through such publications as *News Now* and *PT in Motion*, as well as through the Advocacy link on the national website. The Take Action link in the Advocacy section of the APTA website connects to the members-only Legislative Action Center. This online clearinghouse holds a wealth of information on current physical therapy-related bills before Congress and state legislatures, offers information to quickly identify and contact state and Congressional representatives, and even provides language that can be used in letters to legislators. State chapters also keep members informed through newsletters, and chapter websites may carry legislative information as well.

State and federal governments have a number of official publications and websites regarding pending and recent legislation. For example, the *Congressional Record* publishes a daily record of U.S. House and Senate proceedings. The Library of Congress has extensive federal legislative information available online through its service at https://beta.congress.gov/. Among the information available at this site are the most recent *Congressional Record,* bill texts, committee reports, and summaries of the legislative process.

HOW REGULATIONS ARE MADE

Procedures have also been established for promulgating regulations, which also vary from state to state, and between state and federal governments. In brief, though, an agency must first publish a proposed regulation and give interested parties time to comment on it. This "comment period" gives physical therapy providers an opportunity to educate regulatory bodies on the issues and to influence the form that the final rule will take.[30] At the federal level, proposed and final regulations are published daily in the *Federal Register,* which can be accessed at www.gpoaccess.gov/fr/index.html. All of the federal regulations are compiled and published as the Code of Federal Regulations. State chapter and government publications and websites keep members updated about state regulatory activities as well.

THE COURT SYSTEM

The courts serve a number of functions in our legal system, including clarifying and interpreting statutes and regulations. Thus courts can play a key role in determining how statutes and regulations are ultimately implemented at the state and federal levels. The court system serves as an additional source of law: **common law** is law that has been created by court decisions, written by judges, and handed down.[31] Areas of common law evolve as new court decisions are added to the existing body of law in a particular area and may modify or overrule prior decisions. Certain areas of the law, such as malpractice and negligence, developed primarily through common law, although some states have developed statutory requirements regarding malpractice and negligence.[31] Negligence and malpractice are discussed further in the section on civil law.

CRIMINAL VERSUS CIVIL LAW

The reader should understand that there are different kinds of law. One important distinction is the difference between criminal and civil law. Legal matters will be handled differently, based on this distinction, and the penalties imposed for a finding of wrongdoing also differ.

CRIMINAL LAW

Criminal law involves prosecution in a court of law for acts "done in violation of those duties which an individual owes to the community."[1] Thus crimes are considered to be infractions committed against society, and the state prosecutes these actions on behalf of the public. Crimes today are defined in state and federal statutes, rather than as part of the common law.[1] The consequences of being tried and convicted of, or pleading guilty to, a crime may involve fines, probation, or imprisonment and vary depending on the type of crime committed and the law of the particular jurisdiction involved. For example, the death penalty is legal in certain states, but not others.

Criminal prosecution will not directly affect a provider's license, but may result in referral to a state professional disciplinary agency to initiate such an action, given that most state professional conduct requirements include language that having been found guilty of a crime also constitutes professional misconduct.[27] Earlier in this chapter, an example was given of a therapist prosecuted criminally for Medicare fraud. Other possible sources of criminal liability may involve sexual abuse of patients or, depending on the state law, unlawful practice of a profession. The crime need not relate directly to practice; a crime such as driving under the influence can result in a professional misconduct action.[16] Most states also require applicants for licensure or certification to state under oath, on the application, whether they have ever been convicted of a crime.[32] The same is true when therapists and assistants are periodically required to reregister. Lying on the application or registration forms is also an act of professional misconduct in itself.

Consequently students, and practicing therapists and assistants, must be aware that not only will criminal activity result in criminal liability, it may also complicate the process of obtaining a license or certificate, or may result in loss of license or certification.

CIVIL LAW

Unlike criminal law, **civil law** is concerned with relationships among private parties.[1] Civil actions are also prosecuted in courts of law, but in these cases one private citizen brings a lawsuit against another to seek compensation for injuries received.[16] Unlike in criminal cases, persons found liable in civil cases cannot be punished by the state with fines or incarceration; generally, the remedy available for civil liability is for the defendant to pay money damages to the plaintiff (the person who brings the lawsuit) to compensate that person for injuries shown to be caused by the defendant's actions.[16] A civil lawsuit cannot directly affect a person's professional license, but it may, depending on the nature of the wrong, result in a complaint to the state disciplinary agency to initiate a separate action for professional misconduct. Consider the following: a therapist is supervising a student on affiliation, and the law of the state requires that students be supervised by PTs on-site. The therapist leaves the site, and no other therapists remain on-site, but the student continues to treat patients. If one of those patients were to become injured, not only could he or she file a civil lawsuit, but the patient could also file a professional misconduct complaint against the therapist for failing to properly supervise the student.

Physical therapy providers may be named in civil lawsuits on a variety of grounds, including defamation (saying or writing something untrue that harms another person's reputation), breach of confidence, or breach of contract. The most common grounds for civil actions involving physical therapy providers, however, involve claims of negligence or malpractice.

NEGLIGENCE AND MALPRACTICE

Negligence and malpractice are kinds of **torts**: civil injuries for which the injured party can seek legal help from the courts.[1] **Negligence** is defined as the failure to act as a reasonably prudent person: doing (or failing to do) something that a reasonably prudent person would have done (or would not have done) under similar circumstances.[1] To prove that a therapist was negligent in providing care, a patient would have to prove the following four things in court:

- That the therapist owed the patient a legal duty of care; in other words, that a patient-therapist relationship existed at the time of the injury.
- That the therapist failed to provide the appropriate standard of care at the time of the injury.
- That the patient sustained injuries or damages: physical injuries, financial losses, and so on.
- That the patient's injuries were directly caused by the therapist's failure to provide the appropriate standard of care.[16]

An example of negligence in a physical therapy clinic would be failure to mop up water that had been tracked onto the clinic floor, causing someone to slip, fall, and get injured. This is considered negligence because any reasonably prudent person would have recognized that the water posed a risk of injury and promptly cleaned it up. **Malpractice**, or professional negligence, on the other hand, is the failure to do (or failure to avoid doing) something that a member in good standing in that profession would have done (or avoided doing), which causes subsequent injury to the patient.[1] It is a failure to meet a professional standard of care, a special kind of negligence. An example of malpractice would be a therapist who excessively mobilizes a joint and thereby causes injury. Why is this not negligence? An ordinary reasonably prudent person would not be expected to know whether or how much to mobilize a joint in a given patient. A therapist, as a professional, however, is held to a higher, professional standard of care and is expected to exercise appropriate clinical judgment to avoid patient injury.

Companies that provide liability insurance for PTs and PTAs keep statistics on negligence and malpractice claims. CNA/HPSO, the largest liability insurer for PTs and PTAs in the United States, recently published an analysis of claims against PTs and PTAs insured by them from 2001 to 2010.[33] This resource provides some insight into common types of claims made against physical therapy providers and gives examples of treatment scenarios that resulted in claims against providers. Based on their data, the most common causes behind negligence/malpractice incidents were improper performance of therapeutic exercise, improper use of a physical agent, and improper supervision.

DELEGATION AND SUPERVISION/VICARIOUS LIABILITY

The legal duty to provide a professional standard of care, and the ultimate responsibility for patient care, always remains with the PT. The therapist, therefore, may be held liable for a patient's injury even if the therapist was not directly providing services at that time. The PT bears this liability because a therapist's professional legal duty to the patient includes appropriate decision making regarding delegation and supervision of interventions. As noted earlier, state laws and regulations often spell out the therapist's duties in terms of supervising students and PTAs.[34] PTAs or students on affiliation can be held legally liable for their own errors in clinical judgments; however, the therapist may also be liable if tasks were negligently delegated or supervised.[35] If a therapist determines that delegation is appropriate, the therapist should prevent misunderstandings by always advising the patient of the credentials of the person to whom tasks have been delegated.

Similarly, an employer may be held legally responsible for the negligence or malpractice of employees when it is committed within the scope of their employment duties, regardless of whether the employer was involved in rendering care at the time. This form of liability, known as **vicarious liability** (or *respondeat superior*), is based on the fact that the employer can control the quality of care rendered by controlling the workplace (e.g., policies, hiring).[16] Thus, a therapist who owns a private practice may be held liable for the injuries caused by one of the practice's PTs or PTAs while those employees are treating patients. In contrast, the employer would not be liable for any negligent acts (such as causing a car accident through negligent driving on the way to work) that employees may commit when not performing their professional duties.

RISK MANAGEMENT

Risk management involves coordinated efforts by an organization to reduce the likelihood that the organization will experience physical or financial losses or injuries, particularly those due to civil law claims.[36] Although a full discussion of risk management is beyond the scope of this chapter, PTs are advised to constantly monitor the quality of the services they provide to decrease the risk of loss. In this way, they can avoid or minimize the occurrence of situations that increase the risk of patient or staff injuries and other incidents (e.g., billing errors) that may impose legal or financial liability. In addition, as noted above, they are advised to carry professional liability insurance that would cover the costs of legal fees and settlements or judgments arising from civil liability.[33] (Under ordinary circumstances, however, liability insurance will not cover legal fees for professional misconduct or criminal actions.) Liability insurance carriers, as noted above, also can provide information on risk management strategies for clinicians.

CONTRACT LAW

A **contract** is "an agreement between two or more persons which creates mutual obligations to do or not to do particular things."[1] Contract law is a subset of civil law, and valid contractual obligations can be enforced in court. A full discussion of the various types of contracts encountered by physical therapy providers is beyond the scope of this chapter, but a few of the more prominent ones are mentioned here. For example, although many physical therapy providers are employed without having written contracts, it is extremely important to put the terms of employment arrangements in writing.[37] Therapists may also contract independently to provide particular services for an agency or facility without becoming actual employees. Providers are advised to thoroughly review any contract, preferably with legal counsel, before signing it. Should a provider breach, or fail to fulfill, an employment contract, the employer may seek to enforce it legally. Although providers cannot be forced to stay at jobs against their will, the employer may be entitled to monetary damages as set forth in the contract.[37] For example, some employers may offer to pay moving expenses, tuition reimbursement, or other incentives in return for a provider's agreement to work for the employer for a set period of time. If the provider breaches the agreement by leaving employment early, the employer may be entitled to all or a percentage of the incentives provided, with interest.

Therapists sign agreements with payers, such as insurance companies and managed care organizations (MCOs), to become recognized providers for patients enrolled with or covered by those organizations. It is not uncommon for an MCO to refuse to reimburse or limit reimbursement for services rendered to patients enrolled with the MCO if the provider has not signed an agreement with the organization.[6] When providers have signed agreements with MCOs, the terms may require providers to accept lower rates of reimbursement, or to obtain authorization from the MCO before services are initiated.[6] If a provider does not abide by the terms of the agreement, the payer can deny reimbursement or, if the breach is severe enough, drop the therapist as a recognized provider. Given the complexity of agreements with payers, providers are strongly advised to consult with an attorney to obtain a fair agreement that will adequately cover costs.[38] The reader is reminded, however, that contracts regarding reimbursement do not affect the legality of providing services; if the practice act allows for the provision of the interventions, the provider can often seek reimbursement from other sources (including the patient) if the payer denies reimbursement. Providers must educate their patients, then, about the possibility that the payer may deny reimbursement.

POLICIES

As noted earlier, the term *policy* may refer to public policies or the policies of private organizations; this section will address private policies. APTA, for example, is a private, nongovernmental organization, and its policies do not have the force of law. APTA defines its policies as "Association directives defining operational or administrative activities."[39] Procedures, on the other hand, describe the actions required to achieve a result, such as those needed to implement policies.[39] Private policies affecting physical therapy may be set by other private entities as noted above, such as employers and payers. Private policies, unlike laws, cannot be legally enforced unless set forth in a contract. They do, however, represent the consensus of the members of an organization on a given issue. Consequently, private policies related to physical therapy can influence the relationships between physical therapy providers and private organizations, or they can be used to provide some momentum to effect change within private and public organizations.

AMERICAN PHYSICAL THERAPY ASSOCIATION POLICIES

As noted elsewhere in this text, APTA is the primary professional organization representing the physical therapy profession in the United States. Through the activities of its Board of Directors and House of Delegates, it establishes and annually reviews policies for its members. The policies of APTA address a number of areas relating to practice, from recommendations on documentation to the use of support personnel to national health care policy. Therapists and assistants are encouraged to become active, participating members of APTA in order to ensure that their voices are heard and their efforts can assist the development of APTA policies affecting current and future practice.

Because APTA is a private organization, its policies are binding only on members. These policies can, however, have wide-ranging effects as they drive changes in numerous areas, from scope of practice (through lobbying state legislatures) to reimbursement issues (through dialogue with payers).

Certain policies and interpretive guidelines address practice standards, ethical conduct, and professionalism. These are so fundamental to physical therapy practice that they are collectively known as *Core Documents* (Box 5-1). One example is the *Standards of Practice for Physical Therapy*, "the profession's statement of conditions and performances that are essential for provision of high-quality professional service to society..." (see Chapter 2).[40] Another is *Professionalism in Physical Therapy: Core Values*, adopted in 2003 to assist in the transition to a doctoring profession and to complement the core ethics documents.[41] The two documents that establish standards of ethical conduct for physical therapy providers are the **Code of Ethics for the Physical Therapist** and the **Standards of Ethical Conduct for the Physical Therapist Assistant**. The principles and standards for each of these documents are shown in Boxes 5-2 and 5-3, respectively. These documents are revised periodically and the ethics documents underwent substantial revision (including integration of the core values), in 2010.

Violations of these ethical standards by members can be prosecuted by APTA.[42] A written complaint must first be lodged with the state chapter president (or the national association's Ethics and Judicial Committee [EJC]), who will consult with the state Chapter Ethics Committee (CEC) to determine if the allegations in the complaint describe a violation of the *Code of Ethics* or the *Standards of Ethical Conduct*. If such a determination is made, the chapter president will generally notify the EJC and refer the matter to the CEC for

BOX 5-1 | **Core Documents of the American Physical Therapy Association (APTA)**

- Guiding Principles to Achieve the Vision
- Code of Ethics for the Physical Therapist
- Guide to Professional Conduct
- Standards of Practice for Physical Therapy
- Criteria for Standards of Practice for Physical Therapy
- Guidelines: Physical Therapy Documentation of Patient/Client Management
- Professionalism in Physical Therapy: Core Values
- Standards of Ethical Conduct for the Physical Therapist Assistant
- Guide for Conduct of the Physical Therapist Assistant
- Value-based Behaviors for the Physical Therapist Assistant
- Bylaws of the American Physical Therapy Association
- Standing Rules of the American Physical Therapy Association

5

BOX 5-2

Code of Ethics for the Physical Therapist

Principle 1: Physical therapists shall respect the inherent dignity and rights of all individuals.
(Core Values: Compassion, Integrity)

Principle 2: Physical therapists shall be trustworthy and compassionate in addressing the rights and needs of patients/clients.
(Core Values: Altruism, Compassion, Professional Duty)

Principle 3: Physical therapists shall be accountable for making sound professional judgments.
(Core Values: Excellence, Integrity)

Principle 4: Physical therapists shall demonstrate integrity in their relationships with patients/clients, families, colleagues, students, research participants, other health care providers, employers, payers, and the public.
(Core Value: Integrity)

Principle 5: Physical therapists shall fulfill their legal and professional obligations.
(Core Values: Professional Duty, Accountability)

Principle 6: Physical therapists shall enhance their expertise through the lifelong acquisition and refinement of knowledge, skills, abilities, and professional behaviors.
(Core Value: Excellence)

Principle 7: Physical therapists shall promote organizational behaviors and business practices that benefit patients/clients and society.
(Core Values: Integrity, Accountability)

Principle 8: Physical therapists shall participate in efforts to meet the health needs of people locally, nationally, or globally.
(Core Value: Social Responsibility)

Adapted from American Physical Therapy Association (APTA): Code of ethics for the physical therapist, HOD S06-09-07-12, House of Delegates Standards, Policies, Positions, and Guidelines, Alexandria, VA, 2009, APTA. The full text is available at www.apta.org.

investigation. The member accused of the violation will be notified and given an opportunity to respond. If the investigation shows that the complaint has merit, the CEC will notify the member, who will be given the opportunity to see the evidence involved and has the right to a hearing before the CEC. Based on the evidence, the CEC can either dismiss the complaint or, if there is sufficient evidence against the member, will forward the matter to the EJC of the national organization with recommendations for disciplinary action. The accused member will also be notified. The EJC will then review the matter and determine whether to impose sanctions; those sanctions range from a reprimand to expulsion from the organization. The member may also appeal the decision to the APTA Board of Directors. Any final disciplinary decisions regarding members will then be published by APTA in *Physical Therapy* and/or *PT in Motion*.[42] The APTA action can affect only membership; it has no jurisdiction to levy fines or affect the member's license to practice.

BOX 5-3

Standards of Ethical Conduct for the Physical Therapist Assistant

Standard 1: Physical therapist assistants shall respect the inherent dignity, and rights, of all individuals.

Standard 2: Physical therapist assistants shall be trustworthy and compassionate in addressing the rights and needs of patients/clients.

Standard 3: Physical therapist assistants shall make sound decisions in collaboration with the physical therapist and within the boundaries established by laws and regulations.

Standard 4: Physical therapist assistants shall demonstrate integrity in their relationships with patients/clients, families, colleagues, students, other health care providers, employers, payers, and the public.

Standard 5: Physical therapist assistants shall fulfill their legal and ethical obligations.

Standard 6: Physical therapist assistants shall enhance their competence through the lifelong acquisition and refinement of knowledge, skills, and abilities.

Standard 7: Physical therapist assistants shall support organizational behaviors and business practices that benefit patients/clients and society.

Standard 8: Physical therapist assistants shall participate in efforts to meet the health needs of people locally, nationally, or globally.

Adapted from American Physical Therapy Association (APTA): Standards of ethical conduct for the physical therapist assistant, HOD S06-09-200-18, House of Delegates Standards, Policies, Positions, and Guidelines, Alexandria, VA, 2009, APTA. The full text is available on the APTA website at www.apta.org.

PAYER REIMBURSEMENT POLICIES

A full description of reimbursement policies is included in Chapter 6. They are briefly described here to distinguish them from other types of private policies. Different insurance companies, MCOs, government benefit programs, and other payers have different policies regarding such topics as who can be a provider, what services will be reimbursed and for how much, documentation requirements, and procedures for claims review and appeals for claim denials.[5,6] Physical therapy providers must become familiar with these various policies and adhere to them in order to be reimbursed for their services and/or avoid legal liability. Payer policies may be found in government regulations, insurance company provider agreements, and provider manuals.

Changes in reimbursement policies in recent years have created dilemmas for providers as the temptation exists to allow reimbursement to drive practice. Providers must be actively engaged in dialogue with payers to educate them and ensure that reimbursement policies are adequate to meet patient needs. Providers must be able to advocate successfully on behalf of patients by using such tools as the practice act, the *Code of Ethics,* and research demonstrating the effectiveness of physical therapy services. Therapists and assistants must also become more involved in clinical research to increase the body of knowledge establishing the effectiveness of physical therapy interventions.

EMPLOYER POLICIES

Various employment settings also establish policies and procedures that are specific to that facility or organization. These policies and procedures generally address a wide variety of employment and quality issues, from job descriptions to documentation requirements to infection control and safety issues.[42] It should be noted that the *Standards of Practice for Physical Therapy* require that physical therapy providers have written policies and procedures to ensure the provision of high-quality physical therapy services.[40]

Employer policies can be grounds for disciplinary actions or firing. In addition, inquiries regarding whether facility policies and procedures were followed are often made during legal actions for negligence or malpractice as part of the determination regarding whether the appropriate standard of care was met.[43] Employer policies are not, however, a substitute for professional judgment. As professionals, therapists should not blindly follow policies without question, but should be engaged in active dialogue with their employers to ensure that their policies promote ethical, legal, and effective patient care.

SUMMARY

Government oversight of the physical therapy profession provides practitioners with both opportunities and limitations. This oversight occurs through the enactment of statutes by state and federal legislatures and the development of regulations by state and federal agencies, under the authority delegated to them by the legislature, to fill in gaps in statutes or clarify issues raised in a statute. Physical therapy providers must work with legislators and regulatory bodies to ensure that statutes and regulations accurately reflect the current state of practice and the needs of patients. Court decisions clarify and interpret statutory language and, in the civil law arena, shape practice through the imposition of liability for acts of negligence and malpractice. Therapists may also incur criminal liability if they commit fraud or other criminal acts and can have actions taken against their licenses if they violate state professional conduct rules. Therapists must also understand the legal repercussions of contracts they enter into. Policies adopted by private organizations, such as APTA, can also affect the evolution of physical therapy practice. Examples cited in this chapter indicate how laws, regulations, and policies can have an impact on the practice of physical therapy. Knowledge of and adherence to the applicable laws, regulations, and policies are necessary for safe, legal, ethical, and reimbursable practice.

CASE STUDIES

CASE STUDY ONE

You are a PT operating an outpatient clinic that provides services for patients with a wide variety of needs. One of your patients is a 28-year-old construction worker who injured his knee in a work-related accident. He was referred to your clinic after surgery to repair the anterior cruciate ligament. You have completed your examination and evaluation, generated a diagnosis and prognosis, developed a plan of care, and delegated implementation of the intervention plan to an athletic trainer (ATC) who works for you in your clinic. The patient attends routine therapy visits over the next 2 weeks, but fails to show up for further visits. Calls to the patient are not returned, and communication with his physician fails to explain the patient's apparent decision to terminate therapy. Several months later, legal papers are served at the clinic indicating that a lawsuit has been filed against you. The patient claims that the treatment received reinjured his knee. You discuss the case with the ATC who, after reviewing his notes, can recall no incidents or complaints involving the patient. From conversations with the patient, the ATC had suspicions that the patient was not adhering to activity precautions appropriate for his stage of recovery. However, the ATC did not believe these suspicions were strong enough to share with you or document in the patient's chart. You immediately contact your malpractice insurance carrier and forward all the legal papers and patient records.

An attorney for the insurance company contacts you to discuss the case. Although noting that the patient needs to prove his case to win in court, she states that the failure to follow-up on suspicions regarding the patient's failure to adhere to precautions will hurt your case. In addition, the attorney advises that she has confidentially contacted a representative of your state's physical therapy board, who has advised her that your state law does not permit delegation of physical therapy interventions to ATCs. Given the problems with this case, she notifies you that she will be recommending that the insurance company settle the case.

CASE STUDY ONE QUESTIONS

1. Can the PT be held liable for the patient's injuries in this case? If so, on what grounds? What penalties can be imposed on the therapist for negligence or malpractice?
2. Assume that the PT's conduct also constitutes professional misconduct in this case. What penalties may be imposed on the basis of professional misconduct?
3. Were any policies implicated in this case? Identify possible areas of policy violations.
4. What actions could the PT have taken to minimize liability risks in this case? Who could the PT have consulted?

REFERENCES

1. *Black's law dictionary*, ed 5, St. Paul, MN, 1990, West.
2. Morone J, Kersh R: *By the people: debating American Government,* New York, NY, 2013, Oxford University Press, pp. 609–610.
3. Americans with Disabilities Act of 1990, as Amended. ADA Publications. http://www.ada.gov/pubs/ada.htm. Accessed August 25, 2014.
4. Statute: individuals with Disabilities Education Act. Building the legacy: IDEA 2004. http://idea.ed.gov/explore/view/p/%2Croot%2Cstatute%2C. Accessed August 25, 2014.
5. Medicare program—general information. http://www.cms.gov/Medicare/Medicare-General-Information/MedicareGenInfo/index.html. Accessed August 25, 2014.
6. Sandstrom RW, Lohman H, Bramble JD: *Health services: policy and systems for therapists.* ed 3, Upper Saddle River, NJ, 2014, Pearson Education, Inc., pp 157–172.
7. Dowdal T. Medicare from the start to today. National Bipartisan Commission on the Future of Medicare. http://medicare.commission.gov/medicare/history.htm. Accessed August 25, 2014.
8. The story of medicare: a timeline. http://kff.org/medicare/video/the-story-of-medicare-a-timeline. Accessed August 25, 2014.
9. Health information privacy. http://www.hhs.gov/ocr/privacy/hipaa/understanding/index.html. Accessed August 25, 2014.
10. Drummond-Dye R, Leene G, Crandall D. Health care reform: 2014 progress report. March 2014. http://learningcenter.apta.org. Accessed August 25, 2014.

11. Teitelbaum J, Wilensky S, Reigelman R: *2015 annual health reform update,* Burlington, MA, 2015, Jones & Bartlett Learning.

12. ADA enforcement. United States Department of Justice. http://www.ada.gov/enforce_current.htm. Accessed August 25, 2014.

13. Lowrey A. Study of U.S. health care system finds both waste and opportunity to improve. http://www.nytimes.com/2012/09/12/health/policy/waste-and-promise-seen-in-us-health-care-system.html?_r=0. Accessed November 28, 2014.

14. American Physical Therapy Association Leaning Center. Navigating the regulatory environment: ensuring compliance while promoting professional integrity, part 1. 2014. http://www.apta.org/Courses/Online/NavigatingCompliance/. Accessed November 28, 2014.

15. AlHajal K. Physical therapist gets 10 years for Medicare fraud, must pay $10 million. http://www.mlive.com/news/detroit/index.ssf/2014/01/physical_therapist_gets_10_yea.html. Accessed August 25, 2014.

16. Lewis KD: Jurisprudence essentials. In Nosse LJ, Friberg DG, editors: *Managerial and supervisory principles for physical therapists,* ed 3, New York, NY, 2010, Wolters, Kluwer, pp 151–176.

17. Morone J, Kersh R: By the people: debating. See, for example, the New York state practice act, New York State Education Law Article 136. http://www.op.nysed.gov/prof/pt/article136.htm. Accessed August 25, 2014.

18. Unauthorized practice a crime, New York State Education Law, Article 130, Subarticle 4, Section 6512. http://public.leginfo.state.ny.us/LAWSSEAF.cgi?QUERYTYPE=LAWS+&QUERYDATA=@SLEDN0T8A130*SA4+&LIST=LAW+&BROWSER=BROWSER+&TOKEN=01292688+&TARGET=VIEW. Accessed August 25, 2014.

19. See, for example, American Physical Therapy Association (APTA), Practice Acts by State, http://www.apta.org/Licensure/StatePracticeActs; and Federation of State Boards of Physical Therapy (FSBPT), Licensing Authorities Contact Information, FSBPT website https://www.fsbpt.org/FreeResources/LicensingAuthoritiesContactInformation.aspx. Both accessed August 25, 2014.

20. APTA: *A summary of direct access language in state physical therapy practice acts—January 2014,* 2014. http://www.apta.org/uploadedFiles/APTAorg/Advocacy/State/Issues/Direct_Access/DirectAccessbyState.pdf, Accessed August 25, 2014.

21. Pew Health Professions Commissions: *Reforming health care workforce regulation: policy considerations for the 21st century,* San Francisco, CA, 1995, Pew Research Center.

22. American Physical Therapy Association (APTA). PTA licensure. http://www.apta.org/PTA/Licensure. Accessed August 25, 2014.

23. Federation of State Boards of Physical Therapy (FSBPT). The model practice act for physical therapy, ed 5. https://www.fsbpt.org/FreeResources/RegulatoryResources/ModelPracticeAct.aspx. Accessed August 25, 2014.

24. Carey MP and Christensen MD. Upcoming rules pursuant to the patient protection and affordable care act: Spring 2013 Unified Agenda. Congressional Research Service. January 2, 2014. http://www.ncsl.org/documents/statefed/health/ACA_Sprg2013Agda.pdf. Accessed August 25, 2014.

25. American Physical Therapy Association (APTA). History of medicare therapy caps. http://www.apta.org/FederalIssues/TherapyCap/History. Accessed August 25, 2014.

26. American Physical Therapy Association (APTA). Frequently asked questions: medicare therapy cap—2014. http://www.apta.org/FederalIssues/TherapyCap. Accessed August 25, 2014.

27. See, for example, New York State Office of the Professions, New York's Professional Misconduct Enforcement System. www.op.nysed.gov/opd/. Accessed August 25, 2014.

28. DeSilver D: In late spurt of activity, Congress avoids 'least productive' title . Dec. 29, 2014. http://www.pewresearch.org/fact-tank/2014/12/29/in-late-spurt-of-activity-congress-avoids-least-productive-title/. Accessed May 20, 2015.

29. Shenoy R. Mass. Legislature among states that pass the fewest bills. April 20, 2014. http://necir.org/2014/04/20/mass-legislature-among-states-that-pass-the-fewest-bills/. Accessed August 25, 2014.

30. Office of the Federal Register. A guide to the rulemaking process. https://www.federalregister.gov/uploads/2011/01/the_rulemaking_process.pdf. Accessed August 25, 2014.

31. Budetti PP, Waters TM: *Medical malpractice law in the United States*, 2005. http://kaiserfamilyfoundation.files.wordpress.com/2013/01/medical-malpractice-law-in-the-united-states-report.pdf, Accessed August 25, 2014.

32. See, for example, NY State Office of the Professions, application for physical therapy licensure and first registration. www.op.nysed.gov/prof/pt/pt1.pdf. Accessed August 25, 2014.

33. CNA/Healthcare Providers Service Organization (HPSO). Physical therapy liability: 2001–2010; Jan. 2012. https://www.hpso.com/pdfs/db/CNA_CLS_PTreport_final_011312.pdf?fileName=CNA_CLS_PTreport_final_011312.pdf&folder=pdfs/db&isLiveStr=Y. Accessed August 25, 2014.

34. Welk P: Considerations for physical therapy service delegation, *PT Mag Phys Ther* 16(11):18–21, 2008.

35. See, for example, NY Education Law Section 6736(b)(1) and Section 6738, http://www.op.nysed.gov/prof/pt/article136.htm; and NY code, rules, and regulations, Title 8, Subpart 77, Section 77.6, NY State Office of the Professions website, http://www.op.nysed.gov/prof/pt/part77.htm. Accessed August 25, 2014.

36. Friberg DG: External oversight of health service providers. In Nosse LJ, Friberg DG, editors: *Managerial and supervisory principles for physical therapists*, ed 3, New York, NY, 2010, Wolters Kluwer/Lippincott Williams & Wilkins, pp 211–219.

37. Lewis K: Employment contract: the tie that binds, *PT Mag Phys Ther*, 2006, http://www.apta.org/PTinMotion/2006/10/, Accessed August 25, 2014.

38. Wojciechowski M: *Third-party payers: strategies for private practice PT's, PT Mag Phys Ther*, 2009. April 2009, http://www.apta.org/PTinMotion/2009/4/Feature/ThirdPartyPayers/. Accessed August 25, 2014.

39. American Physical Therapy Association. Standing rules of the American Physical Therapy Association, #21: Definition of association viewpoints and administrative directives. http://www.apta.org/uploadedFiles/APTAorg/About_Us/Policies/General/StandingRules.pdf. Accessed August 25, 2014.

40. American Physical Therapy Association. Standards of practice for physical therapy. http://www.apta.org/uploadedFiles/APTAorg/About_Us/Policies/Practice/StandardsPractice.pdf. Accessed August 25, 2014.

41. American Physical Therapy Association. Professionalism in physical therapy: core values. http://www.apta.org/uploadedFiles/APTAorg/About_Us/Policies/Judicial_Legal/ProfessionalismCoreValues.pdf. Accessed August 25, 2014.

42. American Physical Therapy Association. Disciplinary action procedural document. www.apta.org/uploadedFiles/APTAorg/About_Us/Policies/Judicial_Legal/DisciplinaryActionProceduralDocument.pdf. Accessed August 25, 2014.

43. Page CG: *Management in physical therapy practices*, Philadelphia, PA, 2010, F.A. Davis Company, 73–78.

ADDITIONAL RESOURCES

Purtilo R, Doherty RF: *Ethical dimensions in the health professions*, ed 5, St Louis, MO, 2010, Saunders. The text assumes no formal prior study of ethics. It addresses basic concepts of morality and ethics, applies them to specific dilemmas in health care, and includes a process for ethical decision making. It makes extensive use of case studies and study questions.

American Physical Therapy Association (APTA), House of Delegates Bylaws, Positions, Standards, Policies, Procedures, and Guidelines. Available at http://www.apta.org/policies/. This webpage contains links to standards, policies, and positions adopted by the House of Delegates of APTA and is updated annually. These documents govern the activities of the organization and its members.

**RELATED
WEBSITES**

www.apta.org. Website of APTA. A comprehensive source of information on the profession of physical therapy. Some information is available only to members, but a considerable amount is available to the public, including sections specifically for students and consumers.

www.cms.gov. Site for the CMS, the federal agency within the Department of Health and Human Services that, among other duties, administers the Medicare and Medicaid programs. A free, comprehensive source of information on these programs.

www.fsbpt.org. Home of the Federation of State Boards of Physical Therapy. A free, authoritative source of information on the National Physical Therapy Examination and a clearinghouse for information on licensing within the United States.

www.gpo.gov. Website of the U.S. Government Printing Office. Another free, searchable site with the complete Code of Federal Regulations and Federal Register, as well as federal statutes and pending bills.

https://beta.congress.gov/. Free site maintained by the Library of Congress, with substantial searchable federal legislative information. Information includes the Congressional Record, current bills, and Congressional committee reports, as well as the complete text of all federal statutes.

**REVIEW
QUESTIONS**

1. Describe the differences among (1) a statute, (2) common law, (3) a regulation, and (4) a policy.
2. Give one example of a federal statute and one example of a state statute, and describe how they affect the practice of physical therapy.
3. Describe two ways in which physical therapists and physical therapist assistants could influence public policies that affect physical therapy practice.
4. Describe two types of legal liability that physical therapists and physical therapist assistants could incur if they fail to abide by legal requirements.

R*ight now, we pay too much for too little health care.*
Regina Herzlinger

6 Financing Health Care and Reimbursement in Physical Therapist Practice

Jennifer E. Green-Wilson

KEY TERMS

abuse
access
Accountable Care Organizations (ACO)
Balanced Budget Act of 1997 (BBA)
beneficiary
bundled payment models
capitation
case management
case mix
Centers for Medicare and Medicaid Services
  (CMS)
Children's Health Insurance Program (CHIP)
Children's Health Insurance Program
  Reauthorization Act (CHIPRA)
claims
coinsurance
collaborative care models
consumer-driven health plans
co-payment
covered services
Current Procedural Terminology (CPT) codes
deductible
diagnostic-related groups (DRGs)
durable medical equipment (DME)

employer-sponsored health insurance
entitlement
fee schedule
fee-for-service (FFS)
fraud
gatekeeper
habilitation services
health insurance
health maintenance organization (HMO)
indemnity
independent practice association (IPA) model
insured
insurer
managed care
managed care organization (MCO)
Medicaid
Medicare
Medicare Advantage
Medicare Fee Schedule
Medicare Modernization Act (MMA)
Medicare Part A—Hospital Insurance
Medicare Part B—Supplementary Medical
   Insurance
Medicare Part D
Minimum Data Set (MDS)
open enrollment
Patient-Centered Medical Homes (PCMH)
per diem
pharmaceutical formularies
Physician Quality Reporting System (PQRS)
point-of-service (POS) plan
preferred provider organization (PPO)
premium
primary care provider (PCP)
prospective payment system (PPS)
provider contracting
provider network (panel)
reimbursement
resource utilization groups (RUGs III)

resource-based relative value scale
   (RBRVS)
retrospective reimbursement
risk
shared savings program
staff model
subscriber
third-party payer
usual, customary, and reasonable (UCR)
utilization
utilization review (UR)
waste

LEARNING OBJECTIVES

After reading this chapter, the reader will be able to:

■ Discuss the payment or reimbursement process in health care.
■ Differentiate between retrospective and prospective reimbursement methods.
■ Discuss how risk and health insurance are related.
■ Differentiate between indemnity health insurance and managed care plans.
■ Differentiate among Medicare, Medicaid, and the Children's Health Insurance Program (CHIP).
■ Discuss how health care is financed.
■ Define how managed care organizations control health care costs.
■ State current trends in health care spending.
■ Discuss the Balanced Budget Act of 1997 (BBA) and its impact on physical therapy reimbursement.
■ Discuss recent health care reform initiatives, including the Affordable Care Act of 2010 (ACA).

In the past four decades, major issues in the health care industry have resulted in dramatic changes in how health care is financed, how providers are reimbursed, how employers and consumers share costs, and ultimately how health care is delivered. Costs of health care have skyrocketed. In part, this is because of advances in technology and specialization. In addition, the aging of America has put a strain on Medicare, the government-sponsored health insurance program for older adults. In response to the high cost of health care, health insurance companies and the government have imposed limitations on what and how they will reimburse or pay for health care services and goods. Most of these restrictions were imposed in the 1990s through the expansion of managed care programs in the private sector and the Balanced Budget Act of 1997 in the government sector. Changes in these programs, however, are continuing at a rapid pace. Even more changes are happening and projected as a result of recent health care reform that resulted in President Obama's signing of the Patient Protection and Affordable Care Act (ACA), making it law on March 23, 2010. Providers, including physical therapists (PTs), not only must abide by the limitations or seek reimbursement directly from the patient/client but also are encouraged to assume a role as an advocate for the patient/client, especially during times of health care reform, to ensure appropriate access to care and coverage for health care services.

Financing of health care is a source of great frustration for both the provider and the consumer. Words commonly used to describe the contemporary reimbursement experience include confusing, complex, expensive, competitive, restrictive, exasperating, and ineffective. The need for health care has not changed, but the reimbursement and coverage for these services and goods have changed. Providers must conform to extensive documentation requirements, must respond to constant changes to guidelines, regulations, and payment policies, and have altered their delivery of services in order to be reimbursed. Consumers must pay for the services and goods not covered by the insurance industry and in many cases do not have health insurance because of the expensive premiums.

The current status of financing and reimbursement in health care, as well as how and why they evolved to this point, is described in this chapter. Particular attention is given to the impact on the PT and physical therapist assistant (PTA).

<table>
<tr><td>

HEALTH INSURANCE

</td><td>

Health is unpredictable; it is uncertain if or when a person will become sick or require health care services.[1] The types of health care services a person needs vary greatly from an appointment in a doctor's office to a lengthy hospitalization in an intensive care unit (ICU). The need for catastrophic health care services could obliterate a family's or a person's finances. Therefore, people in the United States purchase health insurance to minimize **risk**, defined in health care as the probability of a financial loss. This purchase is intended to provide "peace of mind" against the high costs of health care.

Health insurance refers to the variety of policies that can be purchased to pay for certain health-related services and goods. Policies range from those that cover the costs of medical, surgical, and hospital expenses to those that meet a precise need, such as covering the costs of long-term care. Typically, to become **insured** (covered by the policy), a **subscriber** (individual who purchases the policy) purchases a health insurance plan from an **insurer** (health insurance company). The subscriber purchases a range of benefits and benefit levels, which are available for a defined period of time, usually 1 year. Benefits are described as **covered services** or those services that are reimbursed by the insurance policy. Some typical covered medical services include inpatient hospital services, outpatient

</td></tr>
</table>

surgery, physician visits (in the hospital), office visits, skilled nursing care, medical tests and X-ray examinations, prescription drugs, physical therapy, and maternity care. Often coverage for some goods, such as **durable medical equipment (DME)**, is limited or not provided under the health insurance plan; in this case, the patient is completely responsible for payment. DME is medical equipment (such as a wheelchair, hospital bed, or ventilator) that a practitioner may prescribe for a patient's use over an extended period.[2]

The need for health insurance developed when, because of technologic advances, specialization, and research, hospitals became entrenched as critical centers for health care. Because individuals and families became dependent on hospitals for health care, they could no longer assume the risk that they could pay if or when hospitalization or sophisticated health care services were needed. In addition, hospitals were no longer able to assume the risk that patients admitted and cared for would pay their bills for services rendered. As a result, health insurance companies developed to fill a need in the health care industry.

FINANCING HEALTH CARE

Health insurance companies do not finance health care. They were established to offer policies that assume risk and to process health insurance claims; both tasks complicated health care transactions and added administrative expenses to the cost of providing health care. Who then finances health care—in other words, who pays for these health insurance policies? Figure 6-1 illustrates the relationship between financing and reimbursement in health care and how this has changed dramatically in the United States over time. In the traditional or first-party system, the individual seeking health care (first party) paid the provider (second party) directly. As health care services and costs increased, health insurance companies and the policies they offered became extensive (see earlier discussion). Individuals could no longer afford to pay for the services or even the policies directly. Employers and the government established programs to contribute to the cost of health insurance. The system shifted to the current or third-party system, in which health insurance companies (third party) are paid for their policies and then, by assuming the role of "administrator," pay providers for health care services.

Fundamentally, health care is financed by the individual directly, the employer, or the government. Figure 6-2 illustrates the percentage of individuals who have insurance provided by each of these sources. Note that this figure is for

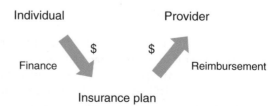

Figure 6-1 ■ The third-party system in the U.S. health care industry incorporates the concepts of finance (who buys insurance) and reimbursement (who pays the provider).

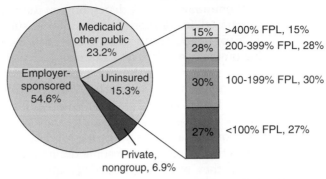

The uninsured population as a share of the nonelderly population and by poverty levels, 2013

268.9 million nonelderly   **41.3 million uninsured**

Figure 6-2 ■ Percentage of individuals who have insurance purchased by themselves (private nongroup), their employers, or the government or not at all. Note that this is for the nonelderly population. In this graph, Medicaid includes the Children's Health Insurance Program and other state programs. FPL = Federal Poverty Level. (Data from *The Uninsured: A Primer - Key Facts About Health Insurance and the Uninsured in America*, December 2014. The Kaiser Commission on Medicaid and the Uninsured/Urban Institute Analysis of 2014 ASEC Supplement to the CPS. http://files.kff.org/attach ment/the-uninsured-a-primer-key-facts-about-health-insurance-and-the-uninsured-in-america-supplemental-tables/ Accessed August 19, 2015.)

the nonelderly population, so the impact of Medicare is limited. In addition, note the significant percentage of individuals who are uninsured. Although health care services may be available, not everyone has **access** to health care, defined as the ability to receive health care services when needed, because of the way the health care system is organized and financed in the United States.

In the private nongroup source of financing health care (see Figure 6-2), the individual purchases a health insurance policy directly from a health insurance company. Acquiring health insurance this way is expensive and not commonly done. In this direct pay approach the individual pays the **premium**, or cost of the insurance, out of pocket.

A second and most common method of financing health care is in an employment-based arrangement (see Figure 6-2). Most employees purchase health insurance through their employers. This is known as **employer-sponsored health insurance** or *group insurance*. Employers offer health insurance coverage as a benefit for their employees, typically those who work full time. Employers are given tax incentives to offer health insurance as a benefit. Essentially, in the group model both employees and employers finance health care. The employers agree to pay all or a certain portion of the premium of a health insurance plan. The employee pays the premiums using payroll deductions combined with the employer's contributions. Each year a period is designated as **open enrollment**, during which an employee has the opportunity to switch to a new health insurance plan based on individual and family needs and health insurance plans available. Once a selection has been made, the subscriber is locked into the choice for a defined period of time, usually 1 year.

Premium costs vary depending on the type of health plan or level of benefits purchased. In addition to the premiums, subscribers and dependents are responsible for financing other health care costs incurred at the point of service depending on the type of health insurance plan purchased; usually these costs are paid out of pocket. These cost commitments can include deductibles, co-payments ("co-pays"), and coinsurances. A **deductible** is the amount that the subscriber incurs before a health insurer will pay for all or part of the remaining cost of the covered services. Deductibles may be either fixed dollar amounts, such as $500, or the value of a particular service, such as 2 days of hospital care. Usually deductibles are linked to some defined time period (e.g., a calendar year) over which they must be incurred. Frequently the insured individual can choose a higher deductible to reduce the monthly premiums for the health insurance policy. **Co-payments** are flat dollar amounts (e.g., $50) a subscriber has to pay for specific health services (e.g., physician office visit) at the time of service. **Coinsurance**, usually expressed as a percentage, is a cost-sharing obligation under a health insurance policy. The subscriber is required to assume responsibility for a percentage of the costs of the covered services (commonly 20%). Box 6-1 provides an example of how these expenses would apply with a typical office visit.

A third and major source of financing health care is the government (see Figure 6-2). The federal government finances the Medicare program, and the federal and state governments finance Medicaid and the Children's Health Insurance Program for each state. In addition, the government funds research efforts through the National Institutes of Health (NIH), the Public Health Service, and other initiatives. Tax dollars collected from individuals and corporations are allocated to finance these programs and services. Worth highlighting, some individuals with low incomes who do not have access to employer-based or other insurance gain coverage through publicly funded programs such as Medicaid and CHIP. Yet more than 41.3 million nonelderly people, more than 15% (about one in six) of the total nonelderly population in the United States, still lacked health

BOX 6-1	Deductibles, Co-payments, and Coinsurance: An Example

An insured individual is covered under a health insurance policy that requires a $1000 deductible, $50 co-pay, and 80/20 coinsurance. The individual sustained a wrist fracture that required casting and is now coming to physical therapy immediately after removal of the cast. At the time of the visit, and at each visit thereafter, the person must pay the $50 co-pay. The individual's health insurance company is responsible for paying 80% of future covered health care expenses, and the individual will be obligated to pay the remaining 20% for each covered health care expense incurred. This will begin only after the individual has paid the deductible, or $1000 in this case, for a specified period of time, usually 1 year.

insurance in 2013 (see Figure 6-2). Nearly all of the elderly are insured by Medicare, yet nearly 640,000 of the elderly were uninsured in 2012.

The **Centers for Medicare and Medicaid Services (CMS)**, under the Department of Health and Human Services, administers the Medicare program and works with each state to administer Medicaid, CHIP, and health insurance portability standards. This agency is the largest purchaser of health insurance in the United States, and its policies have a significant impact on the rest of the health insurance industry.

MEDICARE

Medicare is the federally funded health insurance program that was enacted (as an amendment to the Social Security Act) in 1965 to cover the elderly population (age 65 years and older), persons with end-stage renal disease, and those who are disabled and entitled to Social Security benefits. Medicare provides coverage for more than 49 million beneficiaries.[3] This is an **entitlement** program—that is, Americans 65 years of age and older who have contributed to Medicare through taxes or meet other disability eligibility requirements have the right to the benefits of Part A of this program. An individual entitled to Medicare is known as a **beneficiary**.[4] There are several parts to the Medicare program and they are described below.

Medicare Part A—Hospital Insurance provides mandatory coverage for inpatient hospital care, skilled nursing facility (SNF) services, certain home health services, and hospice care. It is financed by payroll taxes from workers and their employers (each pays 1.45% of the wages or taxable gross; this appears as FICA [Federal Insurance Contribution Act] on the pay stub) and general federal revenues.

Medicare Part B—Supplementary Medical Insurance (SMI) is a voluntary program. Individuals entitled for Medicare Part A have the option to purchase Medicare Part B. Medicare Part B is funded from beneficiary premium payments, matched by general federal revenues. For 2015, most people paid the standard premium amount of $104.90 each month for Medicare Part B with the $147 per year deductible. However, if beneficiaries' modified adjusted gross income as reported on their IRS tax return from 2013 (or 2 years prior) is above a certain amount, they may pay an Income-Related Monthly Adjustment Amount (IRMAA) or an extra charge added to their premium.[5] Medicare Part B helps pay for physician services, outpatient hospital services, select home health services, medical equipment and supplies, and other health services, including physical therapy.

Medicare Part D was enacted as part of the Medicare Prescription Drug, Improvement, and Modernization Act of 2003 (also referred to as the **Medicare Modernization Act or MMA**) and went into effect on January 1, 2006. This federal program subsidizes the costs of prescription drugs and provides more choices in health care coverage (such as Medicare Advantage) for Medicare beneficiaries.

Medicare Advantage is an optional health plan that replaced Medicare +Choice (or Medicare Part C, originally created by the Balanced Budget Act of 1997). Medicare Advantage Plans are plans approved by Medicare, but offered

6

by private insurance companies who are required to follow the rules established by Medicare. Medicare pays the private health plans a fixed amount per member per month for each member who chooses to enroll in a Medicare Advantage plan. Medicare Advantage subscribers may have to pay a monthly premium in addition to the Medicare Part B premium and a fixed co-payment every time they see their primary care provider or specialist (i.e., the specialist co-payment may be higher). This fixed out-of-pocket payment is in contrast to subscribers having to meet a deductible and paying a coinsurance (i.e., 20%) under "traditional" Medicare. Medicare Advantage plans are required to offer a package of benefits, that is, at a minimum, equal to Medicare's and that covers everything Medicare covers, but they do not have to cover every benefit in the same way. For example, Medicare Advantage plans may require higher out-of-pocket costs for some benefits as compared to traditional Medicare (i.e., SNF care), in order to lower their required co-payments for visits to physicians. Or, in some cases, private plans may use some of the excess payments they receive from the government for each enrollee to offer supplemental or expanded benefits, which may include health club memberships and other services not covered by Medicare, such as transportation to and from clinic appointments. Overall, under Medicare Advantage, Medicare beneficiaries gain greater choice and can choose from an array of private health plan options, including managed care arrangements (described later).

MEDICAID

Medicaid is a health insurance program for the indigent population and is funded jointly by state and federal governments. Essentially, each state has its own Medicaid program. States have the authority to determine eligibility standards, set reimbursement rates, and establish specific benefit levels such as the type, amount, duration, and scope of services. In June 2013, 55 million individuals were enrolled in Medicaid; nearly three-quarters of the enrollees were nondisabled, nonelderly individuals. It is important to note that these figures were stated 6 months ahead of the implementation of major coverage expansions and new enrollment standards as part of the Affordable Care Act (ACA). Compared to 2012, enrollment grew by 814,200 or 1.5%. This is the slowest growth rate since the start of the most recent recessionary period, where enrollment growth rates peaked at 7.8% and 7.2% in 2008-2009 and 2009-2010, adding 3.4 million in each period.[6] Nearly 10 million Medicaid beneficiaries are "dual eligibles"—low-income seniors and younger persons with disabilities who are enrolled in both the Medicare and Medicaid programs.[7] Dual eligibles represent approximately 15% of Medicaid enrollees in 2010 and are among the poorest and sickest individuals covered by either Medicaid or Medicare.[7] These individuals are Medicare beneficiaries who have low incomes and limited resources and may be eligible to receive help paying for their Medicare premiums and out-of-pocket medical expenses through Medicaid. In 2009, dual eligible beneficiaries accounted for 33% of Medicare spending while in 2010, 36% of all Medicaid expenditures for medical services were made on their behalf.

THE CHILDREN'S HEALTH INSURANCE PROGRAM

President Obama signed the **Children's Health Insurance Program Reauthorization Act (CHIPRA)** on February 4, 2009, renewing and expanding coverage of the **Children's Health Insurance Program (CHIP)** to nearly 8 million children.[7] CHIP, previously known as the *State Children's Health Insurance Program* (SCHIP), was originally created by the Balanced Budget Act of 1997. CHIP (Title XXI of the Social Security Act) is a state and federal partnership that targets uninsured children and pregnant women in families with incomes too high to be eligible for most state Medicaid programs, but too low to afford private health insurance coverage. Each state, within federal guidelines, determines the design of its individual CHIP program, including eligibility parameters, benefit packages, payment levels for coverage, and administrative procedures.[7] The Affordable Care Act of 2010 maintains the CHIP eligibility standards in place as of enactment through 2019 and also provides an additional $40 million in federal funding to continue efforts to promote enrollment in Medicaid and CHIP.

TRENDS IN HEALTH CARE SPENDING

Figure 6-3 illustrates the spending for health care in the United States in 2012 by source of funding ("where it came from") and type of service delivered ("where it went").

6

Health care spending has grown continually for many years. In August 1997, anticipating that Medicare spending would continue to grow at approximately 9% per year while the general economy would grow at 5% per year, President Clinton passed the **Balanced Budget Act of 1997 (BBA)**.[8] This act eliminated the budget deficit for the first time since 1969. Every segment of the health care industry was affected by the BBA. Many of the cuts in health care spending came as reductions in entitlement spending. For example, some of the imposed reductions—approximately $115 billion for Medicare and $13.6 billion for Medicaid over a 5-year period—reduced Medicare payments to health care providers and hospitals significantly and quickly. It is interesting to note that the impact on outpatient rehabilitation providers was approximately $1.7 million in reimbursement cuts.[8]

Total health expenditures reached $2.8 trillion in 2012, translating to $8915 per person, or per capita (Figure 6-4), and 17.2% of the nation's gross domestic product [GDP; the total dollar value of all goods and services produced in a year in the United States (Figure 6-5)].[9] Specific health care spending trends in several areas include the following: U.S. health care spending growth decelerated in 2012 for the fourth consecutive year, increasing only 3.7% as compared with 6.0% in 2007; hospital spending growth increased 4.9% to $882.3 billion in 2012; spending on physician and clinical services increased 4.6% to $565 billion; spending growth for other professional services, including therapists, reached $76.4 billion, increasing 4.5%; Medicare spending, which represented 20% of national health spending in 2012, grew 4.8% to $572.5 billion; total Medicaid spending grew 3.37% in 2012 to $421.2 billion, an acceleration from 2.4% growth in 2011; private health insurance premiums reached $917.0 billion in 2012, and increased 3.2%, near the 3.4% growth in 2011; and out-of-pocket spending grew 3.8% in 2012 to $328.2 billion, an acceleration from growth of 3.5% in 2011, reflecting higher cost sharing and increased enrollment in consumer-directed health plans.[9]

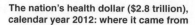

The nation's health dollar ($2.8 trillion), calendar year 2012: where it came from

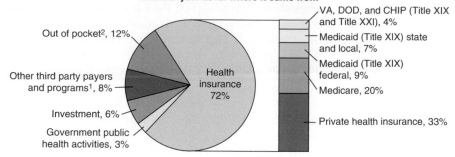

Out of pocket[2], 12%

Other third party payers and programs[1], 8%

Investment, 6%

Government public health activities, 3%

Health insurance 72%

VA, DOD, and CHIP (Title XIX and Title XXI), 4%

Medicaid (Title XIX) state and local, 7%

Medicaid (Title XIX) federal, 9%

Medicare, 20%

Private health insurance, 33%

[1] Includes worksite health care, other private revenues, Indian Health Service, workers' compensation, general assistance, maternal and child health, vocational rehabilitation, Substance Abuse and Mental Health Services Administration, school health, and other federal and state local programs.
[2] Includes co-payments, deductibles, and any amounts not covered by health insurance. Note: sum of pieces may not equal 100% due to rounding.

A

The nation's health dollar ($2.8 trillion), calendar year 2012: where it went

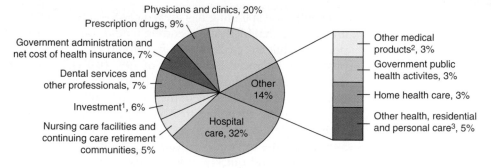

Physicians and clinics, 20%

Prescription drugs, 9%

Government administration and net cost of health insurance, 7%

Dental services and other professionals, 7%

Investment[1], 6%

Nursing care facilities and continuing care retirement communities, 5%

Other 14%

Hospital care, 32%

Other medical products[2], 3%

Government public health activites, 3%

Home health care, 3%

Other health, residential and personal care[3], 5%

[1] Includes noncommercial research (2%), structures and equipment (4%).
[2] Includes durable (1%) and non durable (2%) goods.
[3] Includes expenditures for residential care facilities, ambulance providers, medical care delivered in non-traditional settings (such as community centers, senior citizen centers, schools, and military field stations), and expenditures for Home and Community Waiver programs under Medicaid.
Note: sum of pieces may not equal 100% due to rounding.

B

Figure 6-3 ■ Spending for U.S. health care in 2012. **A,** By source ("where it came from"). **B,** Service provided ("where it went"). (From Centers for Medicare and Medicaid Services [CMS]: *U.S. health care system,* Rockville, MD, CMS, Office of the Actuary, National Health Statistics Group. http://www.cms.gov/Research-Statistics-Data-and-Systems/Statistics-Trends-and-Reports/NationalHealthExpendData/Downloads/PieChartSourcesExpenditures2012.pdf. Accessed October 15, 2014.)

Per capita spending—PPP adjusted

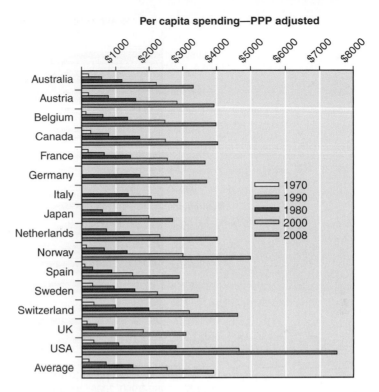

Figure 6-4 ■ Total health care expenditure per capita, U.S. and selected countries, 1970, 1980, 1990, 2000, 2008. PPP=Purchasing Power Parity. (From *Snapshots: Health Care Spending in the United States and Selected OECD Countries*, Menlo Park, CA, 2011, Henry J Kaiser Family Foundation. http://kff.org/health-costs/issue-brief/snapshots-health-care-spending-in-the-united-states-selected-oecd-countries/. Accessed October 15, 2014. Source: Organisation for Economic Cooperation and Development [2010], "OECD Health Data," OECD Health Statistics [database]. doi: 10.1787/data-00350-en. Accessed February 14, 2011.)

Health care spending projections indicate an urgency and necessity of future ongoing health care reform to control health care spending without sacrificing health care quality and access. CMS projects that national health expenditures (NHE) grow at an average rate of 5.7% for 2013-2023, 1.1 percentage points faster than expected average annual growth in the GDP. Expected growth for 2014 is 5.6%, as 9 million Americans are projected to gain health insurance coverage, predominantly through Medicaid or the Health Insurance Marketplaces. Projections indicate that health spending may reach 19.3% as a share of GDP by 2023, up from 17.2% in 2012.[9] Yet some of the health care reform initiatives proposed and being implemented are contentious and are complicating the administrative aspect of health care even further. For example, the passing of the MMA in December 2003 was controversial in projections of cost versus benefits. President Obama signed the Patient Protection and Affordable Care Act into law on March 23, 2010. Although this comprehensive health care reform legislation focuses on

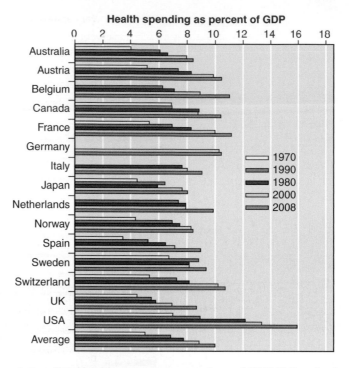

Health spending as percent of GDP

Figure 6-5 ■ Total health expenditure as a share of GDP, U.S. and selected countries, 1970, 1980, 1990, 2000, 2008. (From *Snapshots: Health Care Spending in the United States and Selected OECD Countries*, Menlo Park, CA, 2011, Henry J Kaiser Family Foundation. http://kff.org/health-costs/issue-brief/snapshots-health-care-spending-in-the-united-states-selected-oecd-countries/. Accessed October 15, 2014. Source: Organisation for Economic Cooperation and Development [2010], "OECD Health Data," *OECD Health Statistics* [database]. doi: 10.1787/data-00350-en. Accessed February 14, 2011.)

provisions to expand coverage, control health care costs, and improve the health care delivery system, the overall financial impact, in terms of health care spending, is still relatively unknown.[10]

HEALTH CARE FRAUD, ABUSE, AND WASTE

Unfortunately, the prevalence of health care fraud, abuse, and waste has resulted in the need for federal and state laws, regulations, and other policies to prevent their occurrence.[11] In general, **fraud** is defined as an intentional deception or intentional misrepresentation that a practitioner makes to gain a benefit for which that person is not entitled. Examples of fraud include knowingly billing for services that were not furnished or knowingly altering claim forms to receive a higher payment amount (see Chapter 5 for further description of fraud). **Abuse** involves payment for items or services when there is no legal entitlement to that payment, and the health care provider has not knowingly and/or intentionally misrepresented facts to obtain payment. Given the complexity of payment systems, **waste** is more common than fraud or abuse where waste is defined as the overutilization of services or other practices that, directly or indirectly, result in unnecessary costs to the health care system. Efforts to combat fraud were consolidated and strengthened under the Health Insurance Portability and Accountability Act of 1996 (HIPAA). This act established a comprehensive program to combat fraud committed against all health plans, both public and private. The legislation required the establishment of a national Health Care Fraud and Abuse Control Program (HCFAC), which is designed to coordinate federal, state, and local law enforcement activities with respect to health care fraud and abuse.

REIMBURSE-MENT METHODS IN HEALTH CARE

To this point the focus has been on how health care is financed—that is, who pays for health insurance. The remainder of the chapter shifts to payments to the provider—how does this person or entity get reimbursed or paid for services?

Currently, many factors can hinder or challenge the reimbursement that a PT practice might receive. Therefore, every PT and PTA should be aware of the patient's coverage at the beginning of each episode of care and, without compromising patient care, should integrate any payment limitations into the plan of treatment for the patient.

As consumers we are concerned about the high cost of health care, yet as providers we are concerned about the limited reimbursement for our professional services. As rising health care costs continue to be the focus of health policy debate, limitations on reimbursement continue to be set and reimbursement methods change at a brisk pace. Historically, managing the financial side of the PT practice was left to a select few, so PTs and PTAs spent little time in their formal education experiences and during on-the-job training sessions wrestling with the broader issues of health policy, health care spending, health insurance, and reimbursement. Unfortunately, it is now more difficult to receive a payment after delivering treatment without some delay, denial, or other complication.

Payment levels are seldom equal to a PT's full charge. Therefore, whether operating in a for-profit or not-for-profit environment, providers must understand the intricacies of the reimbursement process so that they can proactively manage it to ensure that high-quality patient care is delivered and all providers, employees, and staff are paid at the end of the day. More than ever, providers need to work vigorously at maintaining a steady cash flow (by ensuring that the money owed to the practice has been collected) for the PT practice so that practice expenses (e.g., salaries) can be paid.

Reimbursement in health care is the process by which health care providers receive payment for their health care services. Because of the way health care is organized in the United States, health care providers are commonly reimbursed by a health insurance company functioning as a **third-party payer** or intermediary (see third-party system in Figure 6-1). As financing methods in health care evolved in response to escalating costs, so did the methods of reimbursement. This shift is described in the following paragraphs.

6

RETROSPECTIVE METHODOLOGY

Historically, health care providers in the United States followed a **retrospective reimbursement** method in which they were paid after health care services were rendered. The insured patient would seek care from the health care provider, the health care provider would provide care to the patient, and then the health care provider would be paid. This method of reimbursement is commonly referred to as **fee-for-service (FFS)**—otherwise known as **indemnity** or *traditional health insurance.* An indemnity insurance contract usually defines the maximum amounts that will be paid for covered services during a defined period of time.

Health insurers with indemnity policies assumed the risk for health care costs and processed the health care **claims** (forms describing the medical condition, services provided, and bill for services). After services were provided, health care providers submitted claims directly to health insurers for reimbursement. Typically, as long as the fees submitted by health care providers for services rendered fell within the **usual, customary, and reasonable (UCR)** range, the claim was paid in full without dispute. Using data collected through community or state surveys of provider charges, health insurers determined their own UCR fees—the maximum charge the insurer will reimburse for a particular health care service. This reimbursement process allowed health care providers to establish their own fees, known as a **fee schedule**, for the specific health care services they provided. Providers had little incentive to limit services or costs.

PROSPECTIVE METHODOLOGY

In an attempt to control rising health care costs, health insurance companies shifted to a **prospective payment system (PPS)**. Prospective payment refers to various methods of paying hospitals, health systems, and organizations, or health care providers in which payments are established in advance. Health care providers are paid these amounts regardless of the costs they actually incur. PPSs establish some control over cost increases by setting limits on amounts paid during a future period. Some PPSs provide incentives for improved efficiency by sharing savings with health care providers who achieve lower than anticipated costs. In retrospective reimbursement, health care providers are reimbursed for actual expenses incurred, whereas in PPSs they are not.

The federal government had a significant influence in the growth of the PPS. The Social Security Amendments of 1983 created a new PPS for hospital inpatients covered under Medicare Part A. The principle of **diagnostic-related groups (DRGs)** was introduced, in which the patient's diagnosis determines the amount the hospital will be paid; the payment is a fixed amount based on the average cost of treating that particular diagnosis. A measure of **case mix** for the institution, or composite of the patients in each DRG, is used to determine reimbursement amounts. The hospital is paid the average cost regardless of length of stay or amount of treatment administered. Therefore, if the patient requires less care or fewer days in the hospital than the DRG average, the hospital makes money. Conversely, if the patient stays in the hospital longer or needs more care than the DRG average, the hospital loses money.

Another action taken by the federal government modified the PPS as it applied to physicians paid for services for Medicare beneficiaries under Part B. A new physician reimbursement method was established by the Omnibus Budget Reconciliation Act of 1989 and became effective in 1992. The **resource-based relative value scale (RBRVS)** replaced the fee-for-service system. RBRVS fees were determined based on three components: the total work completed, costs to practice medicine, and an allowance for malpractice insurance expense.[12] Each health care service was assigned a specified number of relative value units (RVUs); these RVUs were multiplied by a national conversion factor and further adjusted to allow for geographic cost variations. This approach had the effect of containing health care costs because the payment for a given health care service was the same regardless of whether it was performed by a generalist or a specialist physician. This system has become the foundation for the **Medicare Fee Schedule**, which lists payments for thousands of services and is frequently used by third-party payers as one of their key benchmarks to determine payments for all their subscribers (not just Medicare beneficiaries).

Although government intervention had a significant impact on the growth of the PPS, the most influential factor was the development of managed care. The principles of managed care are fairly straightforward, but the methods of implementation are varied and complex. This reimbursement approach is described in the next section.

MANAGED CARE

With health care costs continuing to rise and with global competition becoming fiercer, employers, health care policymakers, and the government needed to cultivate methods to control health care costs while still ensuring high-quality health care. In 1973, the Health Maintenance Organization (HMO) Act was passed. This federal legislation empowered health insurance companies to develop new ways to pay for health care services and goods.[12] The law increased control of the delivery of health care by third-party payers through government-mandated regulations of health care service. The concept of prepaid or fixed payment under a managed care arrangement escalated.

MANAGED CARE ORGANIZATION

In its simplest form, **managed care** consists of two components: a predetermined payment schedule ("discounted fee schedule") established by the insurance company based on utilization data, and a **provider network (panel)** consisting of providers who contract with the insurance company and agree to accept the payment schedule for their services. Subscribers to these health insurance plans generally pay more for services if they are conducted by providers outside the network. Institutions or groups that employ the managed care principles are called **managed care organizations (MCOs)**. Managed care is further characterized by diverse organizational models, distinct methods for reimbursing providers, and various approaches to cost containment. By incorporating these approaches to health care reimbursement, all MCOs restrict access to care in some way in an effort to control utilization, ultimately to decrease costs. Examples of access restrictions include limits on the types of, number of, or payment for services covered. Cost of the insurance may also limit access. Certainly, fixing payment or the number of visits covered without considering the quality or quantity of actual services provided has shifted how health care services are delivered.

Provider networks in MCOs are developed through a process called **provider contracting**. The provider is deemed "on the provider panel" or a "participating provider" if the provider accepts the terms of the insurer's contract (usually after much negotiation) and after the MCO verifies the provider's credentials (using a process called *provider credentialing*). Contract terms outline reimbursement methods, including discounted fees and possible incentives, scopes of services allowed for reimbursement, utilization targets, and other stipulations. Participating providers assume responsibility (share financial risk) with health insurers for a population's health care and health maintenance. The contracting process enables insurers to exert influence or decision-making control over the **utilization**, or delivery and cost, of health care services for a defined period of time.

Currently, the three major types of MCOs (commonly referred to as the "triple option") are HMOs, preferred provider organizations (PPOs), and point-of-service (POS) plans. Basically, these models differ in how tightly the provider panels are controlled. Further descriptions of each of these models follow.

HEALTH MAINTENANCE ORGANIZATION

Health maintenance organizations (HMOs) proliferated with the HMO Act of 1973,[12] which provided loans and grants to form these entities. It also stipulated certain outpatient services that had to be provided, and it required that employers with 25 or more employees offer an HMO option if one was available in the area. Two types of HMOs existed originally: the staff and independent practice association (IPA) models. In the **staff model**, providers are employed (not just under contract) by the HMO that also operates the facilities where the services are provided. The Kaiser-Permanente Health Care System, established in 1938, remains the foremost example of this model. In the **independent practice association (IPA) model**, individual physicians or physician groups form a legal entity that contracts with the HMO to provide services without operating the facilities where the services are provided.[13] This has predominated over the staff model.

PREFERRED PROVIDER ORGANIZATION

The second type of MCO is the **preferred provider organization (PPO)**. A PPO is considered an "open managed care model." In this arrangement, a health insurer or employer negotiates discounted or lower fees with networks of health care providers (doctors, hospitals, and other health care providers) in return for guaranteeing a certain volume of patients. Enrollees in a PPO can elect to receive treatment outside the network but must pay higher premiums, co-payments, or deductibles for it.

POINT-OF-SERVICE PLANS

The third type of MCO, the **point-of-service (POS) plan**, offers both in-network and out-of-network benefits. The greatest level of coverage is available if the insured receives in-network benefits. When an insured receives out-of-network benefits, higher out-of-pocket expenses are incurred. Typically, the insured is responsible for meeting an annual deductible before health care services are reimbursed and for paying a fixed percentage coinsurance amount or co-payment for out-of-network services. The insured may also need to pay the difference between the insurer's payment and the actual charges for services received if the out-of-network health care provider's fees exceed the insurer's acceptable in-network contracted rates.

The types of provider panels determine where and how consumers can access health care. For example, traditional HMOs (the oldest form of managed care) require enrollees to choose a **primary care provider (PCP)** from a "closed panel" of participating providers. A PCP is a generalist physician (family practice, general internal medicine, general pediatrics, and sometimes obstetrics and gynecology for female patients) who provides primary care services. Characteristically in an HMO, PCPs become the **gatekeeper**—the primary coordinator who determines whether the patient needs to see a specialist or requires other nonroutine services. The goal of the gatekeeper is to direct the patient to an appropriate level of service while avoiding unnecessary, possibly duplicative, redundant, and costly referrals to specialists or for specialty services. In other words, the gatekeeper role restricts access to specialty services in an effort to control costs.

The subscriber must make choices regarding the type of managed care plan when purchasing insurance during open enrollment. These purchasing decisions and the amount of choice purchased directly affect a subscriber's potential future cost-sharing obligations. If the consumer stays within the provider network ("in network") to receive health care, the consumer will not incur additional health care costs outside of the agreed-on co-payments and premiums. However, if the consumer desires to purchase the choice to seek health care outside of the network ("out of network"), the consumer would be better off purchasing a PPO or POS plan, rather than a tightly controlled HMO plan.

Cost sharing is a reimbursement strategy adopted by most MCOs. By sharing the cost of health care with health care providers and consumers of health care, MCOs spread the risk or burden of trying to limit the potential for financial loss. Deductibles, co-payments, and coinsurances are examples of specific cost-sharing strategies.

Most managed care plans, especially HMOs, offer preventive health care benefits. Inherent in the foundation of managed care is the emphasis on maintaining wellness or health (hence the term "health maintenance organizations"). Thus, the use of expensive health care services is avoided if a consumer stays healthy (in a state of complete physical, mental, and social well-being).

MCOs use several other strategies to contain costs. These include providing care in the least expensive settings (nursing homes or home care is preferred over hospitals), avoiding the use of expensive emergency rooms in favor of less expensive ambulatory settings such as physicians' offices, and restricting **pharmaceutical formularies**. A pharmaceutical formulary is a list of drugs (usually by generic name) with indications for their use. This list is intended to include a sufficient range of medicines that practitioners can prescribe for all "appropriate" medical treatment. A "closed" formulary provides coverage for a limited set

6

of drugs, whereas a "tiered" formulary rewards patients financially for using generic instead of brand-name drugs.[2]

Cost containment strategies also take the form of defined service review mechanisms, such as **utilization review (UR)** and case management, to ensure that services are efficient and effective. UR is defined as the evaluation of the medically necessary, appropriate, and efficient use of health care services, procedures, and facilities.[13] It can be done on a concurrent and retrospective basis. For example, a UR of a hospital would include a review of admissions, discharges, and lengths of stay. **Case management** provides monitoring and coordination of treatments rendered to patients to control costs and utilization. Usually patients who have chronic disease(s) (e.g., diabetes) are ideal candidates for case management because they frequently require high cost or extensive health care services.

GENERAL ENROLLMENT TRENDS

Employer-sponsored health insurance is the leading source of health insurance, covering about 149 million nonelderly people.[14] In theory, employer-sponsored insurance is a way of "managing care"—linking the delivery of and payment for health care, coordinating the delivery of health care cost effectively, and providing prepaid (fixed) health care services within a defined network of health care providers (e.g., hospitals, physicians, and laboratories) to voluntarily enrolled populations. According to the Kaiser Family Foundation, 58% of covered workers are enrolled in PPOs, whereas 20% of covered workers are enrolled in a high-deductible plan with savings options (HDHP/SO), 13% in an HMO, 8% in a POS plan, and less than 1% in a conventional (also known as an indemnity plan) (Figure 6-6).[14] Enrollment distribution varies by firm size; for example, PPOs are relatively more popular for covered workers at large firms (200 or more workers) than smaller firms (63% vs. 46%) and POS plans are relatively more popular among smaller firms than large firms (17% vs. 4%). Enrollment in HDHP/SOs increased significantly between 2009 and 2011, from 8% to 17% of covered workers, but has plateaued since then (Exhibit E). In 2014, 27% of the firms offering health benefits offer a high-deductible health plan with a health reimbursement arrangement (HDHP/HRA) or a health savings account (HSA) qualified HDHP. In 2014, the average annual premiums for employer-sponsored health insurance were $6025 for single coverage and $16,834 for family coverage (Figure 6-7).[14] Over the past 10 years, the average premium for family coverage has increased 69%.[14] Noteworthy, premiums have increased less quickly over the last 5 years (2009-2014), than the preceding 5-year period or from 2004 to 2009 (26% as compared to 34%). Additionally, average premiums for high-deductible health plans with a savings option (HDHP/SOs) are lower than the overall average for all plan types for both single ($5299) and family coverage ($15,401).

CONSUMER-DRIVEN HEALTH CARE PLANS

Consumer-driven health plans are new health plan arrangements that are receiving increasing attention from invested stakeholders in health care. Consumer-driven health care reflects a new approach for providing health care benefits that combines employer contributions with increased employee choice

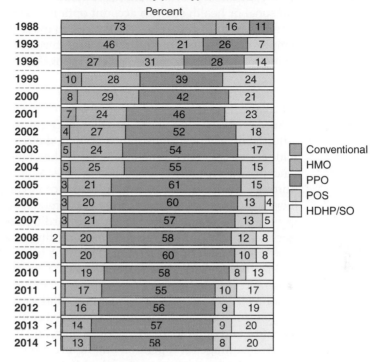

Distribution of health plan enrollment for covered workers, by plan type; 1988-2014

Percent

Year	Conventional	HMO	PPO	POS	HDHP/SO
1988	73		16	11	
1993	46	21	26	7	
1996	27	31	28	14	
1999	10	28	39	24	
2000	8	29	42	21	
2001	7	24	46	23	
2002	4	27	52	18	
2003	5	24	54	17	
2004	5	25	55	15	
2005	3	21	61	15	
2006	3	20	60	13	4
2007	3	21	57	13	5
2008	2	20	58	12	8
2009	1	20	60	10	8
2010	1	19	58	8	13
2011	1	17	55	10	17
2012	1	16	56	9	19
2013	>1	14	57	9	20
2014	>1	13	58	8	20

Figure 6-6 ■ Distribution of health plan enrollment for covered workers by plan type, 1988 to 2014. Figures may not add up to 100% because of rounding. Asterisk indicates that distribution is statistically different from the previous year, shown at $P < 0.05$. (From Employer health benefits: 2014 annual survey, Menlo Park, CA, 2014, Henry J Kaiser Family Foundation. http://kff.org/report-section/ehbs-2014-summary-of-findings/. Accessed October 15, 2014.)

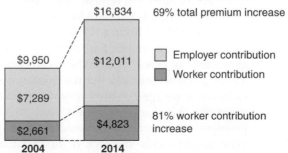

Average annual health insurance premiums and worker contributions for family coverage, 2004-2014

$16,834   69% total premium increase

$9,950 $12,011   ☐ Employer contribution

$7,289   ☐ Worker contribution

$2,661 $4,823   81% worker contribution increase

2004   **2014**

Figure 6-7 ■ Average annual health insurance premium and worker contribution for family coverage, 2004-2014. (From Employer health benefits: 2014 annual survey, Menlo Park, CA, 2014, Henry J Kaiser Family Foundation. http://kff.org/report-section/ehbs-2014-summary-of-findings/. Accessed October 15, 2014.)

and responsibility and increased health plan and provider accountability.[15] Currently, the most prevalent model combines a high deductible (e.g., $1000) with a personal or health savings account option (HDHP/SO). These accounts permit employers, and sometimes employees, to make pretax contributions, which the employees can use to pay for routine medical care, thereby increasing their choice as to how the money will be spent.[14]

HEALTH CARE REFORM

The Patient Protection and Affordable Care Act, simply known as the Affordable Care Act (ACA), signed into law March 23, 2010, aims to increase the quality and affordability of health insurance, contain the rising costs of health care for individuals and the government, and lower the uninsured rate by expanding public and private insurance.[16] Specifically, the ACA increases access to health care through its expansion of health insurance coverage as well as the creation of new insurance safeguards; creates new models of care beyond traditional fee-for-service; shifts payment focus to rewarding providers for the quality of their services; and increases screening and auditing processes to improve the integrity of federal health care programs. The ACA increases access to health care to the uninsured by expanding health insurance coverage through use of the Health Insurance Marketplaces and expansions to Medicaid. Marketplaces act as a resource where individuals, families, and small businesses can learn about options for their health coverage, compare health insurance plans based on costs, benefits, and other features, choose a plan, and enroll in coverage.[17] The Marketplace encourages competition among private health plans.

An important component of the Marketplace is the Essential Health Benefits (EHB) package, which ensures that most health insurance plans offered within the Marketplaces provide a baseline of coverage, benefits, and services, including rehabilitation and habilitation, to their enrollees.[18] Of new interest to the physical therapy profession is the inclusion of **habilitation services** or health care services that help a person keep, learn, or improve skills and functioning for daily living.[19] These services may include physical and occupational therapy, speech-language pathology, and other services for people with disabilities in a variety of inpatient and/or outpatient settings.

Under health care reform, new **collaborative care models** such as **accountable care organizations (ACO)**, **bundled payment models**, and **patient-centered medical homes (PCMH)** are part of the overall approach to transform the health care system and to improve the quality, affordability, and patient experience of care.[16,20] An ACO is an organization of health care providers that agrees to be accountable for the quality, cost, and overall care of Medicare beneficiaries who are assigned to it. Essentially, an ACO is a **shared savings program** for Medicare providers and ACOs are projected to help solve the problem of fragmented, wasteful, and poor-quality care. Also, ACOs are expected to tackle the lack of financial incentives for good health outcomes among Medicare beneficiaries, and the enormous growth in Medicare costs. A bundled payment is a single fee paid related to a treatment or condition.[21] This type of payment model is being used to encourage coordination across providers and to promote more efficient care. A PCMH is an approach in providing comprehensive primary care that facilitates partnerships between individual patients, their personal providers and when appropriate, the patient's family.

The ACA makes additional modifications to payment systems and links payment to quality of care. For example, the Affordable Care Act changes the **Physician Quality Reporting System (PQRS)** in a number of ways, including authorizing incentive payments through 2014 and requiring a penalty, beginning in 2015 for professionals who do not report satisfactorily.

REIMBURSE-MENT IN PHYSICAL THERAPY

Policy changes to control health care spending have affected the practice of physical therapy directly and indirectly for many years. The switch from an FFS or a retrospective reimbursement methodology to a PPS system had a significant impact on the way PTs received payment for their services. This shift in reimbursement forced PTs to look not just at historical costs of providing services (to set fee schedules from year to year), but also at the actual costs of providing care on an ongoing basis. Providers had to implement new approaches to staffing and service delivery to ensure productive, cost-effective care while still maintaining quality.

Managed care has had a dramatic effect on reimbursement and delivery of services in physical therapy. MCOs established limits and other mechanisms to control utilization and cost of health care. In addition to discounted fee schedules, MCOs have required documentation of need ("medical necessity") for physical therapy, a limitation on the number of visits covered, and documentation of functional gains after each physical therapy session. PTs must frequently invest unreimbursable time to advocate for more treatment sessions for individual patients. Documentation requirements across diverse physical therapy practice settings have become more stringent, complex, and labor intensive to improve accountability, causing much friction and sometimes discouragement within the practice of physical therapy. Conflict arises when requirements for documentation become greater and more detailed, yet third-party payers (including CMS) do not reimburse the provider for preparation of the documentation.

Besides discounted fee schedules, other payment mechanisms were created to limit reimbursement for services. Private and managed care insurers pay for a large percentage of inpatient hospital stays on a **per diem** (a prenegotiated, per day, flat or fixed fee) basis. The flat rate covers all services provided in the hospital on a particular day, including physical therapy, regardless of actual time spent with the patient. This payment method requires the provision of care to be time efficient and cost effective.[22] The BBA authorized the implementation of per discharge PPSs for inpatient rehabilitation facilities (IRFs). The IRF PPS uses information from a patient assessment instrument (IRF PAI) to classify patients into groups based on clinical characteristics and anticipated resource needs. Payments are calculated separately for each group, including the use of case- and facility-level modifications.[23] Certain HMOs use a capitated payment method. Under **capitation**, a participating health care provider is paid a fixed amount in advance per member per month (PMPM) in anticipation of future services needed by an enrolled patient. This method involves a significant financial risk to the provider and has not been popular among physical therapists.

The BBA had a widespread impact on reimbursement for health care and physical therapy services. The BBA significantly changed Medicare payment policies for rehabilitation services. Beginning January 1, 1999, an annual $1500 per beneficiary cap for physical therapy (including speech-language pathology services) and for occupational therapy was imposed on Medicare beneficiaries receiving outpatient rehabilitation services. After extensive lobbying by the American Physical Therapy Association (APTA) and other professional organizations, a moratorium on the cap became effective on January 1, 2000 and was extended through 2002. On September 1, 2003, a $1590 cap went into effect, followed by a moratorium on the cap beginning December 8, 2003, through December 31, 2005. This most recent moratorium was a result of the Medicare Modernization Act of 2003. The cap went back into effect January 1, 2006.[24] APTA has advocated strongly against the implementation of this cap, which APTA believes is insufficient to cover the costs of speech and physical therapy (grouped together under one cap). Furthermore, APTA contends that it will disrupt the continuum of care by forcing Medicare patients to change treatment settings so they can continue to receive physical therapy. According to APTA, the $1500 cap (increased to $1940 in 2015) on outpatient rehabilitation services and the SNF (Part A) and home health agency (Part B) PPSs has had an unfavorable impact on the ability of Medicare beneficiaries to access high-quality physical therapy services.

Reimbursement for physical therapy services varies greatly depending on the practice setting, creating more confusion and complexity within the profession. PTs are required to use coding systems to cover a variety of situations. For example, in outpatient physical therapy settings, PTs use **Current Procedural Terminology (CPT) codes** (97000 series; CPT is a registered trademark of the American Medical Association) to indicate what physical therapy services are delivered to patients.[25] In contrast, CMS requires PTs in SNFs to report rehabilitative therapy minutes on the **Minimum Data Set (MDS)**.[25] The MDS is an assessment instrument used in the SNF PPS to classify residents into one of 53 **resource utilization groups (RUGs III)** that categorize patients based on their levels of resources used. The resulting classifications determine payment to the facility. APTA is actively seeking modifications and clarifications to CPT codes and other coding systems to enhance and justify reimbursement for physical therapy services. APTA's goals to reform payment for outpatient physical therapy services include improved quality of care, increased recognition and promotion of the physical therapist' clinical judgment, and the provision of an accurate payment system that ensures the integrity of medically necessary services.[26]

Many of the reimbursement issues created by MCOs have limited access to health care, particularly specialty health care providers. Consequently, PTs faced new challenges, because they have historically been recognized as specialty health care providers. For many years, APTA and PTs nationwide and state by state have been advocating for direct access or patient access to physical therapists' services.[27] Patient access to physical therapists' services without referral means the removal of the physician referral mandated by state law to access physical therapists' services for evaluation and treatment. All 50 states and the District of Columbia allow for evaluation and some form of treatment without physician referral. It is important to note that some states still have time or visit limits or provisions tied to treatment without a referral. Advocating for direct access, however, is not enough. PTs must set patient-centered goals and consider clinical outcomes from the outset. Use of evidence-based practice whenever possible to justify intervention strategies is becoming essential to ensure reimbursement. More than ever, practitioners and physical therapy educators are encouraged to conduct clinical research to augment the bank of existing evidence.

It is essential that PTs in contemporary practice become acclimated to the impact of reimbursement on physical therapy practice. Co-payments for physical therapy services under certain health plans can exceed $60 per visit and additionally can exceed the reimbursement paid by the plan to the provider of care. These high co-payments for physical therapy have been identified as a reason that some consumers currently opt to reduce their frequency of care or forgo medically necessary care. Physical therapists have to ensure that co-pays, coinsurances, and deductibles are collected at the time of service and that they are fair and equitable. Some PTs are adopting first-party payment policies in which they collect payment in full from patients/clients at the time of service, eliminating the need to interface with third-party payers. It is interesting to note that this reimbursement method, generally accepted by consumers for many of the complementary therapies, returns the system to the method so common decades ago. Although the extent of this reimbursement method may never be substantial, it indicates that consumers will pay for what they believe is valuable.

PTs must become invested in the reimbursement or payment processes by other means, including the following:

- Developing effective collection strategies.
- Using and building evidence-based practice to justify interventions.
- Using a standardized documentation language that can be understood by multiple stakeholders in the reimbursement process.
- Understanding costs to provide PT care.
- Advocating to increase the profession's role as primary care practitioners or practitioners of choice.
- Supporting APTA in its efforts to influence payment and health care policy changes.

Furthermore, PTs are encouraged to develop strategies for gaining reimbursement for preventive programs and health care services, an emerging market niche.

SUMMARY

Health care financing and reimbursement originally involved direct transactions between the consumer and provider. Health insurance companies arose to assume the risk of more sophisticated health care and associated costs. The government entered this arena with the Social Security Amendments of 1965, creating the Medicare and Medicaid programs. As health care costs escalated dramatically, new methods of financing health insurance policies and reimbursing health care providers developed. Managed care emerged as the predominant method to control rising health care costs. MCOs took many forms, including

HMOs, PPOs, and POS options. Health insurance companies, through MCOs, were empowered to assume responsibility for decision making to coordinate and control utilization of health care services by limiting reimbursement, covered services, and number of covered visits. Legislation by the federal government and related regulation by CMS introduced several significant changes to health care reimbursement. These included DRGs, RBRVS, and a cap on payments for outpatient physical therapy services for Medicare beneficiaries. Payment policy changes made continuously by CMS and third-party payers create a sense for health care providers that they are trying to stay afloat amidst a reimbursement tidal wave. Curtailing the growth of health care spending has become a major policy priority, as the government, employers, and consumers struggle more and more to keep up with health care costs.

REFERENCES

1. Lee R: *Economics for healthcare managers,* ed 2, Chicago, 2009, Health Administration Press.
2. *Glossary of terms commonly used in health care, ed 2004, Washington, DC, 2004, Academy Health. http://www.academyhealth.org/files/publications/glossary.pdf.* Accessed October 15, 2014.
3. Centers for Medicare and Medicaid Services: Medicare coverage general information, Baltimore, MD. https://www.cms.gov/home/Medicare.asp. Accessed October 15, 2014.
4. Bodenheimer T, Grumbach K: *Understanding health policy: a clinical approach,* ed 6, New York, 2012, Lange Medical Books/McGraw-Hill.
5. Medicare: your costs at a glance. http://www.medicare.gov/your-medicare-costs/costs-at-a-glance/costs-at-glance.html. Accessed October 10, 2014.
6. Kaiser Family Foundation: Medicaid enrollment: June 2013 data snapshot, Menlo Park, CA.
7. Kaiser Family Foundation: Dual eligibles: Medicaid's role for low income Medicare beneficiaries—December 2010, Menlo Park, CA. http://kff.org/medicaid/fact-sheet/dual-eligibles-medicaids-role-for-low-income-2/. Accessed October 15, 2014.
8. The Balanced Budget Act: How it affects physical therapy, Alexandria,VA, American Physical Therapy Association. www.apta.org/AM/Template.cfm?Section=Home&CONTENTID=22156&TEMPLATE=/CM/Contentdisplay.cfm. Accessed October 11, 2014.
9. *Highlights-National Health Expenditures, Baltimore, 2012, Centers for Medicare and Medicaid Services. https,//www.cms.gov/NationalHealthExpendData/Downloads/highlights.pdf.* Accessed October 10, 2014.
10. The Henry J. Kaiser Family Foundation: Summary of the Affordable Care Act, 2013. http://kff.org/health-reform/fact-sheet/summary-of-the-affordable-care-act/. Accessed October 15, 2014.
11. American Physical Therapy Association (APTA): *Preventing fraud, abuse, and waster: a primer for physical therapists, Alexandria, VA, 2014, APTA. http://www.apta.org/Integrity/Primer/. Accessed October 1, 2014.*
12. Sultz H, Young K: *Health Care USA: understanding its organization and delivery,* ed 7, Sudbury, MA, 2011, Jones and Bartlett Learning.
13. Shi L, Singh D: *Delivering health care in America: a systems approach,* ed 6, Sudbury, MA, 2014, Jones and Bartlett.
14. Henry J: *Kaiser Family Foundation: employer health benefits: 2014 annual survey summary of findings,* Menlo Park, CA, 2014, Henry J. Kaiser Family Foundation.
15. Wojciechowski M: The future of physical therapy as shaped and defined by patients, *PT Mag Phys Ther* 13(2):46–52, 2005.
16. American Physical Therapy Association (APTA): Health care reform. http://www.apta.org/HealthCareReform/. Accessed October 15, 2014.
17. Health Insurance Marketplace. https://www.healthcare.gov/glossary/health-insurance-marketplace-glossary/. Accessed October 15, 2015.
18. American Physical Therapy Association (APTA): Essential health benefits (EHB). www.apta.org/ehb. Accessed October 15, 2014.
19. American Physical Therapy Association (APTA): Collaborative care. http://www.apta.org/CollaborativeCare/. Accessed October 15, 2014.

20. Kaiser Family Foundation: *The uninsured: a primer—key facts about health insurance on the eve of coverage expansions, Menlo Park, CA, 2015, Kaiser Family Foundation. http://kff.org/uninsured/report/the-uninsured-a-primer-key-facts-about-health-insurance-on-the-eve-of-coverage-expansions/.* Accessed October 15, 2014.
21. PT in Motion (APTA): Contemporary topics in health care: bundling, April 2010. http://www.apta.org/PTinMotion/2010/4/Feature/Bundling/. Accessed October 15, 2015.
22. Private insurance, payment by treatment setting, Alexandria, VA, American Physical Therapy Association. http://www.apta.org/Payment/PrivateInsurance/. Accessed October 15, 2014.
23. Inpatient Rehabilitation Facility PPS Overview, Baltimore, MD, Centers for Medicare and Medicaid, U.S. Department of Health and Human Services. http://www.cms.gov/Medicare/Medicare-Fee-for-Service-Payment/InpatientRehabFacPPS/index.html. Accessed October 15, 2014.
24. Medicaid and CHIP: The Children's Health Insurance Program (CHIP). Centers for Medicare and Medicaid Services, Baltimore, MD. https://www.healthcare.gov/medicaid-chip/childrens-health-insurance-program/. October 15, 2014.
25. American Physical Therapy Association (APTA): *The reimbursement resource book,* Alexandria, VA, 2005, APTA.
26. American Physical Therapy Association (APTA): Payment reform, physical therapy classification and payment system (PTCPS). http://www.apta.org/PTCPS/. Accessed October 15, 2014.
27. American Physical Therapy Association (APTA): *Legislation aims to increase access to physical therapist services by eliminating physician referral requirement, Alexandra, VA, 2009, APTA http://www.prnewswire.com/news-releases/legislation-aims-to-increase-access-to-physical-therapist-services-by-eliminating-physician-referral-requirement-61666592.html.* Accessed October 15, 2014.
28. Centers for Medicare and Medicaid Services: Medicare part B premium costs in 2014, Baltimore, MD. http://www.medicare.gov/your-medicare-costs/part-b-costs/part-b-costs.html. Accessed October 15, 2014.

6

REVIEW QUESTIONS

1. How is prospective reimbursement different from retrospective reimbursement?
2. What does it mean to be "insured" in health care?
3. How does a person become insured for health care in the United States?
4. How is risk in health care linked to health insurance?
5. How has managed care attempted to control health care costs?
6. How has the BBA affected physical therapy reimbursement?
7. What role does APTA play in physical therapy reimbursement?
8. What strategies can PTs use to enhance reimbursement?
9. What role does the government play in financing health care in the United States?
10. What role does the consumer play in financing his or her own health care?
11. In what ways can PTs and PTAs assume an advocacy role for their patients/clients, especially during times of health care reform?

*T*herapeutic communication requires learning a new skill, but more than that, it requires unlearning habitual, nonhelpful ways of interacting.
Carol M. Davis, PT

7

Communication in Physical Therapy in the Twenty-First Century

Helen L. Masin

CHAPTER OUTLINE

WHAT IS COMMUNICATION?
  Verbal and Nonverbal Communication
  Reading
  Writing
  Listening
  Electronic Communication

PROFESSIONAL BEHAVIORS AND COMMUNICATION

BUILDING AFFECTIVE COMMUNICATION SKILLS

COMMUNICATING EFFECTIVELY IN A MULTICULTURAL HEALTH CARE ENVIRONMENT

COMMUNICATING WITH PEOPLE FROM CULTURES DIFFERENT FROM YOUR OWN
  High-Context Assumptions
  Low-Context Assumptions
  Culture of Medicine

COMMUNICATING WITH PEOPLE WHO HAVE SPIRITUAL OR RELIGIOUS TRADITIONS THAT ARE DIFFERENT FROM YOUR OWN

COMMUNICATING WITH PEOPLE WHO SPEAK LITTLE OR NO ENGLISH

COMMUNICATING WITH PEOPLE WHO COME FROM GENERATIONS DIFFERENT FROM YOUR OWN

COMMUNICATING WITH PEOPLE WHO HAVE VISUAL IMPAIRMENTS

COMMUNICATING WITH PEOPLE WHO HAVE AUDITORY IMPAIRMENTS

COMMUNICATING WITH PATIENTS/ CLIENTS, CAREGIVERS, AND FAMILIES

COMMUNICATING WITH OTHER MEMBERS OF THE HEALTH CARE TEAM

COMMUNICATING THROUGH DELEGATION

COMMUNICATING AS A STUDENT IN THE CLASSROOM AND CLINICAL EXPERIENCES

ELECTRONIC COMMUNICATION ACROSS GENERATIONS

SUMMARY

CASE STUDIES

REFERENCES

ADDITIONAL RESOURCES

KEY TERMS

affective domain

beginning professional behaviors

cultural continuum

culture of medicine

developing professional behaviors

entry-level professional behaviors

haptics

high-context assumptions

internal dialogue

LAMP document

low-context assumptions

mirroring and matching

oculesics

post-entry-level professional behavior

professional behaviors

proxemics

rapport—cultural, verbal, and behavioral

self-assessment

LEARNING OBJECTIVES

After reading this chapter, the reader will be able to:

■ Define the components of communication.

■ Recognize the role of the affective domain in communication.

■ Use rapport in building effective communication.

■ Recognize effective communication in a multicultural health care environment.

■ Discuss high- and low-context communication assumptions.

■ Recognize the culture of medicine.

■ Discuss differences in communication across generations.

■ Recognize differences in religious, spiritual, agnostic, and atheistic orientations.

■ Respond effectively to patients/clients with visual or auditory impairments or both.

■ Respond effectively to patients/clients and their caregivers and families.

■ Respond effectively with other members of the health care team.

■ Develop effective communication as a student in both the classroom and the clinic.

■ Recognize the role of electronic communication in education and health care.

Physical therapy practitioners of the twenty-first century agree that communication is integral to the successful practice of physical therapy. The purpose of this chapter is to provide you with both a theoretical and practical background for developing the communication skills you will need to become an effective physical therapist (PT) or physical therapist assistant (PTA) in the twenty-first century. In the spirit of communication, this chapter is written in a more personal tone. Reflective questions and actions are embedded throughout the chapter (rather than placed at the end) to promote a more direct consideration of the theory or application of the skill and the art of therapeutic communication.

In the year 2000, the American Physical Therapy Association (APTA) defined a clear vision for the profession in the twenty-first century (Box 7-1; see also Box 1-5 for the complete version).[1] Although it was superseded by a new Vision Statement in 2013 (see Box 1-7), "Vision 2020" as it was commonly known, had a significant impact on goals and action in practice, education, and research as well as professional behaviors.

Similar values and behaviors are recognized by the section on Health Policy and Administration of APTA in the development of Leadership, Administration,

BOX 7-1

American Physical Therapy Association Vision Sentence for Physical Therapy 2020

Physical therapy will be provided by physical therapists who are doctors of physical therapy, recognized by consumer and other health care professionals as the practitioners of choice to whom consumers have direct access for the diagnosis of, interventions for, and prevention of impairments, functional limitations, and disabilities related to movement, function, and health.

From American Physical Therapy Association (APTA): APTA Vision Sentence for Physical Therapy 2020 and APTA Vision Statement for Physical Therapy 2020, HOD P06-00-24-35, House of Delegates Policies, Positions, and Guidelines, Alexandria, VA, 2009, APTA.

Management, and Professionalism (LAMP) skills set forth by the section.[2] These skills are promoted in a **LAMP document** and annual LAMP Summit meeting. In the core values and beliefs of the 2002 LAMP Summit, all PTs, not just managers, must have LAMP skills to become effective professionals.

In the rapidly changing health care environment, LAMP skills affect the physical therapy profession's ability to influence large organizations such as local, state, and national agencies. LAMP skills are the basis for developing such leadership behaviors as networking and political activism, which promote the growth of the profession.

In the educational environment, LAMP skills can best be integrated into the educational experience when they are woven throughout the curriculum. Academic and clinical faculty can model the LAMP skills in the classroom and thereby provide students with role models for learning these behaviors in both the classroom and the clinic.

A Delphi study by Lopopolo, Schafer, and Nosse revealed that the top-ranked LAMP skills identified by respondents were communication, professional involvement and ethical practice, delegation and supervision, stress management, reimbursement sources, time management, and health care industry scanning.[3] All of the respondents were experienced managers and members of APTA who were familiar with the content of the LAMP skills. Of the top-ranked LAMP categories, communication had the highest median score and was, therefore, the most important category. The findings indicated that beginning PTs need "extensive knowledge" of communication techniques and should be "skilled" in applying these techniques in a clinical environment. These skills are essential in both the clinical management and the patient care aspects of physical therapy. To develop the knowledge and skill essential in communication you need to appreciate what is involved in effective communication.

WHAT IS COMMUNICATION?

What does communication mean to you? Write down your definition of communication before reading further.

As defined in Merriam Webster Online, communication is "the act or process of using words, sounds, signs, or behaviors to express or exchange information or to express your ideas, thoughts, feelings, etc., to someone else."[4] There are many types of communication skills, including skills in verbal, nonverbal, reading, writing, listening, and electronic communication and social media. Communication can occur between individuals, within an individual, or among a group of people.

VERBAL AND NONVERBAL COMMUNICATION

What happens during communication between individuals? Both verbal and nonverbal elements of communication occur simultaneously. You can hear what each person is saying when individuals talk to each other. You can observe their body language and note whether what they are saying matches their body language. The verbal and nonverbal systems together transmit a message.

Think of a recent conversation you had with a friend. What did the friend say to you? What did his or her gestures and facial expressions convey to you? Were the verbal and nonverbal messages similar? How do you know?

Communication may occur within an individual, and this is called **internal dialogue**.[5] It is "heard" only by the individual himself or herself and may affect his or her nonverbal communication to other people. Internal dialogue may occur when the individual is alone, with another person, or in a group of people.

Think of a time when you were meeting with your academic advisor. You were listening to her words, but you also "heard" yourself talking to yourself about what you wanted to do over the weekend. The professor noticed that you were not attending to the conversation, but she did not know what was causing your lack of attention. Your lack of attention may affect your interactions with her in future conversations. What assumptions might she have made regarding your lack of attention? How do you know?

Communication may also occur in a group. In a group interaction, multiple speakers may be conveying information both verbally and nonverbally.

Think of a time when you were listening to a professor lecture about a topic in physical therapy. The professor asks several questions of the class. Some students are enthusiastically raising their hands to answer, but others appear to be dozing. What assumptions do you think the professor might make regarding the differing communications by these students? How do you know?

Communication occurs every time we interact with one another. Communication occurs whether or not words are spoken. One cannot *not* communicate.

Think of a time when you met someone but did not speak to him or her. What assumptions did you make about that person? What cues did you notice about the person to make those assumptions?

READING

Reading is a critical communication skill that enables you to evaluate professional literature and use the findings in your practice. Your reading and understanding of medical information about your patient/client are essential for developing effective physical therapy evaluations and interventions. In addition, your ability to read, understand, and use information from current literature will enhance the quality of care you provide.

WRITING

Writing is an essential communication skill for clinical care, as well as communication with other professionals and peers. Your accurate writing skills often determine whether you will be reimbursed for your services by third-party payers. Claims may be denied because of inadequate documentation. Whether you are writing a clinical evaluation for reimbursement or an article for a peer-reviewed journal, your writing skills reflect your ability to effectively communicate your findings to your readers.

LISTENING

Listening is a foundational communication skill for your success as a professional. Whether you are actively listening when interviewing a client or listening to a colleague request your input, your ability to listen actively will let the speaker know that you have understood his or her intended meaning. According to Davis, active listening requires practice and is not easy. It contains three elements: restatement, reflection, and clarification.[6] Restatement involves repeating the words of the speaker as you have heard them. Reflection involves verbalizing both the content and the implied feelings of the sender. Clarification involves summarizing or simplifying the sender's thoughts and feelings and resolving unclear verbalizations by the sender.

ELECTRONIC COMMUNICATION

Electronic communication has become a mainstay form of communication. This includes not only email and social media, but in health care as well using an Electronic Health Record for documentation. The interest and comfort in the use of electronic communication and social media vary with age. These are discussed in relation to generational expectations later in this chapter.

As a physical therapy professional, you can develop skill with all six types of communication. You can benefit from understanding the impact of verbal and nonverbal communication on yourself, your colleagues, your patients, and their families. In addition, you can enhance your skills in reading, writing, listening, and electronic communication. According to Davis, communication by practitioners may enhance or detract from their therapeutic presence in their interactions.[6] As a practitioner, you can learn the communication skills that enhance your therapeutic presence and thereby promote healing.

Visualize yourself as a student at your first clinical experience. You are meeting with your first client for the first time. What types of communication occur between you and this new client? How do you know?

PROFESSIONAL BEHAVIORS AND COMMUNICATION

The original research on professional behaviors of students as they progress through their clinical experiences was conducted by use of a Delphi study with clinical educators from the University of Wisconsin in Madison. Clinical educators were asked to identify the behaviors essential for physical therapy professionals that were not explicitly part of the profession's core of knowledge and technical skills, but were required for success in the profession. Ten essential skills were identified. Each of these behaviors can be related to the development of effective communication skills. Through mastering each of these behaviors, you demonstrate the behaviors of a physical therapy professional and thereby enhance your communication with your clients, their families, and your colleagues.[7]

This research has recently been updated to address the changing scope of the physical therapy profession in response to increased autonomy and the new graduates from the Millennial generation (born 1980-2000). The 10 **professional behaviors** (formerly known as generic abilities) have remained the same as those identified in the original research; however, the rank order has changed, and they are now referred to as *professional behaviors for the twenty-first century* (Boxes 7-2 and 7-3).[8] These behaviors have also been recommended as essential for the development of LAMP skills for practicing clinicians.[2]

BOX 7-2

Professional Behaviors

Critical thinking—The ability to question logically; identify, generate, and evaluate elements of logical argument; recognize and differentiate facts, appropriate or faulty inferences, and assumptions; and distinguish relevant from irrelevant information. The ability to appropriately utilize, analyze, and critically evaluate scientific evidence to develop a logical argument, and to identify and determine the impact of bias on the decision-making process.

Communication—The ability to communicate effectively (i.e., verbal communication, nonverbal communication, reading, writing, and listening) for varied audiences and purposes.

Problem solving—The ability to recognize and define problems, analyze data, develop and implement solutions, and evaluate outcomes.

Interpersonal skills—The ability to interact effectively with patients, families, colleagues, other health care professionals, and the community in a culturally aware manner.

Responsibility—The ability to be accountable for the outcomes of personal and professional actions and to follow through on commitments that encompass the profession within the scope of work, community, and social responsibilities.

Professionalism—The ability to exhibit appropriate professional conduct and to represent the profession effectively while promoting the growth/development of the Physical Therapy profession.

Use of constructive feedback—The ability to seek out and identify high-quality sources of feedback, reflect on and integrate the feedback, and provide meaningful feedback to others.

Effective use of time and resources—The ability to manage time and resources effectively to obtain the maximum possible benefit.

Stress management—The ability to identify sources of stress and to develop and implement effective coping behaviors; this applies for interactions for: self, patient/clients and their families, members of the health care team, and in work life scenarios.

Commitment to learning—The ability to self-direct learning to include the identification of needs and sources of learning; and to continually seek and apply new knowledge, behaviors, and skills.

Adapted from May W, Kontney L, Iglarsh A: Professional Behaviors for the 21st Century, 2009–2010. Unpublished research project.

BOX 7-3

Levels of Professional Behaviors for Students and Professionals in Communication

Beginning Level

■ Demonstrates understanding of the English language (verbal and written); uses correct grammar, accurate spelling and expressions, and legible handwriting.

■ Recognizes impact of nonverbal communication in self and others.

■ Recognizes the verbal and nonverbal characteristics that portray confidence.

■ Utilizes electronic communication appropriately.

Intermediate Level

■ Utilizes and modifies communication (verbal, nonverbal, written, and electronic) to meet the needs of different audiences.

■ Restates, reflects, and clarifies message(s).

■ Communicates collaboratively with both individuals and groups.

■ Collects necessary information from all pertinent individuals in the patient/client management process.

■ Provides effective education (verbal, nonverbal, written, and electronic).

Entry level

■ Demonstrates the ability to maintain appropriate control of the communication exchange with individuals and groups.

■ Presents persuasive and explanatory verbal, written, or electronic messages with logical organization and sequencing.

■ Maintains open and constructive communication.

■ Utilizes communication technology effectively and efficiently.

Post entry-level

■ Adapts messages to address needs, expectations, and prior knowledge of the audience to maximize learning.

■ Effectively delivers messages capable of influencing patients, the community, and society.

■ Provides education locally, regionally, and/or nationally.

■ Mediates conflict.

Adapted from May W, Kontney L, Iglarsh A: Professional Behaviors for the 21st Century, 2009–2010. Unpublished research project.

BUILDING AFFECTIVE COMMUNI-CATION SKILLS

Three domains of learning have been described. The cognitive domain involves knowledge, application, analysis, synthesis, and evaluation and deals with didactic learning.[9] The psychomotor domain involves perception, guided response, complex overt response, and adaptation, and deals with "hands-on" skills.[10] Skills in the **affective domain** are considered among the most difficult to teach because this domain deals with attitudes, values, and character development, which influence all the other professional skills.[11] This also applies to communication skills. Communication falls within the affective domain.

The mastery of affective behaviors develops over time. May and colleagues described **beginning, developing, entry-level,** and **post entry-level professional behaviors** related to the generic abilities in their initial research.[7] In the updated research, the 10 behaviors still have specific behaviors associated with performance at each level of development; however, the descriptors for the levels have changed to beginning, intermediate, entry-level, and post entry-level behaviors. The current levels start with the beginning level, in which behaviors are consistent with those of a learner in the beginning of the professional phase of physical therapy education and before the first significant clinical experience. This is followed by the intermediate level, in which behaviors are consistent with those of a learner after the first significant clinical experience. The third level is entry level, in which the behaviors are consistent with those of a learner who has completed all didactic work and is able to independently manage a caseload with consultation as needed from clinical instructors (CIs), coworkers, and other health care professionals. The fourth level is post entry level, in which the behaviors are consistent with those of an autonomous practitioner beyond entry level (see Box 7-3).[8]

Because many beginning PTs and PTAs are young adults, they are learning attitudes, behaviors, values, and character attributes that lay the foundation for their professional development.[12] According to Davis, when students fail to acquire the behaviors on their own, faculty members should assist them in developing these behaviors.[6] When students face challenges in the affective domain, faculty may assist them in learning professional behaviors through **self-assessment** using the professional behaviors and guided discovery during advisory sessions with a faculty member.[13]

Faculty can also assist students in developing their affective communication skills by teaching them how to recognize and use rapport in their interactions. When building rapport, the professional must be aware of both verbal and nonverbal components of communication (Table 7-1).[14] These are further described later.

In verbal communication, you can recognize a variety of communication patterns by listening to the speaker.[14] The language patterns of the speaker may help you to identify his or her learning style. For example, a speaker may say "that

7

Table 7-1
Verbal and Nonverbal Components of Communication

Verbal Components	Nonverbal Components
Language	Gesture
Pacing	Posture
Tonality	Haptics
Intent	Proxemics
Speed of communication	Oculesics

sounds good" when hearing about the prescribed exercise program. This suggests an auditory learning pattern. Auditory learners may prefer to learn the exercises by hearing you describe how to perform them. The pace of the speaker might include long or short pauses between words or thoughts. The tonality of the speaker might be high pitched and nervous or low pitched and calm. The intent of the speaker might be to request help or demand service. The speed of the communication might be fast, slow, or variable. Through paying attention to these patterns, you can build rapport by matching the client's verbal pace, tonality, intent, and speed.

In nonverbal communication you can recognize the gestures, postures, haptics, proxemics, and oculesics of the speaker.[14] **Haptics** involve the use of touch as part of a communication pattern. For some people, touching during speaking is an important cue. Others might consider touching to be rude. **Proxemics** is the distance between the speaker and the listener. Appropriate distance between speaker and listener varies depending on the cultural background of the speaker. **Oculesics** is the use of eye contact or gaze aversion. In some groups direct eye contact is a sign of respect for the speaker, whereas in other groups gaze aversion signals respect. As a professional you must learn the nonverbal cues that specifically apply to the patients you serve.

Rapport is an important characteristic of communication. **Rapport** is defined as an interaction marked by mutual collaboration and respect, but not necessarily indicating agreement.[5] When people are in rapport, they have behavioral patterns that become similar in nature.

The first of the three primary types of rapport is **cultural rapport**, which is established by using the form of dress or greeting appropriate to the setting. For example, you might wear a lab coat in an acute care clinical setting, but a polo shirt and khaki pants in an outpatient orthopaedic clinical setting. You might use a traditional greeting style appropriate for the culture of your patient, such as touching the patient's cheek or shaking hands with the patient (Figure 7-1).

Remember a clinical situation in which you thought your clothing was appropriate for the particular clinical setting. How did you know?

The second type of rapport is **verbal rapport**. This is established when you use the same or similar descriptive phrases and conversation content as the person with whom you are speaking. For example, you might work with a client who asks to "see you do the exercises" before performing them. You might respond by "showing" the patient/client how to do the exercise and using verbal language patterns related to visual descriptors, such as "How does this look to you?"

Remember a situation in which you were talking with a patient/client and the conversation seemed to flow very easily. What type of language patterns was the patient/client using? What type of language patterns were you using?

The third type of rapport is **behavioral**. This is established when you **mirror** the posture and body movements of the person with whom you are speaking. You may also match the person's voice tonality and tempo. For example, you might be working with a toddler in an early intervention program for your pediatric clinical rotation. You could squat or kneel at the eye level

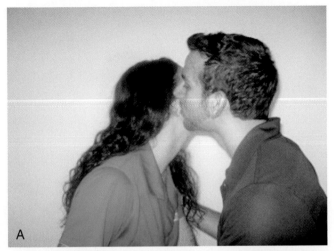

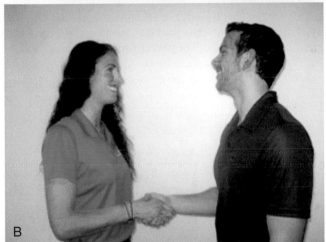

Figure 7-1 ■ Cultural rapport. **A,** Both participants use a common Latin American greeting of touching each other on the cheek. The participants are "in sync" and building rapport with each other. **B,** Both participants use a common North American greeting of shaking hands. The participants are "in sync" and building rapport.

of the toddler to build behavioral rapport. Another example might be matching the posture while the person is sitting in a chair (Figure 7-2). To break rapport, you can mismatch the posture of the listener by not mirroring it (Figure 7-3).

Remember a situation in which you talked to a patient/client in a wheelchair. Did you change your posture so that you were at the level of the patient/client's eyes? Did changing your posture affect your communication with that patient/client?

Through matching the cultural, verbal, and behavioral patterns of another person, the professional can build rapport in the interaction. Rapport is closely related

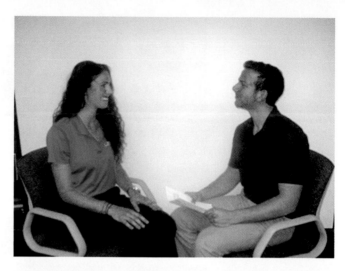

Figure 7-2 ■ Building behavioral rapport. The speaker seated on the left matches the body posture and eye contact of the listener seated on the right. The participants are "in sync" and building rapport with each other.

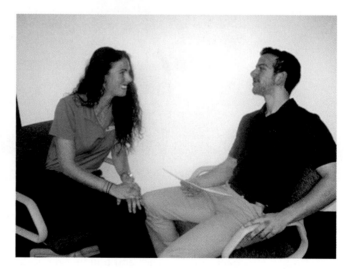

Figure 7-3 ■ Breaking behavioral rapport. The speaker on the left leans forward while the listener on the right leans back and pulls away. The speaker is breaking rapport with the listener. They are "out of sync," and rapport is being broken.

to the communication process. Studies have shown that people who assume like postures are judged to have a higher rapport with each other than those who do not have similar postures. Through enhancing rapport, the clinician builds a collaborative relationship characterized by mutual respect and harmony. When you coordinate your nonverbal behavior with that of others, you indicate to them that

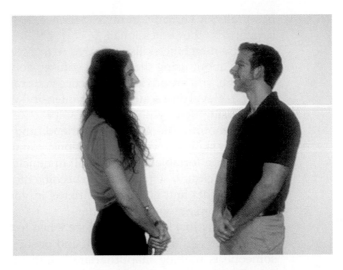

Figure 7-4 ■ Building behavioral rapport. The speaker standing on the left matches the posture, eye contact, and facial expression of the listener standing on the right. They are "in sync" and building rapport.

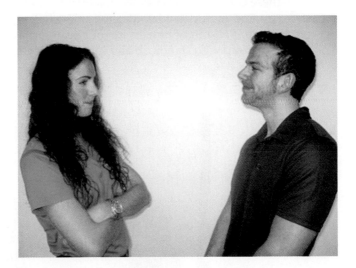

Figure 7-5 ■ Breaking behavioral rapport. The speaker standing on the left breaks rapport by crossing her arms while speaking when the listener on the right is standing with his hands clasped in front. They are "out of sync," and rapport is being broken.

you are listening to them and want to hear more. Interpersonal interactions with positive emotions and attention enhance the total experience of rapport. Good rapport is often described as harmonious or "in tune," (Figure 7-4) whereas poor rapport is described as awkward or "out of sync" (Figure 7-5).[15]

When students first learn about rapport and matching, they sometimes express concern that the person will notice that they are being matched posturally or verbally. In my experience, individuals are rarely aware of being matched by the professional.

To use matching skills, you need to feel comfortable with yourself. If you are anxious about using these skills, your anxiety may be conveyed to the listener. Therefore, you are advised to practice your rapport skills in low-stress situations (at the 1-3 level on a scale of 1-10 in intensity) with classmates, family, and friends before using them with clients. Also practice your matching skills during low-stress communications with your friends and family. Once you feel comfortable with your skills in low-stress situations, you may practice at higher levels. When you feel comfortable using the skill in nonclinical situations, you can apply the skill in the clinical setting. As you become more skilled at recognizing and interpreting verbal and nonverbal patterns in yourself and others, these skills will become more automatic for you.

Students must learn to recognize when to break rapport in a challenging situation. You can mismatch verbal and postural patterns to break rapport when someone is making inappropriate comments or sexual overtures. If you are seated, you might stand and assertively state that the comments of the patient/client are not acceptable in the clinical environment and that you cannot continue treatment unless the inappropriate comments cease. As you learn to use these communication skills effectively, you will demonstrate your professionalism and maturity when dealing with challenging situations. For example, in a group, you might remain in your seat and avoid eye contact with someone in the group who stands up and makes inappropriate comments during a meeting (Figure 7-6).

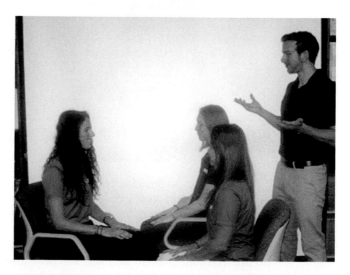

Figure 7-6 ■ Rapport with a group. The speaker seated on the left is matching the posture of the participants seated on the right and mismatching the posture of the participant standing on the right. The speaker is "in sync" with those seated and "out of sync" with the participant who is standing.

**COMMUNI-
CATING
EFFECTIVELY
IN A MULTI-
CULTURAL
HEALTH CARE
ENVIRONMENT**

As a PT or PTA in the twenty-first century, you will be working with patients/clients and families from a wide variety of ethnicities, generations, religious beliefs, sexual orientations, and socioeconomic backgrounds. Their at-risk status and physical or mental capabilities will differ. Effective communication skills can assist you in working optimally with patients/clients from a diversity of cultures, beliefs, and sociocultural groups.

According to Pellegrino, the definition of a professional is a person who puts the good of those he or she serves ahead of self-interest.[16] As a professional PT, you assume responsibility for modifying your behavior to meet the needs of your client. Students may find this challenging if they have not lived or worked in settings where there is diversity. To put the good of those served ahead of your own self-interest, you can learn to acknowledge and appreciate the beliefs, attitudes, and behaviors of clients from a variety of backgrounds. You can learn the skills to become culturally competent in your knowledge, attitudes, and behaviors when working with clients and colleagues whose culture is different from your own.

Cultural competence is defined as having the set of behaviors, attitudes, and policies that come together in a health care system, agency, or individual practitioner in order for that system, agency, or practitioner to function effectively in cross-cultural interactions.[17] In the affective domain this includes awareness of the impact of sociocultural factors, acceptance of responsibility for understanding the cultural dimensions of health and illness, willingness to make clinical settings more accessible to patients of all cultures, appreciation of the heterogeneity that exists within and across cultural groups, recognition of one's own personal biases and reactions, and appreciation of how one's personal cultural values, assumptions, and beliefs affect clinical care.[18] PTs and PTs are expected to provide culturally competent care as described in one of the Guiding Principles to Achieve the Vision (companion document to the Vision Statement for the Physical Therapy Profession), Consumer-centricity: "The physical therapy profession embraces cultural competence as a necessary skill to ensure best practice in providing physical therapist services by responding to individual and cultural considerations, needs, and values."[42]

Levels of sensitivity to cultural behaviors have been described as a **cultural continuum**.[19] The cultural continuum is a theoretical model that describes six stages of culturally related behaviors, including (cultural) destructiveness, incapacity, blindness, precompetence, competence, and proficiency (Table 7-2). Students may find themselves at different levels of the cultural continuum as they develop their professional skills.

I have an interesting anecdote regarding the stage of cultural blindness. When I taught the cultural continuum to a group of health care professionals several years ago, one of the participants made an important observation about the term "cultural blindness." As a person who was blind himself, he suggested that the term be changed from *cultural blindness* to *cultural neutral*. He pointed out that our use of language itself may indicate our bias or stereotype toward a group of people.

There are indications that the health care community is becoming more sensitive to cultural competence. According to Leavitt, "In my opinion, which is based on my 30 years of experience in this area, many physical therapists—and health care institutions—today are progressing from cultural blindness (neutral) to cultural precompetence."[20] Health care institutions have begun to

Table 7-2 Stages of the Cultural Continuum	
Stage	Description
Cultural destructiveness	People are treated in a dehumanizing manner and denied services on purpose.
Cultural incapacity	Health care system is unable to work with patients from other cultures effectively, and patients are treated with biases, paternalism, and stereotypes.
Cultural blindness (neutral)	Health care system is based on a presumption that all people are the same and that biases do not exist. Services are ethnocentric and encourage assimilation.
Cultural precompetence	Health care system is using appropriate response to cultural differences, weaknesses are acknowledged, and alternatives are sought.
Cultural competence	Cultural differences are accepted and respected. There is continuous expansion of cultural knowledge, and resources and services are continuously adapted. There is constant vigilance regarding the dynamics of cultural differences.
Cultural proficiency	Cultural differences are highly regarded. The need for research on cultural differences is acknowledged, and new approaches are developed to promote culturally competent practice.

From Leavitt RL: *Cross-cultural rehabilitation: an international perspective*, London, 1994, Saunders.

recognize the roles that racism and health care disparities play in access to appropriate health care. Indeed, the Office of Minority Health has updated the national standards for the provision of culturally and linguistically appropriate services (CLAS) in health and health care and developed a blueprint for advancing and sustaining CLAS policy and practice.[21] These standards are designed to encourage health care organizations and employees to provide more culturally competent services, recognizing the needs of culturally and linguistically different individuals and their families.

Reflect on the six stages of cultural competence. Where would you place yourself on the cultural continuum? What skills do you need to learn to enhance your cultural competence? What resources are available to assist you?

COMMUNICATING WITH PEOPLE FROM CULTURES DIFFERENT FROM YOUR OWN

Anthropologists and linguists have long recognized the critical role that culture plays in developing our relationships with those whose culture is different from our own. Anthropologist and linguist Michael Agar stated that "communication in today's world requires culture. Problems in communication are rooted in who you are in encounters with a different mentality, different meanings, a different tie between language and consciousness. Solving the problems inspired by such encounters inspires culture."[22] As PTs and PTAs, we work with individuals from a diversity of cultures in the broadest sense of culture. This includes individuals with differences in ethnicity, gender, disability, socioeconomic status, sexual orientation, religion, philosophy, and health care expectations. Each of these differences requires us to develop our cultural competence in order to enhance our effectiveness in working with these patients/clients and colleagues.

The first step in enhancing cross-cultural communication is recognizing your own cultural beliefs, attitudes, and behaviors as well as the beliefs, attitudes, and behaviors of your profession. You can reflect on your family history and cultural ties and how these affect your life and assumptions about others. For example, your culture may place a high value on direct eye contact or on gaze aversion during verbal interactions with authority figures. You can reflect on the culture of your profession and how this culture influences your behavior as a professional. For example, the biomedical Western culture places high value on direct and linear verbal communication. The second step is educating yourself and appreciating the differences in the cultural community in which you work.

A theoretical tool that can help you appreciate cultural differences is the concept of high- and low-context cultural assumptions and understanding how these assumptions may influence the beliefs, attitudes, and behaviors of you and your clients.[23] Context in communication refers to what gives "meaning" during a communication. In appreciating contextual assumptions, the clinician learns to appreciate the different cues that create meaning in the culture of the patient/client. For example, in certain cultures, direct eye contact conveys respect between the speaker and the listener. In other cultures, gaze aversion by the listener conveys respect for the speaker. These cues vary in different cultural groups. The culturally competent practitioner learns to recognize these verbal and nonverbal cues and how to respond appropriately.

HIGH-CONTEXT ASSUMPTIONS

High-context or collectivistic assumptions assume that the group is more important than the individual. The communication style is indirect, and spiral and circular logic is used. Meaning is assumed based on implicit cues, such as where the communication occurs rather than what is said. Nuances in the communication such as posture, eye gaze, and gestures are considered important. The communication is influenced by what the listener already knows rather than what the speaker is saying.

Is your communication style high context? How do you know? Think about people you know who use high-context assumptions in their communication with you. How do those assumptions affect your communications with them?

LOW-CONTEXT ASSUMPTIONS

Low-context or individualistic assumptions assume that the individual is more important than the group. The communication style is direct, linear, and logical. The meaning is based on explicit cues—that is, "what is said is what is meant." Communication is less dependent on contextual cues or nuances. It is influenced by what the speaker is saying rather than what the listener already knows.

Is your communication style low context? How do you know? Think about people you know who use low-context assumptions in their communication with you. How do those assumptions affect your communications with them?

7

CULTURE OF MEDICINE

High- and low-context assumptions in communication impact the **culture of medicine**. Biomedical Western medicine operates primarily from low-context assumptions in communication. Kleinman, a medical anthropologist and physician, stated that it is the professional's responsibility to understand the family's explanatory model (their beliefs, based on their culture) of the cause, onset of symptoms, pathophysiology, course of sickness, and treatment for the problem being addressed.[24] He stated that the explanatory model of the family may differ from that of the medical caregivers, which can lead to miscommunication and hamper health care.

If the patient/client being served also operates from low-context assumptions, the chance of miscommunication is reduced. If the patient/client operates from high-context assumptions, however, miscommunication is more likely. The story of Lia Lee in Anne Fadiman's ethnographic book *The Spirit Catches You and You Fall Down* dramatically portrays the life-threatening problems that may result when cross-cultural miscommunication occurs.[25] Lia Lee was a toddler from the Hmong culture in Cambodia who emigrated to California with her parents and older siblings. She was treated for a severe seizure disorder at Merced County Hospital in California. Her physicians prescribed medication to manage her seizures, but her family was not comfortable with administering the drugs to their daughter for a variety of reasons related to Hmong cultural norms.

In the explanatory model of the physicians, the seizures were caused by abnormal electrical discharges in her brain that could be reasonably managed by antiseizure medications. However, in the explanatory model of the family, the seizures were caused when Lia experienced soul loss—a spiritual explanation in the Hmong culture. Because the family viewed the problem from a spiritual perspective, they called on a spiritual healer or shaman to perform healings for Lia in their home. Although the family still administered the antiseizure medications, they had difficulty doing this according to the expectations of the Western medical doctors. For the Lee family, the concept of telling time by the clock was unfamiliar. They were used to telling time by the activity of the day—waking in the morning, working during the day, and eating when hungry rather than using a clock to determine their activities. The biomedical assumptions about a regular schedule for the administration of medicine based on clock time were unfamiliar to the family.

Beyond this individual example, the entire Hmong community operated from high-context assumptions. Decisions were made by the extended family and the Hmong community and not just the nuclear family. The medical community operated from low-context assumptions and neither recognized the nuances in communication nor the importance of the extended family and the Hmong community in decision making. Unfortunately, there was little understanding of the explanatory models on either side. Without the acknowledgment and appreciation of these critical differences, Lia's care was compromised. At one point, she was removed from her home by the State of California and placed in foster care. For the Lee family this was a terrible blow, because children are deeply adored in the Hmong culture. Because of the high context or collectivistic orientation of the Hmong culture, removal of a child from her home was a tragedy for the whole community. Her mother became depressed, and other family members experienced emotional distress. Although Lia was eventually reunited with her family, her seizures became worse, and severe cognitive and motor deficits developed.

In subsequent interviews by Fadiman with the medical providers, the staff said that they had done everything they could to help Lia and her family. In retrospect, however, they recognized that they had not understood the cultural issues that resulted in continued miscommunications. Since the publication of Fadiman's book in 1997, several educational institutions for medical professionals have made the book required reading to educate students about the critical impact of effective cross-cultural communication in health care.[26]

If you work in a community in which your colleagues and staff come from cultures different than your own, your colleagues can serve as cultural informants for you. They can inform you about the beliefs, attitudes, and behaviors expected by the patients/clients of their cultures.

Through educating yourself and appreciating cultural differences, you can learn to recognize differing explanatory models and differing contextual styles. By recognizing these differences, you may prevent miscommunication that might hamper your delivery of care.

Can you think of a time in which you have experienced a cross-cultural miscommunication? How did you know? Did you resolve it effectively?

When working with individuals from a culture different from your own, you should avoid stereotyping based on ethnic and cultural expectations. Differences among members of the same ethnic or cultural group may be as great as those among individuals of different ethnic and cultural groups. For example, a client who moves to the United States from Honduras may be similar to or different from another person who arrives from Honduras at the same time. Although they share a nationality, they may differ significantly in such sociocultural variables as religion, socioeconomic status, and sexual orientation. Each individual has a unique cultural experience. As a health care provider, you can use your verbal and nonverbal communication skills to determine how the individual perceives himself or herself and adapt your evaluation and intervention accordingly.

COMMUNICATING WITH PEOPLE WHO HAVE SPIRITUAL OR RELIGIOUS TRADITIONS THAT ARE DIFFERENT FROM YOUR OWN

As mentioned in the case of Lia Lee earlier, her family believed that her seizures were related to "soul loss," which is a spiritual interpretation of her seizures.[25] Because the family valued this spiritual interpretation, they used a shaman to assist them in addressing Lia's soul loss. This spiritual approach was not familiar to the medical doctors at Merced Hospital. Perhaps if the medical doctors had understood the significance of the shaman's spiritual intervention for the family, they might have developed a more trusting relationship with the Lee family. In response, the family may have been more willing to combine the biomedical Western approach with the spiritual approach. This may have facilitated a more favorable outcome for Lia and her family.

Our patients and clients continue to become increasingly diverse. In order to provide patient-centered care, we must also be aware of our own religious, spiritual, atheistic, or agnostic background and that of our patients, because these beliefs can affect patient outcomes. PTs and PTAs can self-assess their own spiritual perspective using the OPEN assessment tool. PTAs can use a psychosocial screening tool such as the HOPE assessment to determine a patient's spiritual background.[27] Through these tools, the PT gains insight into the belief systems of patients related to their healing. In addition, PTs and PTAs can learn more about the religious, spiritual, atheistic, or agnostic background of different groups by exploring the available training resources related to spirituality and health.[27,28]

A patient's positive attitude can enhance positive health outcomes. The evidence from more than 850 research studies indicates that there is a connection between faith and better physical and mental health.[27] It appears that spiritual and religious beliefs are foundational in maintaining a patient's sense of hope. As PTs and PTAs, we must know our own comfort level with these spiritual, religious, atheistic, or agnostic issues and recognize that the more we know, the better we can assist ourselves and our patients.

COMMUNICATING WITH PEOPLE WHO SPEAK LITTLE OR NO ENGLISH

Another communication issue that commonly presents problems in health care delivery is language. Whenever possible, you should use a trained medical interpreter to communicate with clients whose language is different from yours.[29] Although younger children in the family may be able to translate, it is preferable not to have them translate, because the topics being discussed may contain sensitive health information inappropriate for children.[21] When you do use a medical interpreter to translate, however, you can build rapport with the client by matching the posture and eye contact of the client rather than that of the interpreter. In this way, you are building rapport at the nonverbal level with the client even if you are unable to speak his or her language.

Be sure to work with the family decision maker. In some cultures, the decision maker may be a family elder or member of the extended family rather than the client.

Be open to working collaboratively with culturally accepted caregivers such as the shaman in the Hmong community. You can build rapport with the patient/client and the family by recognizing and appreciating their cultural norms for healing. By integrating their practices with yours (as long as they are not dangerous to the client), you acknowledge the cultural beliefs of the patient/client and family. As a result, they may be more willing to follow your recommendations.

When working with a medical interpreter, you may notice that the response given by the interpreter is shorter or longer than the statements translated for you. This may be a result of differences in high- and low-context communication styles. If the family uses circular and spiral communication, the medical interpreter may modify the circular communication and provide you with a more linear and logical interpretation, or vice versa for the family.

You may decide to ask the medical interpreter to provide you with the literal translation if you feel that you are not getting the meaning you expect from the interpretation. By watching the body language of the family, you may notice when the information being translated does not reflect the meaning intended by the family and you may ask for a more literal translation.

Remember that language does not equal culture. You may be conversant in a language different from your own, but you may not be aware of cultural norms in different ethnic groups in which the same language is spoken. There may be different cultural interpretations of the same word that would require knowledge of the culture to understand. For example, in British English, the noun "boot" means the trunk of a car. In American English, the noun "boot" means a type of footwear. Because of differences like these, it is optimal to work with a trained medical interpreter who is multicultural as well as multilingual.

When teaching at the Children's Hospital in Montevideo, Uruguay, several years ago, I had an experience that taught me that language does not equal culture. I was demonstrating a facilitation technique with an infant in front of several hundred staff members in the hospital auditorium. Because I studied Spanish in Miami, I used terminology that is common in Caribbean Spanish. My teachers had warned me that there are certain words in Caribbean Spanish that are not acceptable in South American Spanish. When I asked the child to "take the toy" in Caribbean Spanish, the auditorium went totally silent. One could hear a pin drop in the room. I knew that I must have used one of those words. The translator immediately ran onstage and corrected me. What I had said in Caribbean Spanish was considered extremely rude in South American Spanish. Since that time, I check with my local hosts and attempt to avoid similar mistakes!

COMMUNICATING WITH PEOPLE WHO COME FROM GENERATIONS DIFFERENT FROM YOUR OWN

PTs and PTAs interact with individuals in a diversity of generations from pediatrics to geriatrics. To communicate effectively across generations, you will find it helpful to understand and appreciate the differing traits of each generation.

In the United States today, the four primary generations receiving health care are the Traditionalists, Baby Boomers, Generation Xers (GenXers), and Millennials. Each generation has characteristics that influence its behaviors and communication styles (Table 7-3).[30]

Traditionalists may be dealing with a wide variety of health disorders, including hearing and visual impairments, hypertension, and heart disease. They may have other chronic diseases that may impair their physical, cognitive, or sensory abilities. They may be taking a variety of medications.[30]

Think of someone you know who could be described as a Traditionalist. Does he or she demonstrate the characteristics described in the previous paragraph? How are they similar to or different from your own?

Baby Boomers are "sandwiched" between their adolescent children and their elderly parents and may be experiencing stress from caregiving as well as coping with age-related disorders themselves.

Table 7-3
Characteristics of Generations in the United States

Generation	Size	Birth Years	Traits	Rewards	Preferred Feedback
Traditionalists	75 million	Before 1946	Patriotic, loyal, fiscally conservative, faith in institutions	Satisfaction of a job well done	No news is good news
Baby Boomers	80 million	1946-1964	Competitive, question authority, desire to put their own stamp on things, "sandwiched" (see text)	Money, title, recognition	Once a year whether you need it or not
Generation Xers	46 million	1965-1981	Eclectic, resourceful, self-reliant, distrustful of institutions, highly adaptive, skeptical	Freedom is the ultimate reward	"So, how am I doing?"
Millennials	76 million	1982-2000	Globally concerned, integrated, cyber literate, media savvy, realistic, environmentally conscious	Work that has meaning for me	From a virtual coach with the push of a button

Modified from Lancaster L, Stillman D: *Bridging generation gaps in today's workplace.* Presented at APTA Combined Sections Meeting, Tampa, FL, 2003.

Think of someone you know who could be described as a Baby Boomer. Does he or she demonstrate the characteristics described in the previous paragraph? How are they similar to or different from your own?

Generation Xers enjoy being up-to-date with the latest and greatest technology. They value new learning as a reward.

Think of someone you know who could be described as a Generation Xer. Does he or she demonstrate the characteristics described in the previous paragraph? How are they similar to or different from your own?

Millennials multitask, doing things simultaneously, and they prefer regular feedback.

Think of someone you know who could be described as a Millennial. Does he or she demonstrate the characteristics described in the previous paragraph? How are they similar to or different from your own?

As a physical therapy provider, you may be working with individuals from each of these generations. Remember that there are exceptions within each of these categories. Treat each person individually regardless of his or her category. You can recognize the characteristics related to rewards and feedback for each person. You can use that information to enhance your communication when working with individuals from different generations.

COMMUNICATING WITH PEOPLE WHO HAVE VISUAL IMPAIRMENTS

According to the 2012 National Health Interview Survey, 20.6 million American adults who are 18 or older reported having vision loss.[31] Vision loss refers to people who reported having trouble seeing even when wearing glasses or contact lenses as well as those who reported being blind or unable to see at all. These impairments can range from mild to severe and may include cataracts, glaucoma, or macular degeneration. As a physical therapy provider, you may have patients/clients with visual impairments.[32] When speaking or listening to someone who is visually impaired, you can introduce yourself and others by name when you enter the room. When speaking, you can use everyday words, including "see" and "look." You can ask the person if he or she would like assistance if you need to move from one place to another.

If you are writing a home program, the type should be in a large font with high contrast between the foreground and the background. If the program is handwritten, print or block lettering but not script should be used. Text using both uppercase and lowercase letters is easier to read. Check into printing the program in Braille. You can learn about computer technology for the blind and assist your client in accessing the information. Refer your client to services for individuals with visual impairment in your community.

COMMUNICATING WITH PEOPLE WHO HAVE AUDITORY IMPAIRMENTS

According to a 2011 study by Lin et al, about one-fifth of the U.S. population 12 years and older have hearing loss severe enough to make communication difficult.[33] These may range from mild loss of sensitivity to total hearing loss. The largest group experiencing hearing loss consists of individuals over the age of 65.[32] When listening to or speaking with someone who is deaf or hard of hearing, ask what you can do to improve your communication with him or her. You may change your position so that you face the person directly or look directly at the person to provide a clear view of your lips. A light touch on the shoulder will get the person's attention when you want to communicate. Articulate clearly and use natural tones. Shouting may reduce the effectiveness of a hearing aid. If possible, avoid areas that have distracting sounds in the background. Be sure to confirm that the person understood what you said by having the person repeat what was understood in his or her own words.

For written communication, write clearly and simply using everyday words. If the individual has both visual and auditory impairments, use a large font with high contrast between foreground and background. If you recommend instructional videos, make sure they have subtitles.

If you are working with a hearing-impaired patient/client, you can help him or her to access the text-telephone device (TTY) system for telephone communications. When using interpreters, have a certified deaf interpreter to deliver important information and make sure the client feels comfortable with the interpreter.

COMMUNICATING WITH PATIENTS/CLIENTS, CAREGIVERS, AND FAMILIES

Remember to create a positive environment for the patient/client and caregivers or family. You can use your verbal and behavioral rapport skills to enhance the communication process. Be sure to introduce yourself and address the patient/client by name. Ask the patient/client how he or she prefers to be addressed. Limit your teaching objectives, and teach only manageable amounts at a time. Ask the patient/client for his or her goals, and link those with your goals.

Make your communication clear and simple. Use lay terminology rather than medical jargon. Watch the patient's/client's body language for signs of understanding or lack of understanding. If you notice confusion, ask what is unclear and then explain it in a different way.

Use a variety of ways to get your message across. Some patients/clients prefer written programs, others prefer demonstration, and still others prefer to watch a DVD. Offer information regarding community agencies and support groups that may assist the patient/client after the physical therapy visit.

Verify that your message was understood by having the patient/client repeat back to you what the person understood in his or her own words. Have the patient/client demonstrate the activities you have taught so that you can offer constructive feedback for improving his or her exercise form or skills.[32] By incorporating communication skills in your patient/client interactions, you will enhance the quality of the physical therapy services you provide.

COMMUNICATING WITH OTHER MEMBERS OF THE HEALTH CARE TEAM

As a PT or a PTA, you will be interacting with a wide variety of health care providers and will serve as a member of the health care team. You can learn about other disciplines as part of your preservice education, by observing other disciplines at work, or by studying about disciplines other than your own.

PTs not only work closely with PTAs, but also collaborate with occupational therapists, speech-language pathologists, nutritionists, psychologists, nurses, physicians, social workers, audiologists, respiratory therapists, and other professionals. Through collaboration with other disciplines, you learn from other team members about additional information and resources that may enhance the outcome for your client. For example, you may have a client who has been reluctant to participate in physical therapy. Through collaboration with the psychologist, you may learn about psychological barriers that could impede the patient/client from participating in physical therapy. The psychologist may suggest strategies you can use to address those barriers with your client.

Team meetings require good communication skills. Interdisciplinary team meetings are often conducted in hospital and rehabilitation settings. You may be called on to report your findings related to a patient's/client's movement dysfunction. Your verbal and behavioral rapport skills may assist you in promoting communication among all team members. Curtis identified eight behaviors that may assist you in developing effective interdisciplinary collaboration (Box 7-4).[34] When team members follow these guidelines, the patient outcomes may be enhanced as a result of the successful collaboration of the team members.

COMMUNICATING THROUGH DELEGATION

As a PT, you will supervise and interact with a wide variety of individuals. They may include PTAs, physical therapy aides, transport staff, and administrative staff.

As a professional, you must know the legal boundaries regarding supervision and delegation in your state. Once you are familiar with the physical therapy practice act in your state, you will be able to delegate accordingly. Because members of the support staff provide service under your supervision and license, your communication skills are critical to the success of your delegation and

BOX 7-4

Behaviors to Assist in Interdisciplinary Collaboration

- Making an effort to involve all team members in communication at meetings and in written communications.
- Recognizing the perspective of other team members.
- Acknowledging the contribution of others.
- Scheduling meetings at reasonable times for all members.
- Acknowledging your own biases or stereotypes when working with other team members.
- Breaking down role conflicts.
- Knowing your professional identity.
- Focusing on the outcome.

From Curtis K: *Physical therapy professional foundations*, Thorofare, NJ, 2002, Slack.

supervision. You can use your verbal and behavioral rapport skills to enhance the effectiveness of your communication with your support staff.

COMMUNI-CATING AS A STUDENT IN THE CLASSROOM AND CLINICAL EXPERIENCES

Development of your professional communication skills begins in the physical therapy classroom. Faculty members model professional behaviors for students in the classroom by demonstrating professional behaviors. They demonstrate commitment to learning by continually seeking new knowledge and understanding through review of current literature and attendance at continuing education courses. Interpersonal skills are modeled when they communicate respectfully with students and colleagues in and out of the classroom. Communication skills are modeled when faculty members demonstrate appropriate listening skills while answering questions posed by students and colleagues. Faculty demonstrates appropriate reading and writing skills in their syllabi, course assignments, and research resources. They model appropriate and respectful verbal and nonverbal communication when speaking with students and colleagues. Effective use of time and resources is demonstrated by planning, implementation, and evaluation of their course content. Faculty demonstrates the use of constructive feedback by acknowledging student queries regarding exams and assignments in a timely and respectful manner. Problem-solving skills are demonstrated when a variety of possible solutions related to course content are considered and course content is updated based on current research. Faculty shows professionalism by dressing appropriately for both classroom and lab sessions. They participate in APTA and often serve as elected officers in their chosen specialty areas. They model responsibility by being punctual, following through on commitments to students and colleagues, and assuming leadership roles in the profession. They model critical thinking by critiquing hypotheses and ideas and challenging students to think critically in the classroom. Effective stress management is demonstrated when preventive approaches to stress management are used, such as establishing a support network for self and students. By observing these professional behaviors in faculty members, students have an opportunity to recognize the importance of the behaviors and reflect on their own behaviors as compared with those of their faculty role models.

7

For students, the classroom provides an opportunity to practice their professional skills in a safe environment with constructive feedback from both faculty and peers. Through self-assessing your professional behaviors using the professional behaviors in your classes and receiving constructive feedback from the faculty and peers, you develop your professional skills from the outset of the curriculum. You may receive grades for your professional behaviors as part of your class participation, your timely completion of assignments, and your affective behaviors during practical examinations.[12]

As a student PT or a student PTA in the clinical setting, you have an opportunity to apply the professional behaviors learned in the classroom setting in the clinical environment. The student PT is required to practice under the direct supervision of a licensed PT who serves as a CI. PTAs may serve as CIs for student PTAs. If you experience challenges with your professional behaviors in the clinical setting, faculty can assist you in modifying these challenging behaviors by having you self-assess using the professional behaviors taught in the classroom setting. A faculty advisor may help you to change your challenging behaviors based on your self-assessment and the assessment of your CI. In this way, you learn to self-correct and develop your professional behaviors with the guidance of your CI and your faculty advisor.[13]

ELECTRONIC COMMUNICATION ACROSS GENERATIONS

Today's GenX and Millennial students are comfortable with electronic communication, which includes e-mail, texting, social networking, and blogging. These students have been described as "digital natives," whereas Traditionalists and Baby Boomers are considered "digital immigrants."[35] The use of digital media can be perceived as both a blessing and a curse in education and health care. It can be a blessing when information needs to be transmitted quickly and efficiently. It can be a curse when the message is misinterpreted and feelings are hurt.

Educators who are neither GenXers nor Millennials may experience challenges when working with students who use digital media but who may not recognize the problems that can occur with its use. Students may feel frustrated when the faculty does not respond to their requests as quickly as they are used to with their peers. Educators have little guidance about preventing misuse of electronic media and ensuring standards for professional conduct. For example, e-mail and texting are two-dimensional communication.[36] According to Mehrabian, 60-90% of communication is nonverbal,[37] so e-mail and texting are missing more than half of the information being transmitted! Because the sender does not see the receiver, the communication can be misinterpreted and conflict can arise. A student may send an e-mail to a faculty member about an emotionally charged issue that the student would be reluctant to discuss if the meeting were face to face. Faculty who are Traditionalists and Baby Boomers may feel uncomfortable with the informal tone of e-mail communication from students. Because the receiver cannot observe the facial expression, tonality, pacing, gesture, or pitch of the e-mail or text, miscommunication can occur.

It is critical that educational institutions develop policies and procedures regarding the proper and professional use of digital communication. It is also critical that educators address unprofessional digital behavior as soon as it occurs. One medical school advises students to "think before you post."[38] Legal challenges have arisen because of e-mails that were forwarded inadvertently to the wrong person and jeopardized someone's professional reputation.

The APTA has developed standards of conduct for the use of social media by physical therapists, physical therapist assistants, and students. It is critical that these individuals be knowledgeable about policies on social media as established by employers, educational institutions, or clinical training sites.[39]

Social media includes tools and platforms that are used to produce, publish, and share online content and interact with others. These include blogs, podcasts, videos, microblogs, wikis, and more. In 2009, 79% of American adults used the Internet and 46% of online American adults used a social networking site including Facebook, MySpace, or LinkedIn. These social media sites can produce both serious professional and legal concerns when they overlap. Currently, the problem has increased, because different generations perceive personal information differently. Welk, a PT and attorney, recommends that clinicians, "ask yourself if what you are putting on your social media site is professional and whether it exemplifies the professional image you want to have out there."[39] Each clinician must determine the professional image she or he wants to project using e-mails, texts, photos, and videos. Since electronic communication occurs online, it can impact patient safety and privacy as well as the clinician's professional image. Anything that is posted electronically is considered public and permanent. Each clinician must remember to keep federal regulations regarding protecting patient information in mind at all times (see description of the Health Insurance Portability and Accountability Act [HIPAA] in Chapter 5). In an article titled, Professionalism and Social Media, Bemis-Dougherty recommended Seven Steps to Safer Social Networking (Box 7-5).[40]

Think of a time when you sent an e-mail or text that was clear to you but was misinterpreted by the receiver. What was the outcome? How did you resolve the situation?

BOX 7-5

Seven Steps to Social Networking

- Avoid becoming online "friends" with patients/clients.
- Avoid including information gained from online social networking regarding your patient as part of the patient/client management process.
- Avoid including information gained from online social networking regarding students' performance in clinical education.
- Use caution when posting and disclosing personal information on social networking sites.
- Check the social networking site's privacy settings, and control who can access your online profile.
- Avoid "venting" on blogs or social networks.
- Have a strategy regarding social networking and commit to it.

From Professionalism and Social Networking. www.apta.org/PTinMotion/2010/6/Feature/ ProfessionalismandSocialNetworking. Accessed September 29, 2014. Reprinted from http:// www.apta.org, with permission of the American Physical Therapy Association, Copyright © 2015 American Physical Therapy Association.

Finally, recent research indicates that multitasking decreases one's efficiency.[41] Contrary to what popular media tell us, researchers have found that the mental balancing necessary to multitask robs areas of our brains that are needed for memory and learning. It appears that electronic communication has begun to alter our attention span. Our brains are rewiring for speed instead of mindfulness.[41] Because health care requires us to be mindful in patient care, we must assess how electronic communication affects us and our patients and be diligent in ensuring that it is used for the highest good of all concerned.

SUMMARY

PTs and PTAs use a variety of communication behaviors that may enhance their effectiveness in the clinical and educational settings. Several research studies indicate that communication is one of the most important skills used by physical therapy professionals.[2,3] Communication skills include the ability to listen, read, write, and use electronic communication effectively. They also include effective verbal and nonverbal skills in interactions with clients, families, colleagues, supervisors, and support staff. Cultural, verbal, and behavioral rapport skills can be learned and implemented in the classroom and the clinic to enhance communication effectiveness. Strategies are discussed for communicating effectively with diverse groups, including:

- Individuals who come from cultures different from your own.
- Individuals who speak little or no English.
- Individuals who come from a generation different from your own.
- Individuals who have visual impairments.
- Individuals who have hearing impairments.
- Patients/clients and caregivers.
- Health care team members.
- Support staff.
- Faculty and clinical supervisors.
- Those who use electronic communication.

Students first learn these professional communication behaviors in their physical therapy classes and apply the behaviors with their faculty and peers. By practicing these behaviors during classroom experiences, students are better prepared to develop them as they proceed from beginning skills as students to post-entry-level skills as they become physical therapy providers.

CASE STUDIES

CASE STUDY ONE

You are a PT student working in an early intervention program in Miami, Florida. You have been assigned to evaluate a 2-year-old boy with Down syndrome whose family recently immigrated to Miami from Nicaragua. The family is very concerned because their son is not yet walking. You do not speak Spanish, and you are expected to complete the evaluation with the child and the family.

What professional behaviors will you use to enhance your communication with this family?

CASE STUDY ONE ANSWERS

1. Request a bicultural and bilingual medical interpreter for the examination and evaluation.
2. Use your behavioral rapport skills with the family when the interpreter is translating.
3. Speak with cultural informants in your clinical setting who are knowledgeable about Nicaraguan culture.
4. Seek written or Web resources to learn more about Nicaraguan culture.
5. Request a medical interpreter to translate for you.[29]
6. Contact your CI for assistance if the family has difficulty in understanding your examination, evaluation, or intervention suggestions.

CASE STUDY TWO

You are a PT or PTA student completing your clinical experience at an inpatient rehabilitation hospital. Your CI has given you feedback at your midterm evaluation that your nonverbal communication indicates that you are disinterested and aloof when working with patients. You are upset because you were not aware that you were conveying disinterest or aloofness toward patients. Your CI stated that she observed you standing about 10 feet away from her patients with your arms folded across your chest when she was treating them. She stated that other staff members had noticed similar nonverbal patterns when you observed their patient treatments.

What professional behaviors will you use to enhance your communication in this situation?

CASE STUDY TWO ANSWERS

1. Meet with your CI and ask for specific constructive feedback related to your nonverbal behaviors. Explain that you had not realized how your nonverbal behavior had been perceived.
2. Take responsibility for the behavior and indicate your willingness to modify your behavior appropriately.
3. Contact the academic coordinator of clinical education (ACCE) at your institution and request her assistance in remediation for your nonverbal skills.
4. Complete a self-assessment of your communication and interpersonal skills using the professional behaviors.
5. Meet with your CI and the ACCE to compare your self-assessment with the assessment of your nonverbal communication by the CI.
6. Develop a plan for modifying your nonverbal behavior with the assistance of the CI and the ACCE.
7. Modify your behavior by implementing your verbal and behavioral rapport skills.
8. Meet with your CI and ACCE to evaluate your new behavior after a week.

REFERENCES

1. Vision 2020, American Physical Therapy Association. http://www.apta.org/Vision2020/. Accessed November 20, 2014.
2. Lopopolo R, Schafer S: Re-conceptualizing the role of leadership, administration, management, and professionalism (LAMP) in physical therapy practice, *Health Policy Resour* 4(2):1–4, 2004.

3. Lopopolo RB, Schafer DS, Nosse LJ: Leadership, administration, management, and professionalism (LAMP) in physical therapy: a Delphi study, *Phys Ther* 84:137–150, 2004.
4. Merriam Webster Online. www.merriam-webster.com/dictionaery/communication. Accessed November 25, 2014.
5. Konefal J: *Neurolinguistic psychology practitioner manual,* Miami, 2002, University of Miami.
6. Davis CM: *Patient practitioner interaction: an experiential manual for developing the art of health care,* ed 3, Thorofare, NJ, 1998, Slack.
7. May WW, Morgan BJ, Lemke JC, et al.: Model for ability-based assessment in physical therapy education, *J Phys Ther Educ* 9(1):3–6, 1995.
8. May W, Kontney L, Iglarsh A: Professional behaviors for the 21st century, 2009-2010. Unpublished research project.
9. Bloom BJ: *Taxonomy of educational objectives: the classification of educational goals: handbook I: cognitive domain,* New York, 1956, David McKay.
10. Simpson EJ: *The classification of education objectives in the psychomotor domain,* Washington, DC, 1972, Gryphon House.
11. Krathwohl DR, Bloom BS, Masa BB: The need for classification of affective objectives. In Bloom BJ, editor: *Taxonomy of educational objectives, handbook II: affective domain,* New York, 1964, David McKay.
12. Masin HL: Education in the affective domain: a method/model for teaching professional behaviors in the classroom and during advisory sessions, *J Phys Ther Educ* 16(1):37–45, 2002.
13. Masin HL: Integrating the use of the generic abilities, clinical performance instrument, and neurolinguistic psychology processes for clinical education intervention, *Phys Ther Case Rep* 3 (6):258–266, 2000.
14. O'Connor J, Seymour J: *Introducing neurolinguistic programming,* London, 2011, Conari Press.
15. Bernieri B, Rosenthal R: Interpersonal coordination: behavior matching and interactional synchrony, *Fundamentals of nonverbal behavior,* Cambridge, England, 1991, Cambridge University Press.
16. Pellegrino ED: What is a profession? *J Allied Health* 12(3):168–176, 1983.
17. Cross T, Bazron B, Dennis K, et al.: *Toward a culturally competent system of care,* Washington, DC, 1989, CAASP Technical Assistance Center, Georgetown University Child Development Center.
18. American Physical Therapy Association (APTA): *Cross cultural and international special interest group: draft of guidelines for cultural competency in the affective domain,* Missoula, MT, 2000, APTA.
19. Leavitt RL: *Cross cultural rehabilitation: an international perspective,* London, 1994, Saunders.
20. Leavitt RL: Developing cultural competence in a multicultural world, part I, *PT Mag Phys Ther* 10 (12):36–48, 2002.
21. National Standards for Culturally and Linguistically Appropriate Services is Health and Health Care: A blueprint for advancing and sustaining CLAS Policy and Practice, April 2013, Office of Minority Health, US Dept of Health and Human Services.
22. Agar M: *Language shock—understanding the culture of conversation,* New York, 1994, Perennial.
23. Graham M, Miller D: Cross cultural interactive preference profile, *The 1995 annual: vol 1, training,* San Diego, CA, 1995, Pfeiffer.
24. Kleinman A: Concepts and a model for the comparison of medical systems as cultural systems, *Soc Sci Med* 12:85–93, 1976.
25. Fadiman A: *The spirit catches you and you fall down—a Hmong child, her American doctors, and the collision of two cultures,* New York, 1997, Farrar, Strauss, Giroux.
26. Taylor JS: Confronting culture in medicine's culture of no culture, *Acad Med* 78:555–559, 2003.
27. Coyne C: Addressing spirituality issues in patient interventions, *PT Mag Phys Ther* 13:38–44, 2005.
28. Culture, Faith Traditions, and Health. www.csh.umn.edu/modules/culture/. Accessed October 8, 2014.
29. Lattanzi JB, Masin HL, Phillips A: Translation and interpretation services for the physical therapist, *HPA Resour* 6:4, 2006.
30. Lancaster L, Stillman D: *When generations collide: who they are, why they clash, how to solve the generational puzzle at work,* New York, 2002, HarperCollins.
31. Facts and Figures on Adults with Vision Loss. www.AFB.org/info/blindness-statistics/adults/facts-and-figures/2351. Accessed September 17, 2014.

32. Osborne H: *Overcoming communication barriers in patient education,* Gaithersburg, MD, 2001, Aspen.

33. Lin FR, Niparko JK, Ferrucci L: Hearing loss prevalence in the US, *Arch Int Med* 171 (20):1851–1852, 2011.

34. Curtis K: *Physical therapy professional foundations,* Thorofare, NJ, 2002, Slack.

35. Digital nation: life on the virtual frontier. www.pbs.org/wgbh/pages/frontline/digitalnation/view. Accessed October 8, 2014.

36. Hickson GB, Pichert JW, Webb LE, et al.: A complementary approach to promoting professionalism: identifying, measuring and addressing unprofessional behaviors, *Acad Med* 82:11, 2007.

37. Mehrabian A, Ferris S: Decoding of inconsistent communications, *J Pers Soc Psychol* 6(1):109–114, 1967.

38. Farnan JM, Paro JA, Higa JT, et al.: The relationship status of digital media and professionalism: its complicated, *Acad Med* 84:11, 2007.

39. Standards of Conduct in the Use of Social Media, American Physical Therapy Association. http://www.apta.org/uploadedFiles/APTAorg/About_Us/Policies/Ethics/StandrdsConductSocialMedia.pdf#search=%22standards%20in%20conduct%20in%20the%20use%20of%20social%20media%22. Accessed November 20, 2014.

40. Professionalism and Social Networking. www.apta.org/PTinMotion/2010/6/Feature/ProfessionalismandSocialNetworking. Accessed September 29, 2014.

41. Freeman J: *The tyranny of email,* New York, 2009, Scribner, pp. 141–142.

ADDITIONAL RESOURCES

Ethnomed: *Ethnic medicine from Harborview Medical Center,* 2005. Available at, www.ethnomed.org. Accessed October 8, 2014.

Leavitt RL: *Cultural competence—a lifelong journey to cultural proficiency,* Thorofare, NJ, 2010, Slack, Inc. This is a comprehensive text for allied health professionals that provides the reader with tools to acquire the knowledge, attitudes, and skills to become a culturally proficient practitioner in our increasingly diverse world.

Spector RE: *Cultural diversity in health and illness,* ed 6, Upper Saddle River, NJ, 2004, Pearson, Prentice Hall. This is a comprehensive text for nursing professionals dealing with the complexities of working with people from diverse cultural backgrounds. It includes resources for developing knowledge, attitudes, and skills related to health and illness in the American Indian and Alaska Native population, black population, Hispanic population, and white population. It includes data resources and networks for selected health organizations.

7

Practice

8

Physical Therapy for Musculoskeletal Conditions

Hilary B. Greenberger and Barbara C. Belyea

KEY TERMS

accessory motion
active-assisted range of motion
active-free exercises
active range of motion (AROM)
active-resisted exercise
activities of daily living (ADL)
aerobic training
aquatic physical therapy
balance
bursitis
clinical practice guidelines
closed kinetic chain exercise
core strengthening
cryotherapy
dysfunction
electrical stimulation
flexibility
flexibility exercise
fluidotherapy
fracture
functional exercise
goniometer
goniometry
history
hot pack
hydrotherapy

hypermobile joint
hypomobile joint
joint mobilization
manual muscle testing (MMT)
massage
muscle endurance
muscular strength
muscular power
myofascial release
nerve entrapment
objective examination
open kinetic chain exercise
outcome measure
palpation
paraffin treatment
passive range of motion (PROM)
range of motion (ROM)
range-of-motion exercise
resistance exercise
resisted test
short-wave diathermy
soft tissue mobilization
special tests
sprain
strain
strength
subjective examination

tendinitis
tendinopathies
tendinosis
thermal agent
ultrasound
whirlpool

LEARNING OBJECTIVES

After reading this chapter, the reader will be able to:

- List common conditions seen in musculoskeletal physical therapy.
- Identify the components of an initial musculoskeletal examination.
- Define and give examples of the various tests and measures used in physical therapy for musculoskeletal conditions.
- List the general goals of a therapeutic exercise program.
- Describe the various types of therapeutic exercises.
- Describe various physical agents used to address musculoskeletal problems.

Conditions that affect the musculoskeletal system are the primary domain of physical therapists who specialize in orthopaedic physical therapy. One of the largest clinical specialties within the physical therapy profession, orthopaedic physical therapy encompasses a wide array of therapeutic techniques and philosophies of treatment. Physical therapists (PTs) and physical therapist assistants (PTAs) in the field of orthopaedics work in a variety of clinical settings and treat patients of diverse ages, focusing on the prevention and rehabilitation of musculoskeletal injuries. This chapter describes the types of patients with whom an orthopaedic PT would work and presents some commonly used examination tests and measures and interventions.

GENERAL DESCRIPTION

Although the clinical interests or approaches to patient care may be diverse, the common thread throughout physical therapy for musculoskeletal conditions is the focus on a patient's function. By examining the patient's functional abilities, the PT determines the cause and extent of any limitations and restrictions in desired activities, and works with the patient/client to return the individual to his or her preinjury level of function in the shortest time possible.[1] A person's function can be affected when a disruption occurs in the musculoskeletal system.

This disruption may be the result of traumatic or repeated stress to tissue, structural imbalances of muscle or bone, congenital conditions, surgery, or degenerative changes in the body. **Dysfunctions** of the musculoskeletal system often result in symptoms of pain, stiffness, edema (swelling), muscle weakness or fatigue, or loss of **range of motion** (**ROM**; movement at a joint).

To conduct a comprehensive examination, establish an accurate diagnosis, and develop an appropriate plan of care, therapists must have an extensive understanding of anatomy, biomechanics, pathokinesiology, and exercise physiology. They must also be knowledgeable in the application of a variety of interventions and be able to make clinical decisions using the best available evidence in order to implement a plan of care that is appropriate for each individual patient situation. Effective communication skills are also critical for PTs and PTAs so they can establish good rapport with patients and provide the necessary education to gain the patient's adherence to the plan of care.

DEVELOPMENT

Several factors contribute to the continued growth of musculoskeletal physical therapy. New contributions to the scientific literature provide therapists with evidence supporting diagnostic tests, prognostic factors, and various interventions that allow for evidence-based clinical decision making. In response to the overwhelming amount of physical therapy research, the American Physical Therapy Association (APTA) recently developed PTNow,[2] a website designed to help clinicians access the latest literature. This includes orthopaedic **clinical practice guidelines**, which allow therapists to have rapid access to synthesized research findings related to diagnosis, prognosis, and interventions, as well as case studies, clinical summaries, tests and measures (including videos), and searching functions. Easy access to these materials enables therapists to readily translate research findings into the clinic. The development of sophisticated technology and new intervention techniques has also provided new diagnostic and treatment options for PTs who evaluate and treat this patient population. Changes in lifestyle have also contributed to the growth of orthopaedic physical therapy. Increasing participation in physical fitness by the general population has resulted in an increase in musculoskeletal disorders caused by overuse or traumatic injuries, while the increasing prevalence of obesity has created a need for interventions and patient education regarding the impact of obesity on the musculoskeletal system. The increased use of computers and other technical equipment requiring repeated motions has also had an impact on the incidence of overuse injuries in the upper extremity. Individuals who must sustain postures at a computer or operate machinery while performing repeated motions with their hands may be at risk for the development of muscle injury or nerve entrapment requiring intervention by a PT. An increase in life span has also resulted in the growth of this area of physical therapy, as people are living longer, more active lives and experiencing symptoms related to degenerative changes in their bodies.

A great deal of similarity exists between orthopaedic physical therapy and sports physical therapy. In both areas, the focus of rehabilitation is to regain optimum function and return the patient to the previous level of activity. A sports PT must, therefore, incorporate sport-specific activities into the treatment program

8

to make sure that the patient/client can meet the physical demands of the sport with respect to strength, endurance, balance, speed, and coordination. An orthopaedic PT may work with athletes, but may also treat individuals with a variety of musculoskeletal conditions that are not related to sports activities.

COMMON CONDITIONS

Within the broad scope of musculoskeletal physical therapy, a variety of patient problems may be treated. These problems include injuries sustained through sports participation, work-related injuries, conditions resulting from orthopaedic surgical procedures, trauma, and degenerative changes that accompany the aging process. As previously stated, patients with musculoskeletal conditions may report pain, swelling, weakness, or loss of motion resulting from stress to the musculoskeletal system. This stress may include damage to bones or soft tissue such as muscles, tendons, joint capsules, ligaments, bursae, cartilage, and fascia in the extremities or spine.

OVERUSE INJURIES

Repeated stress to the musculoskeletal system can cause overuse injuries that may result in pain, inflammation, and dysfunction. The following examples are some common conditions caused by overuse.

BURSITIS

Bursitis is an inflammation of bursae, which are fluid-filled sacs located throughout the body that decrease friction between structures. Bursae become irritated and painful when they are repeatedly pinched between two structures. A common example of this mechanism of injury occurs at the shoulder; the subacromial bursa may be pinched during repeated movements when the shoulder is in an overhead position, such as when painting, reaching, or throwing.

TENDINOPATHY

Tendons are the structures that connect muscle to bone, and can become injured with repeated use or rapid overstretching of muscles. Disorders of tendons (**tendinopathies**) can be the result of inflammation (**tendinitis**) or degenerative changes caused by overuse (**tendinosis**). Tendinopathies usually result in painful movements and are frequently seen in the patellar tendon at the knee in people who perform repeated jumping (e.g., dancers, basketball players), at the elbow in people who do repeated or sustained gripping activities (e.g., carpenters, tennis players), or at the thumb with excessive smartphone use. Excessive overload of a tendon can also result in a partial or complete tear of the tendon, which is commonly seen in the ankle (Achilles rupture) or elbow (biceps rupture) and may need to be surgically repaired.

NERVE ENTRAPMENT

Pressure on a nerve, causing **nerve entrapment**, may result from a variety of sources and usually causes symptoms of tingling, pain, weakness, or any combination of these. A common condition of nerve compression at the wrist is referred to as *carpal tunnel syndrome*. Patients with carpal tunnel syndrome usually complain of numbness and pain in the hand and fingers, which commonly results from repeated activities with the wrist in a flexed position (e.g., musicians, computer keyboard operators).

TRAUMATIC INJURIES

Musculoskeletal injuries may also occur as a result of direct trauma. Bones, muscles, ligaments, and other soft tissues may be injured when they sustain a direct blow or when they are placed under excessive stretch. The following are just a few of the common conditions that can result from direct trauma to the musculoskeletal system.

LIGAMENT SPRAIN

Ligaments are supporting structures at joints that serve to stabilize the joint and prevent excess movement. When ligaments are overstretched, their fibers can tear and cause pain and instability at the joint. A common site of **sprain** is at the ankle when the lateral (outside) ligaments are overstretched. This injury occurs when a person lands on the foot with the ankle in an inverted (turned-in) position. Another common site of ligament sprain is the anterior cruciate ligament (ACL) at the knee. Injuries to this ligament are usually the result of a cutting or twisting movement of the knee when the foot is planted, commonly occurring in sports that require jumping or quick changes in direction, such as soccer or volleyball.

FRACTURE

Direct trauma to bone can result in a break, or **fracture**, of the bone. Fractures can occur in any bone in the body, but are commonly seen at the wrist or the hip after falls. Older adults are particularly prone to fractures because of changes in the structure of their bones resulting from inactivity, inadequate nutrition, and degenerative conditions. Fractures are best diagnosed through the use of radiographs.

MUSCLE STRAIN

A sudden contraction of a muscle or excessive stretch of a muscle can cause tearing of the muscle fibers, known as a **strain**. Muscle strains can occur in any area of the body and can range in severity. A strain of the rotator cuff muscles at the shoulder can result in shoulder pain and weakness when lifting the arm, and cervical strains may be the result of a sudden trauma to the neck, as with a whiplash injury.

SURGICAL CONDITIONS

Individuals who have had surgery are another group of patients commonly seen by an orthopaedic PT. Injuries resulting from repeated stress, acute trauma, or disease processes may require surgical intervention for appropriate healing. The following are examples of orthopaedic surgery in which patients can benefit from physical therapy intervention to reduce pain and regain motion and strength, which will allow optimal function.

TOTAL JOINT ARTHROPLASTY

Painful movement caused by degenerative changes at joint surfaces can be alleviated through surgical replacement of the joint surfaces. Joints most commonly replaced are weight-bearing joints, primarily the hips and knees. A variety of metal alloy, ceramic, and plastic implants are used to effectively replace degenerated joint surfaces. Physical therapy intervention is necessary postoperatively for the patient to regain maximum strength and function and to receive education regarding postoperative management to prevent complications such as dislocation.

AMPUTATION

Surgical amputation is the removal of a portion of an extremity because of trauma, inadequate blood flow, or the presence of a malignant growth. Inadequate circulation can be a result of disease processes such as diabetes mellitus or peripheral vascular disease, whereas a growth may indicate the presence of cancer. Postoperative physical therapy often includes exercises to maintain strength in the remaining portion of the limb, functional training with a prosthesis, and activities to improve overall fitness and well-being.

MEDICAL CONDITIONS

Numerous medical conditions may also affect the musculoskeletal system, resulting in pain, weakness, or loss of function. Systemic diseases such as rheumatoid arthritis, obesity, or cancer may cause impairments that disrupt the musculoskeletal system and result in functional challenges that can be addressed by the orthopaedic PT.

PRINCIPLES OF EXAMINATION

Working with a patient with a musculoskeletal condition requires the PT to have a comprehensive understanding of anatomy, pathology, biomechanics, and pathokinesiology. The first step in understanding the needs of a patient is to perform a thorough examination. Reexaminations are performed throughout the rehabilitative process to monitor patient progress toward established functional goals.

This section describes the following components of an initial examination: patient/client history, systems review, and tests and measures performed by the PT. The history is part of the **subjective examination** (verbal descriptions of the condition), whereas the remaining parts constitute the **objective examination** (quantitative measurements to determine the status of the body and condition).

PATIENT/CLIENT HISTORY

The **history** involves gathering information about the current and past health status of the patient related to why the patient/client is seeking the services of a PT.[3] The information may be obtained by interviewing the patient or the patient's family, by accessing the patient's medical record, and by consulting with other members of the patient's health care team. The history is qualitative information based on the patient's perception of the problem and is, therefore, included in the "S" portion of the SOAP note (see Chapter 2).

The role of the therapist during the interview is to guide the patient through pertinent questions about the patient's musculoskeletal condition. This interaction allows the therapist to develop a rapport with the patient and to understand the patient's insight into and opinion of the problem. The interview also assists the therapist in appropriately directing the remainder of the examination. Often, the patient interview will give the therapist ample information to make a list of possible differential diagnoses that is then further refined during the remainder of the examination. Questions asked during the interview include information about the onset of the condition, current symptoms, previous physical therapy treatments, past medical history, and lifestyle and health habits pertaining to work and recreation. Box 8-1 lists typical questions asked during the patient interview.

In addition to these questions specific to the patient's reason for seeking physical therapy, the therapist should perform a *review of systems* (ROS) in order to identify symptoms that may have been overlooked in the history and to screen for medical conditions that may require referral to other health care providers.[4] The ROS is usually performed by using checklists of common symptoms typically associated with various systems of the body (e.g., cardiovascular/pulmonary system, gastrointestinal system).

For more specific information about the location of symptoms, the patient is often asked to draw the location of the symptoms on a body chart (Figure 8-1).

BOX 8-1

Questions Typically Asked During the Patient History Component of an Initial Physical Therapy Examination

1. What brings you to physical therapy today?
2. What do you feel is your primary problem? Is it stiffness? Pain? Weakness? Instability?
3. Was the onset of the problem slow or sudden? Was the problem caused by a specific incident or mechanism of injury?
4. Have you ever had this problem before? If so, were you treated for it? How long did it take to recover?
5. What provokes your symptoms? What relieves your symptoms?
6. Are your symptoms worsening or improving?
7. Are your symptoms constant or intermittent?
8. Can you describe your pain? Does your pain spread to other parts of your body?
9. What is your occupation?
10. What activities are you unable to do because of your symptoms?
11. Have you had any radiographs ("X-rays") taken or diagnostic tests performed?
12. Are you currently taking any medication for this problem?
13. How is your general health?
14. Is there anything else you would like to tell me that I have not asked and that would be pertinent to your problem?

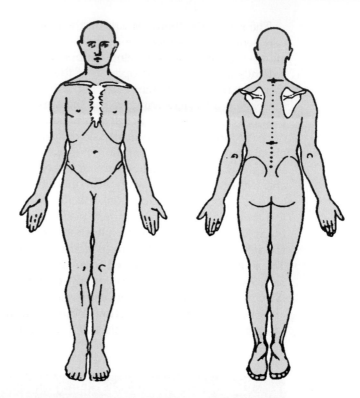

Figure 8-1 ■ Body chart to indicate areas of pain. The patient is asked to indicate areas of pain with Xs, areas of numbness with slashes, and areas of tingling with plus signs.

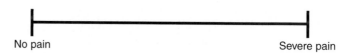

No pain   Severe pain

Figure 8-2 ■ Visual analog scale. On the line provided, the patient is asked to mark the degree of pain experienced.

Pain scales may also be used to gauge the amount of pain the patient is experiencing (Figure 8-2). On completion of the history taking, the therapist should have gained information regarding the description and location of symptoms, nature of the disorder (acute vs. chronic condition), behavior of the symptoms (what activities make the symptoms either better or worse), health risk factors that may be present, and limitations in activities the patient may be experiencing.

SYSTEMS REVIEW

The objective portion of the examination refers to quantitative or qualitative measurements that are taken by the PT. This portion of the examination begins with a systems review and is included in the "O" section of the SOAP note (see Chapter 2). The systems review includes a brief examination of the other systems of the body related to physical therapy (e.g., cardiovascular/pulmonary, neuromuscular, and integumentary) and information about the patient's cognition, communication, and preferred learning style.[3] The information gathered during the systems review assists the therapist in developing an appropriate, individualized plan of care and may further identify health problems that may require consultation with or referral to another health care provider. In a patient with a musculoskeletal condition, common systems reviews may include monitoring of heart rate, blood pressure, height and weight, assessment of skin integrity, and a gross assessment of joint ROM, strength, and coordinated movements.

TESTS AND MEASURES

During the tests and measures portion of the examination, specific numbers or grades may be assigned (quantitative measurement), as is the case with ROM or strength measurements. At other times, parts of the examination are performed by observing and describing patterns of movement, deformities, or both (qualitative measurement). The purpose of the tests and measures is to establish baseline values and observations that assist in establishing a diagnosis and can be used for comparison after a single treatment or a series of treatments. The PT can then make appropriate changes in the plan of care based on the amount of progress or lack of progress found with repeated tests and measures.

This section briefly describes some of the tests and measures performed in an orthopaedic physical therapy setting. The purpose is to familiarize introductory level students with common terms used when working with a patient who has a musculoskeletal problem.

OBSERVATION
Observation is the "looking" phase of the examination. It may begin in the waiting room, where the therapist can observe the patient's general attitude, posture, and willingness to move. A perfunctory gait assessment may be made as the patient enters the examination area. Once the patient is appropriately undressed, a more detailed inspection can be made, including observation of obvious deformities such as an abnormal curvature of the spine, joint subluxations (a condition in which a joint partially dislocates), asymmetric body contours, swelling, and color and texture of the skin. Many musculoskeletal injuries are a result of or are exacerbated by poor sitting and standing postures. Therefore, particular attention is paid to the standing and sitting postures of the patient.

ACTIVE RANGE OF MOTION
Active range of motion (AROM) refers to the ability of the patient to voluntarily move a limb through an arc of movement. AROM provides the therapist with information regarding the quality of the movement (smooth vs. rigid movement), the willingness of the patient to move the limb, any pain produced during movement, and whether the patient has any limitations in the motion as compared with the unaffected side. An example of AROM of the shoulder in multiple planes is provided in Figure 8-3.

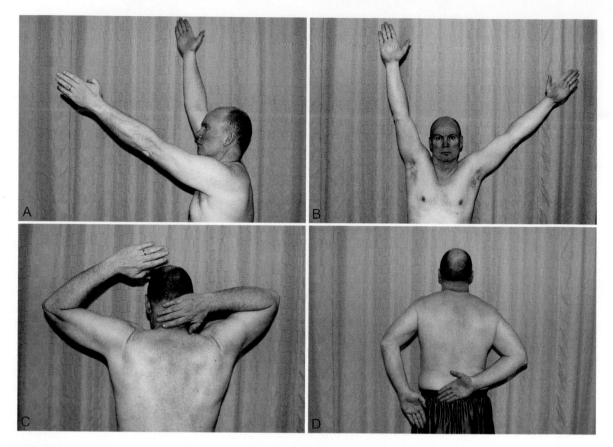

Figure 8-3 ■ Examination of active range of motion at the shoulder; note the decreased range of motion in the left shoulder. **A,** Shoulder flexion. **B,** Shoulder abduction. **C,** Shoulder external rotation. **D,** Shoulder internal rotation. (Courtesy Mark Hine.)

PASSIVE RANGE OF MOTION

Passive range of motion (PROM) refers to the amount of movement at a joint that is obtained by the therapist moving the segment without assistance from the patient. In some instances, because of injury or prolonged immobilization, a joint may have less motion than is considered functional. A joint in this condition is referred to as a **hypomobile joint**. In other cases, such as a joint subluxation, the joint may have excessive motion and is referred to as a **hypermobile joint**. PROM also gives the therapist an indication of the degree and pattern of pain, as well as the "feel" of the movement.

Many methods may be used to measure and document AROM and PROM. The most common measurement technique, **goniometry**, is performed with a **goniometer** and measures joint angles. Examples of goniometers are shown in Figure 8-4. The amount of motion available at any joint depends on the structure of the joint. In addition, normal values for joint ROM depend on several factors,

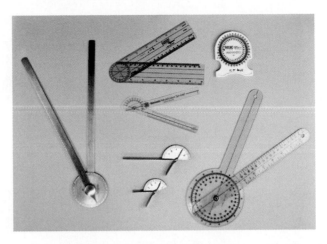

Figure 8-4 ■ Variety of goniometers to measure joint angles. The size and type vary to measure long and short limb segments and the cervical region. (Courtesy Mark Hine.)

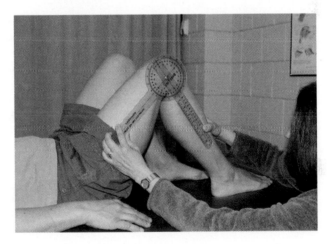

Figure 8-5 ■ Physical therapist conducting a goniometric measurement of knee flexion. (Courtesy Mark Hine.)

including the patient's age and gender. Typically, the therapist compares ROM values of the affected joint with those on the unaffected side. Figure 8-5 shows a PT measuring PROM of a patient's knee flexion.

STRENGTH

Strength can be defined as the amount of force produced during a voluntary muscular contraction. This contraction may be performed statically (no motion) or dynamically (through an assessment of ROM). When one is assessing the status of the muscles and tendons, a quick **resisted test** is used. This test allows the therapist to determine the general strength of a muscle group and assess whether the muscle contraction produces pain. If the resisted test shows that a muscle or

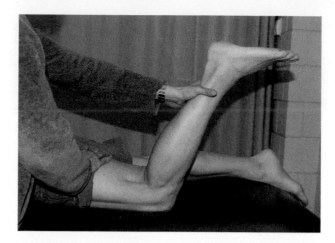

Figure 8-6 ■ Physical therapists commonly perform manual muscle tests to determine muscle strength. Pictured is the manual muscle test for the hamstring musculature. (Courtesy Mark Hine.)

muscle group is weak or painful, further testing may be performed to isolate the specific muscle. To isolate and test specific muscles, **manual muscle testing (MMT)** is performed (Figure 8-6). MMT allows the therapist to assign a specific grade to a muscle. This grade is based on whether the patient can hold the limb against gravity and how much manual resistance can be tolerated. Several systems of grading are widely used. One of the most common grading systems was initially described by Robert Lovett, MD, and later modified by Henry Kendall, PT, and Florence Kendall, PT.[5] This key to muscle grading is outlined in Table 8-1.

With the development of sophisticated technical equipment, many other methods are now available to measure strength, including handheld dynamometers and computerized instruments such as isokinetic devices. These devices allow the therapist to obtain strength curves of isolated muscles, as well as specific force values.

FLEXIBILITY

Flexibility refers to the ability to move a limb segment through a specific ROM. The amount of flexibility at a given joint depends on two factors. First, the soft tissue surrounding the joint must be pliable to allow movement between the joint surfaces. This feature is referred to as *accessory motion* of the joint. **Accessory motion** is the ability of the joint surfaces to glide, roll, and spin on each other. Second, muscles crossing the joint must be able to lengthen an appropriate extent to allow adequate motion to occur. For example, the ability to bend over and touch the toes while keeping the knees straight depends on the flexibility of the back and posterior hip muscles, as well as the ability of the spinal vertebrae to move.

Appropriate flexibility or balance of muscles is a key component of proper posture and body mechanics. Many musculoskeletal problems seen by clinicians

Table 8-1
Key to Manual Muscle Testing Grades

	Function of the Muscle	Grade	Symbols	Symbols
No movement	No contraction felt or seen in the muscle	Zero	0	0
	Tendon becomes prominent or feeble; visible movement of the part	Trace	T	1
Supported in horizontal plane	Moves through partial range of motion	Poor−	P−	2−
	Moves through complete range of motion	Poor	P	2
	Holds against slight pressure in test position Moves through partial range of motion against gravity	Poor+	P+	2+
	Gradual release from test position	Fair−	F−	3−
	Holds test position (no added pressure)	Fair	F	3
	Hold test position against slight pressure	Fair+	F+	3+
Tests in the antigravity position	Holds test position against slight to moderate pressure	Good−	G−	4−
	Holds test position against moderate pressure	Good	G	4
	Holds test position against moderate to strong pressure	Good+	G+	4+
	Holds test position against strong pressure	Normal	N	5

Modified from Kendall FP, McCreary EK, Provance PG, et al: *Muscles: testing and function,* ed 5, Baltimore, 2005, Lippincott Williams and Wilkins.

can be linked to muscle imbalances that have caused movement dysfunctions.[6] For example, if the muscles surrounding the shoulder do not act synergistically (because of lack of flexibility), compensation might occur at joints distal and proximal to the shoulder, such as the elbow and cervical spine.

A PT may perform a number of tests to determine flexibility. One common test for the lower extremity is the 90/90 straight leg raise (Figure 8-7). This test objectively measures flexibility of the hamstring muscles, located on the posterior aspect of the thigh.

FUNCTIONAL TESTS

The ultimate goal of therapy is to return the patient to the previous level of activity, which may include anything from the ability to go grocery shopping independently to returning to athletic competition. With some types of injuries, a return to the previous level of activity is not feasible. In these cases, the ultimate goal would be to return the individual to the highest level of function achievable.

8

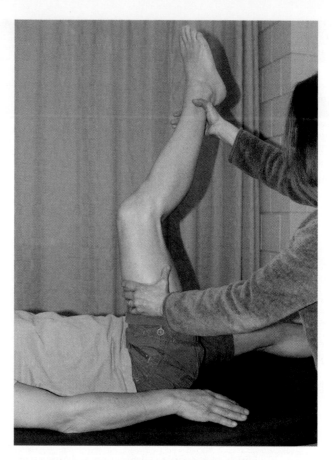

Figure 8-7 ■ Example of a test for flexibility: the 90/90 straight leg raise. (Courtesy Mark Hine.)

Traditionally, functional assessment has referred to such activities as the patient's bed mobility, transfers between a variety of surfaces (e.g., moving from a sitting position in a wheelchair to a standing position), and ability to perform **activities of daily living (ADLs)**, such as hair combing, dressing, and bathing. PTs may spend a large percentage of their time during the initial examination assessing the patient's ability to perform these ADLs. Box 8-2 lists examples of ADLs.

Individuals who wish to return to activities other than ADLs require more aggressive types of functional testing. Examples of these types of functional tests are hop tests, jump tests, lunge tests, excursion tests, and balance tests. Gary Gray and others have described these and other types of functional tests in detail.[7,8]

OUTCOME MEASURES

Outcome measures are standardized instruments that measure an individual's actual or perceived activity limitations and participation restrictions, and/or an individual's quality of life or health status. These instruments are typically closed-ended questions completed by the patient and scored by the PT. Scores

BOX 8-2	*Examples of Activities of Daily Living*

Eating
- Eat with spoon.
- Eat with fork.
- Cut with knife.
- Open milk carton.
- Pour liquid.
- Drink from cup.

Dressing and Undressing
- Reach clothes in closet.
- Put on shoes.
- Manage zippers.
- Remove coat.

Bathing and Grooming
- Turn on faucet.
- Wash hands.
- Dry with towel.
- Manage cosmetics.
- Brush teeth.

Bed and Bathroom
- Get out of bed.
- Transfer to toilet.
- Reach objects on nightstand.
- Sit up in bed.

Transfer and Ambulatory Activities
- In and out of bus.
- In and out of car.
- Safe outdoor ambulation.
- Endurance.

Other Activities
- Propel wheelchair forward.
- Propel wheelchair backward.
- Manage elevator.
- Hold book.
- Dial a telephone.
- Use scissors.

8

can then be used to assess the initial degree of limitation as well as changes in ability or health status before and after treatment. Examples of common outcome measures include the Oswestry Low Back Disability Questionnaire, the Medical Outcomes Study 36-Item Short Form (SF-36), the Patient-Specific Functional Scale (PSFS; Box 8-3), and the Lower Extremity Functional Scale (Table 8-2).

BOX 8-3

Patient-Specific Functional Scale (PSFS)

The patient is asked to list up to five activities that he or she is having difficulty in performing because of his or her injury or condition. The patient is then asked to rate these activities on a scale of 0-10, where 0 indicates the patient is unable to perform the activity and 10 indicates he or she is able to perform the activity at the same level as before the injury or condition. Scores are based on either the sum of the scores or the average of the ratings.

Table 8-2
Lower Extremity Function Scale

We are interested in knowing whether you are having any difficulty at all with the activities listed below *because of your lower limb problem*. (Circle one number on each line.)

Activities	Extreme Difficulty or Unable to Perform Activity	Quite a Bit of Difficulty	Moderate Difficulty	A Little Bit of Difficulty	No Difficulty
Any of your usual work, housework, or school activities	0	1	2	3	4
Your usual hobbies, recreational or sporting activities	0	1	2	3	4
Getting into or out of the bath	0	1	2	3	4
Walking between rooms	0	1	2	3	4
Putting on your shoes or socks	0	1	2	3	4
Squatting	0	1	2	3	4
Lifting an object, such as a bag of groceries from the floor	0	1	2	3	4
Performing light activities around your home	0	1	2	3	4

Continued

Table 8-2
Lower Extremity Function Scale—cont'd

Activities	Extreme Difficulty or Unable to Perform Activity	Quite a Bit of Difficulty	Moderate Difficulty	A Little Bit of Difficulty	No Difficulty
Performing heavy activities around your home	0	1	2	3	4
Getting into or out of a car	0	1	2	3	4
Walking two blocks	0	1	2	3	4
Walking a mile	0	1	2	3	4
Going up or down one flight of stairs	0	1	2	3	4
Standing for 1 hour	0	1	2	3	4
Running on even ground	0	1	2	3	4
Running on uneven ground	0	1	2	3	4
Making sharp turns while running fast	0	1	2	3	4
Hopping	0	1	2	3	4
Rolling over in bed	0	1	2	3	4
Column totals:					
Score: ____/80					

Modified from Stratford PW, Binkley JM, Watson J, Heath-Jones T: Validation of the LEFS on patients with total joint arthroplasty. Physiother Can. 52:97, 2000.

SPECIAL TESTS
Special tests are used to examine specific joints to indicate the presence or absence of a particular problem. The purpose of these tests is to confirm or reinforce a physical therapy diagnosis. Because so many special tests are available for each joint, only those that appear to be indicated based on the results of tests and measures are performed. Examples of special tests are those that examine nerve compression (Phalen's test; Figure 8-8, *A*), shoulder impingement (Hawkins test; Figure 8-8, *B*), and ligamentous knee injuries (Lachman test; Figure 8-8, *C*).

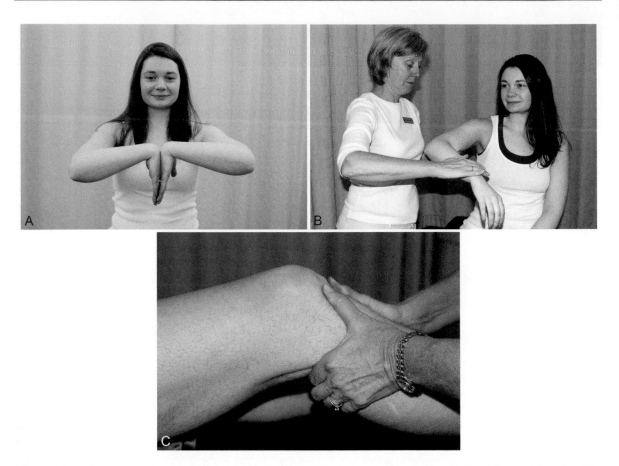

Figure 8-8 ■ Examples of special tests. **A**, Phalen's test for nerve compression. **B**, Hawkins test for shoulder impingement. **C**, Lachman test for anterior cruciate ligament instability. (Photos courtesy Mark Hine.)

PALPATION

A comprehensive understanding of anatomy is essential for any PT. In the clinical situation the therapist uses the sense of touch, known as **palpation**, to assess what is occurring below the skin and what musculoskeletal structures are involved in an injury. When palpating an area of the body, the therapist is feeling for areas of pain and tenderness, areas of restriction, swelling, and proper orientation of structures.

OTHER DIAGNOSTIC PROCEDURES

Depending on the patient's clinical presentation, other examination procedures may need to be performed to provide a more complete assessment of the patient. If the patient has had neurologic damage, full sensory testing may be indicated. Additional tests for patients with cardiovascular/pulmonary conditions may include an assessment of lung capacity. Some of these tests are presented in more detail in Chapters 9 and 10.

Diagnostic ultrasound (also referred to as diagnostic musculoskeletal ultrasound or MSK US) is a relatively new tool that can be used to provide additional information about the status of a patient's musculoskeletal tissues.[9] MSK US utilizes sound waves that reflect off of tissue interfaces to produce an image, which can be useful in identifying abnormalities in musculoskeletal structures. The patient may need to be referred to other medical personnel for additional diagnostic imaging techniques, such as plain film radiographs (X-rays), computed tomography (CT) scans, and magnetic resonance imaging (MRI). Current practice emphasizes the importance of a PT incorporating the results of medical imaging into the clinical decision-making process.

PRINCIPLES OF EVALUATION, DIAGNOSIS, AND PROGNOSIS

Based on evaluation of the findings from the comprehensive examination, the PT identifies the patient's impairments, activity limitations, and participation restrictions and then determines the diagnosis and prognosis. Once the problems have been identified, the therapist and patient develop goals to address each problem. Common short-term goals are to decrease pain and edema and increase strength and motion. The ultimate long-term goal for patients with musculoskeletal dysfunctions is to achieve an optimal level of function, whether that means returning to work, resuming athletics, or performing daily activities independently. Therapeutic goals should include how each goal is to be measured and the expected time frame to achieve each goal. Once goals have been established, the therapist develops a plan of care designed to achieve these outcomes.

The plan of care is based on determining which interventions will most effectively improve a patient's function. The process begins by identifying the relevant evidence in the literature, combined with the therapist's clinical expertise and preferences of the patient. Numerous intervention options and rehabilitation approaches are available to the orthopaedic PT. Some therapists focus their treatment approaches on exercises, whereas others incorporate manual techniques or physical agents. Often a combination of techniques is appropriate when designing a comprehensive plan to address the needs of a patient with a musculoskeletal dysfunction. When selecting a plan of care, the therapist must consider the goals of the patient and the desired outcome of therapy.

PRINCIPLES OF INTERVENTION

The following discussion of intervention options introduces the reader to the typical indications and uses of various techniques. The techniques described include patient/client instruction, biophysical agents, manual techniques (including soft tissue and joint mobilization), therapeutic exercise, and home exercise programs. These are presented in the order in which they appear in the Guide to Physical Therapist Practice 3.0.[3] The reading list at the end of the chapter gives sources for in-depth information regarding the application of these and other interventions used in musculoskeletal physical therapy.

PATIENT/CLIENT INSTRUCTION

As mentioned earlier in the chapter, communication is a critical component of the orthopaedic physical therapy experience. The therapist's depth of knowledge and effectiveness in performing and interpreting the examination and the variety of treatment options available are of little value if the therapist cannot share this information effectively with patients and encourage their active participation in the rehabilitation process. The patient and therapist must work as a team and focus on common goals and sharing of information to achieve optimal results.

The PT and PTA are responsible for educating the patient about his or her diagnosis and about exercises to perform at home, postures or positions to avoid during daily activities at work or home, and strategies to prevent the dysfunction from recurring (Figure 8-9). To communicate effectively, the therapist must create a treatment atmosphere that takes into account the patient's values and goals and must also provide the necessary information in a clear, easily understood manner.

It is important for the PT and PTA, when working with a patient, to treat the whole person rather than just the injured area. Each patient comes to physical therapy with a different set of values, different expectations, and a different cultural background. All these factors must be considered if the patient is to be successfully and effectively treated as an individual.

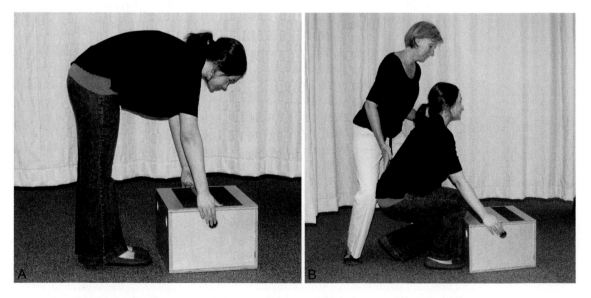

Figure 8-9 ■ Patient education is essential to rectify improper habits regarding body movement and posture. **A,** Improper lifting can result in straining of lower back muscles and ligaments. **B,** Instruction in proper lifting techniques can prevent injuries to the back. (Courtesy Mark Hine.)

BIOPHYSICAL AGENTS

Many biophysical agents are available for PTs to incorporate into the plan of care when treating patients with musculoskeletal problems. Biophysical agents may be classified by the tissue's response to treatment (e.g., thermal changes caused by heating or cooling agents) or classified based on the type of energy used by the agent (e.g., ultrasound, electrotherapy). Biophysical agents can be used to address a variety of impairments; their therapeutic benefits include pain management, increased flexibility, improved ROM, increased muscle strength, and wound healing. The decision to include biophysical agents as a direct intervention is based on a thorough examination of the patient's symptoms, the desired outcomes of therapy, and the therapist's knowledge of the physiologic and clinical effects of each biophysical agent. Table 8-3 lists common biophysical agents used in physical therapy according to their physical effects and includes their physiologic effects and clinical indications.

Table 8-3
Summary of Common Biophysical Agents Used in Physical Therapy

Physical Effect	Biophysical Agents	Physiologic Effects	Clinical Indications
Superficial heat	Hot packs Paraffin Fluidotherapy Whirlpool	Increases blood flow Increases metabolism: promotes healing and removal of waste products Decreases pain Decreases stiffness	Pain Joint stiffness
Deep heat	Ultrasound Short-wave diathermy	Increases blood flow Increases metabolism: promotes healing and removal of waste products Decreases pain Decreases stiffness	Muscle spasm Pain Joint stiffness
Cold	Ice packs Ice massage Cold whirlpool Cold compression	Decreases blood flow Decreases metabolism Decreases edema Decreases pain	Acute injury Swelling Pain Muscle spasm After exercise
Electrical stimulation	Transcutaneous electrical nerve stimulation (TENS) Iontophoresis Electrical stimulation for wound healing Neuromuscular electrical stimulation (NMES)	Decreases pain Decreases inflammation Promotes wound healing Reeducates muscles Decreases spasticity	Pain Inflammation Wounds Nerve regeneration Muscle weakness and imbalance

8

THERMAL AGENTS

When human tissue sustains an injury, an automatic response is initiated in an attempt to heal the tissue and return it to its preinjured state. These naturally occurring processes are referred to as *inflammation* and *repair*.[10] The inflammation and repair stages of tissue healing can be altered through the use of thermal agents or electrical stimulation. **Thermal agents** are used to modify the temperature of surrounding tissue and result in a change in the amount of blood flow to the injured area. Besides vascular changes, temperature changes affect the metabolism of the surrounding tissue, in addition to altering neuromuscular and connective tissue. Through the use of therapeutic changes in temperature, the healing process can be accelerated and the injured tissue restored to optimal strength and integrity.

The extent of the therapeutic changes caused by an alteration in tissue temperature depends on the intensity of the thermal agent applied, the length of time the tissue is exposed to the agent, and characteristics of the tissue being treated. The therapist must continually monitor and reexamine the patient to ensure that the thermal agent selected is appropriate and that the treatment outcomes are being achieved.

Thermal agents can be classified as those that provide superficial heat, deep heat, or cold. Superficial heat modalities create an increase in blood flow to cutaneous tissue close to the surface of the skin and are effective in reducing pain and stiffness, increasing ROM, and promoting healing.[11] Examples of superficial heat agents include hot packs, paraffin, fluidotherapy, and whirlpools.

A **hot pack** is a pouch available in various shapes that is filled with silica gel and soaked in thermostatically controlled water (Figure 8-10). Hot packs are applied to the affected body part with layers of towels to prevent overheating (see Figure 2-3C). **Paraffin treatment** involves dipping a patient's involved

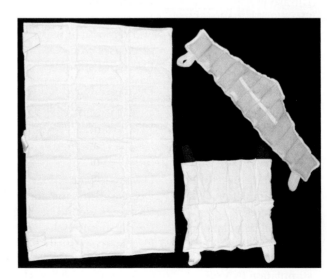

Figure 8-10 ■ Variety of hot packs to apply superficial heat to different body areas. (Courtesy Mark Hine.)

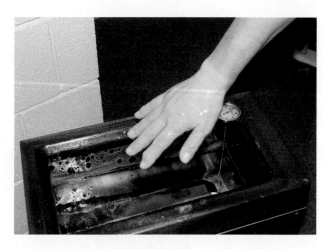

Figure 8-11 ■ Paraffin tank to apply paraffin to a hand. (Courtesy Mark Hine.)

extremity (usually hands or feet) into a mixture of melted paraffin wax and mineral oil that is maintained at a temperature of approximately 135 °F (Figure 8-11). The heat from the paraffin produces the relaxing and pain-reducing effects of other superficial heat treatments and leaves the skin feeling warm and soft, which increases comfort when ROM exercises are performed.

Fluidotherapy is the use of a self-contained unit filled with corncobs finely chopped into a sawdust-type substance. The particles are heated to the desired temperature and circulated by air pressure around the involved body part. In addition to receiving the effects of heating, the patient can exercise while the treatment is in progress.

Deep heat modalities produce physiologic effects similar to those of superficial heat agents, but at a greater tissue depth. Therefore, patients with deep muscle or joint dysfunction may receive more therapeutic benefit from the application of deep heat than from a superficial heating agent. Deep heat modalities include ultrasound and short-wave diathermy. Thermal **ultrasound** is the therapeutic application of high-frequency sound waves that penetrate tissue and increase tissue temperature to promote healing and reduce pain (Figure 8-12). Similar results are achieved with **short-wave diathermy**, which is the use of electromagnetic energy to produce deep therapeutic heating effects.

In contrast to heating agents, therapeutic cold (**cryotherapy**) may be applied to decrease tissue temperature. Temperature differences produced by the application of cold agents cause a decrease in blood flow and metabolism, which results in a decrease in swelling and pain. Cryotherapy is the physical agent of choice for patients who have acute injuries with clinical symptoms of swelling or pain or both (see Figure 2-3D). Cold may also be incorporated into a treatment protocol after exercise to help reduce postexercise soreness. Cryotherapy may take the form of commercial cold packs, ice massage, or cold used in conjunction with compression.

8

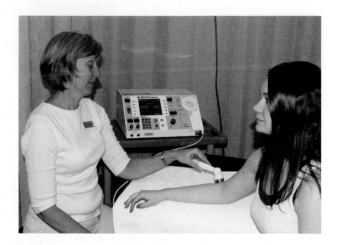

Figure 8-12 ■ Application of ultrasound to produce deep heat in the shoulder region. (Courtesy Mark Hine.)

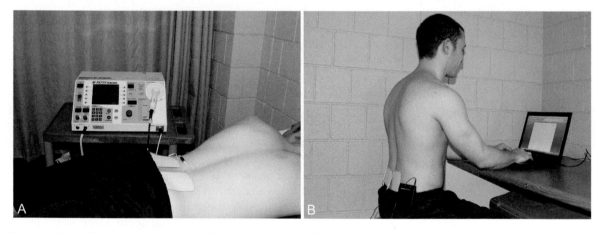

Figure 8-13 ■ Use of transcutaneous electrical nerve stimulation (TENS) for the treatment of pain in the low back region. **A**, Clinical unit. **B**, Portable unit. (Courtesy Mark Hine.)

A **whirlpool** can be used to provide superficial heat or therapeutic cold (cold whirlpool). The body part is immersed in a tank of water. Various sizes of tanks are available, ranging from a small tank for the distal ends of extremities to a full-body tank known as a *Hubbard tank*.

ELECTRICAL STIMULATION
PTs and PTAs may use **electrical stimulation** as part of their plan of care to achieve therapeutic results. With the use of electrical stimulation units, electrodes are placed on the skin at specified locations to stimulate nerves, muscles, and other soft tissues in an attempt to reduce pain and swelling, increase strength and ROM, and facilitate wound healing (Figure 8-13).[12] The therapist must have

a clear understanding of the desired effects of the electrical stimulation intervention and have knowledge of the appropriate parameters to use with regard to treatment intensity, voltage, and current type. Common electrotherapy applications are listed in Table 8-3.

OTHER BIOPHYSICAL AGENTS

Additional biophysical agents that may be used in the treatment of patients with musculoskeletal dysfunction include mechanical traction, hyperbaric oxygen, biofeedback, LASER therapy, and extracorporeal shockwave therapy (ESWT). ESWT is a noninvasive modality that uses high-pressure sonic waves that penetrate through human tissue.

These modalities achieve therapeutic benefit through mechanisms different from those of thermal or electrical agents, but they may also be used to decrease a patient's pain, promote healing, or improve strength or motion in an attempt to maximize function.

MANUAL THERAPY TECHNIQUES

PTs working with patients who have musculoskeletal dysfunction always have two tools at their ready disposal—their hands. Whether palpating a structure during an examination, providing manual force for a patient to resist against when performing strengthening exercises, or performing a mobilization to increase ROM, a therapist's hands are important therapeutic instruments. A variety of manual techniques are frequently used by orthopaedic PTs, and many of these techniques are the subject of current clinical research to validate and clarify their purpose and clinical efficacy.

For the purpose of this text, manual techniques are divided into two categories: soft tissue and joint mobilization. A discussion of specific procedures and the schools of thought behind the various techniques is beyond the scope of this text. The reading list at the end of this chapter provides further information regarding this topic.

SOFT TISSUE MOBILIZATION

Soft tissue mobilization includes a variety of "hands-on" techniques designed to improve movement and function by restoring extensibility to tight tissue. The techniques are designed to decrease pain or swelling and relax muscle or fascia tension to create proper postural alignment and optimal muscle function.

Two common forms of soft tissue mobilization are **massage** and **myofascial release**. Massage involves the systematic use of various manual strokes to produce certain physiologic, mechanical, and psychological effects. Swedish massage strokes promote relaxation by decreasing pain or swelling, relieving tension, and improving the metabolism of surrounding tissue. More vigorous massage strokes may be used before physical activity to stimulate and prepare the muscles for exertion. Another soft tissue technique, known as *transverse friction massage*, is useful for promoting proper healing and improving the flexibility and function of soft tissues such as muscles, ligaments, and tendons.[13]

Myofascial release involves manual stretching of the layers of the body's fascia, which is connective tissue that surrounds muscle and other soft tissue in the body (see Figure 2-3B).[14] Myofascial release techniques are reported to soften and reduce restrictions in muscles and fascia that are limiting normal movement.

JOINT MOBILIZATION

In contrast to soft tissue mobilization, which focuses on stretching or relaxing soft tissue, **joint mobilization** techniques are used when a patient's dysfunction is the result of joint stiffness or hypomobility (limited motion). Based on knowledge of the anatomy of joint surfaces and the findings from joint examination, the therapist applies specific passive movements of varying amplitude to a joint, in either an oscillatory (rhythmic, repeated movements) or a sustained manner. Joint mobilization techniques are used to reduce pain and stiffness affecting movement and restore normal joint motion.

THERAPEUTIC EXERCISE

Therapeutic exercise forms the core of most rehabilitation programs.[3] This foundation is based on scientific principles and the knowledge that the human body has the ability to react and respond to physical stresses placed on it. In particular, the muscular and cardiovascular/pulmonary systems are adaptable, depending on the stresses and forces placed on them. When these systems are stressed with a program of progressive exercise, positive changes such as improvement in strength and endurance occur. Similarly, the effects of abnormal stresses, such as prolonged bed rest, can lead to detrimental changes, including osteoporosis and muscle atrophy.

The goals of therapeutic exercise are not only to facilitate and restore normal function in an individual, but also to prevent an initial injury, educate the patient on how to prevent recurrence of an injury, and help maintain normal function. These goals are based on the results of the patient's examination and assessment of needs.

The level of sophistication of an exercise program should not be determined by the type of equipment the clinic has. Some of the most sophisticated exercises can be performed with inexpensive equipment. With creativity, various pieces of equipment can be adapted to incorporate many of the goals of therapeutic exercise. This section describes a variety of therapeutic exercise techniques that may be used with a patient who has a musculoskeletal dysfunction. These techniques include exercises to improve ROM, strength, flexibility, balance and coordination, cardiovascular endurance, and function.

RANGE-OF-MOTION EXERCISE

As mentioned earlier in the chapter, **range-of-motion exercise** can be categorized into two types: passive and active. PROM may be provided manually by the therapist or mechanically by a machine. This type of exercise might be used with (but is not limited to) patients who are restricted to bed rest or have paralysis of one or more limbs. It may also be used when AROM is contraindicated. AROM can be subdivided into active-assisted movement, active-free movement, and active-resisted movement. When performing **active-assisted**

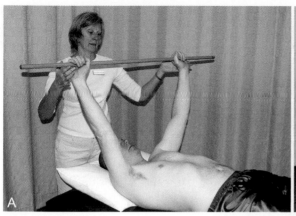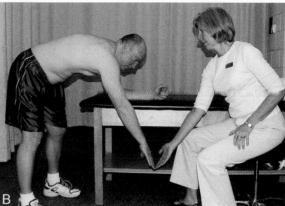

Figure 8-14 ■ Range-of-motion exercises are used to maintain or improve joint motion. **A**, A dowel can be used to perform simple active-assistive range-of-motion exercises for the shoulder. **B**, Pendulum exercises are effective active-free exercises and require no special equipment. (Courtesy Mark Hine.)

range of motion, the patient may be assisted either manually or mechanically if the prime muscle mover is weak (Figure 8-14, *A*). Pendulum exercises in which the patient does not receive any support or resistance are an example of **active-free exercises** (Figure 8-14, *B*). In **active-resisted exercises** an external force resists the movement. The last category includes a variety of techniques, several of which are described in the next section.

RESISTANCE EXERCISE

Resistance exercise is a form of active movement in which some form of resistance is provided. The goals of a resistance exercise program are to increase muscular strength, endurance, and power. **Muscular strength** is the maximal amount of tension an individual can produce in one repetition. **Muscle endurance** is the ability to produce and sustain tension over a prolonged period. **Muscle power** is the amount of work produced by the muscle in a given amount of time. If the goal is to increase strength, the program would concentrate on low repetitions with heavy resistance. If the goal is to increase endurance, the exercise program would concentrate on using low resistance for high repetitions. When the goal is to increase power, the exercise program would consist of explosive high-intensity muscle activity such as jumping. The type of exercise performed depends on the types of activities to which the patient is planning to return. When designing a program, the therapist must consider the type or types of resistance exercises on which the patient should concentrate. Resistance exercise can be categorized into three types: isometric, isotonic, and isokinetic. Definitions and examples of these types are outlined in Table 8-4. Typically, a combination of all three types of exercises is necessary to perform any type of functional activity.

Resistance can be applied either manually by the therapist or mechanically by the use of equipment. Manual resistance can be applied to isolated muscle

8

Table 8-4
Classification of Resisted Exercises

Type of Exercise	Definition	Example
Isometric	Muscle contraction without visible joint movement	Pushing against a wall
Isotonic concentric	Muscle contraction that produces or controls joint motion, resulting in muscle shortening	Flexing elbow with dumbbell in hand (biceps brachii muscle)
Isotonic eccentric	Muscle contraction that produces or controls joint motion, resulting in muscle lengthening	Extending elbow with dumbbell in hand (biceps brachii muscle)
Isokinetic	A concentric or eccentric muscle contraction that occurs at a constant speed	Knee extensions using an isokinetic device

groups (as is the case with MMT positions) or to patterns of movement that involve several muscle groups. An example of the latter is a technique called *proprioceptive neuromuscular facilitation*, which is described in Chapter 9. The use of manual resistance offers many advantages, the primary one being that the therapist can control the amount of resistance provided. This advantage is particularly useful when working with patients in the early stages of rehabilitation when ROM may need to be limited or the patient can tolerate only mild to moderate resistance. The disadvantage of manual resistance is the difficulty in quantifying the amount of resistance provided. Inability to accurately document the resistance makes it difficult for another therapist to replicate the same force on that patient.

Many pieces of equipment can be used when applying mechanical resistance, from an inexpensive strip of elastic tubing to expensive and highly technologic isokinetic equipment. Other common and frequently used equipment in the clinic includes free weights exercise machines and pulley systems (Figure 8-15).

CORE STRENGTHENING
Core strengthening refers to the strengthening of the deep postural muscles of the lumbar and cervical spine. The premise behind core strengthening is that it helps provide stability to proximal structures, allowing for appropriate movement patterns in the distal extremity. A number of core conditioning exercise classes such as Pilates and tai chi emphasize core strengthening during functional movement. Examples of core strengthening for the lumbar spine are shown in Figure 8-16.

FLEXIBILITY EXERCISE
Patients recovering from a musculoskeletal injury frequently have decreased flexibility in the muscles crossing the involved joint. Conditions that may produce decreased flexibility include prolonged immobilization and tissue trauma. Many times, prior limitations in flexibility contributed to or were the primary

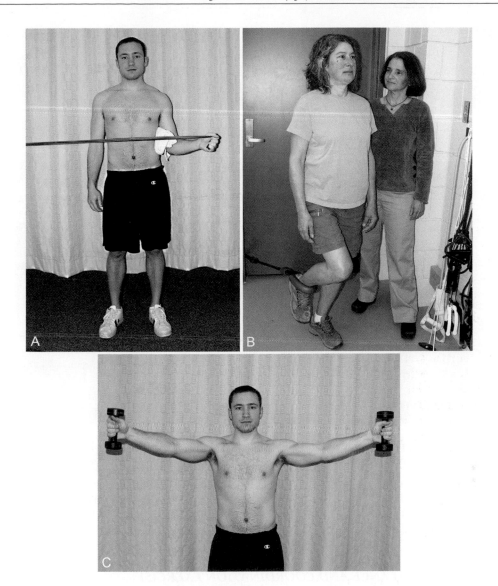

Figure 8-15 ■ Different methods of using mechanical resistance for exercise. **A** and **B**, Elastic tubing is easy and convenient. **C**, Free weights are readily available to produce mechanical resistance. (Courtesy Mark Hine.)

cause of the injury. Therefore, **flexibility exercise** is an important component to address with the patient.

Soft tissue, such as muscle, has the ability to change length or adapt over time with stress. Although a variety of techniques can be used to increase flexibility, no consensus has been reached on the most effective way to stretch. Furthermore, a stretching technique that works well for one patient may be ineffective for another.

Stretching techniques can be performed passively with an external force applied either manually or mechanically. Stretching can also be performed by

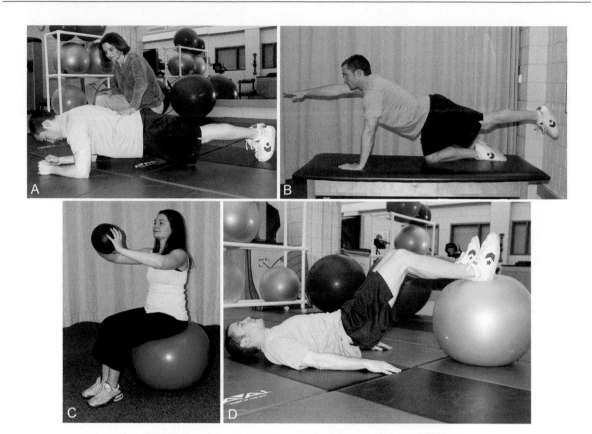

Figure 8-16 ■ Examples of core strengthening exercises for the lumbar spine. **A**, The plank position. **B**, The quadruped position. **C**, Seated on an exercise ball. **D**, Bridging on an exercise ball. (Courtesy Mark Hine.)

actively inhibiting the shortened muscle. This technique, called *contract-relax*, requires that the shortened muscle actively contract before a stretching force is applied.

BALANCE AND COORDINATION EXERCISE

Loss of balance is an impairment that PTs frequently address in a rehabilitation program. **Balance** refers to the ability to maintain body position in equilibrium.[15] Proper balance requires the nervous and musculoskeletal systems to interact with the environment to control body position. After injury, if these systems are not properly integrating information, loss of balance and coordination may result. Several clinical tests are used to assess a patient's balance, and numerous exercises and equipment can be used to facilitate proper balance. One popular piece of equipment seen in the clinic is a BOSU balance trainer (Figure 8-17). The patient may be progressed from double-leg to single-leg stance. The exercise can be made more challenging by having patients close their eyes and by incorporating upper extremity movement with and without weights.

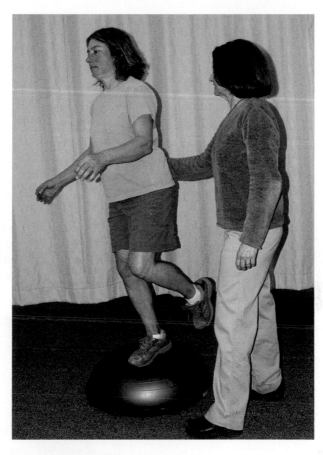

Figure 8-17 ■ BOSU balance trainer can be used for balance exercises. (Courtesy Mark Hine.)

CARDIOVASCULAR ENDURANCE TRAINING

Cardiovascular or **aerobic training** is exercise performed over a long period at low intensity. Aerobic exercise typically involves large muscle groups used in a rhythmic type of activity. Many modes of exercise are available to improve cardiovascular endurance, including walking, running, stair climbing, cycling, cross-country skiing, and swimming. The PT will choose the most appropriate exercise modality for the patient. For example, a patient who is recovering from a low back injury and has difficulty sitting may participate in a walking program rather than a cycling program. See Chapter 10 for a more detailed description of cardiovascular exercise.

FUNCTIONAL EXERCISES

As mentioned earlier in this chapter, the ultimate goal in physical therapy is to allow the patient to return to the previous level of function or highest level of function achievable. Therefore, exercises mimicking functional movements and activities must be incorporated into the rehabilitation program. A **functional**

exercise incorporates strength, flexibility, balance, and coordination. Incorporating all these factors allows patients to return to function with confidence because they know that they performed the same or similar exercises in the clinic.

The use of closed kinetic chain exercises allows the patient to incorporate these functional movements. A **closed kinetic chain exercise** is an exercise in which movement at one joint affects movement at other joints. This occurs when the distal segment is not free to move. For example, when a person squats, the foot is fixed to the ground, and movement occurs simultaneously at the ankle, knee, and hip joints. This is in contrast to an **open kinetic chain exercise** in which the end limb segment is free. An example of an open chain exercise is the seated leg extension machine frequently seen in fitness centers. Because the lower extremity typically functions with the foot on the ground, closed chain exercises are particularly important in the rehabilitation of the lower extremity. Therefore, exercises involving the movement of joints while the foot is on the ground facilitate movement that mimics function (Figure 8-18). Closed kinetic chain exercises are also used with patients with upper extremity injuries, particularly those with shoulder dysfunctions. An example of an upper extremity closed kinetic chain exercise is a push up.

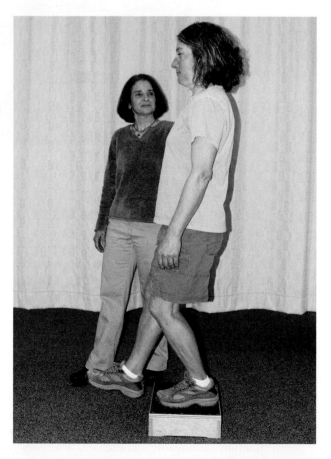

Figure 8-18 ■ Functional exercises, such as descending a step, are designed to mimic daily activities. (Courtesy Mark Hine.)

AQUATIC THERAPY

The use of water for therapeutic benefit dates back to the ancient Greeks and Romans, who used therapeutic baths for relaxation and pain reduction.[16] "Pool therapy" developed in the 1920s in the United States as part of the rehabilitation program for children with poliomyelitis (see Figure 1-4). As polio declined with the introduction of vaccines, so did the therapeutic use of pools. Since that time, the popularity of **aquatic physical therapy** has grown significantly and has been shown to be beneficial for a variety of orthopaedic dysfunctions. The uniqueness of the aquatic environment for therapeutic purposes resulted in the APTA establishing, in 1992, the Aquatic Physical Therapy Section.

The Aquatic Physical Therapy Section offers a comprehensive description of this form of therapy (Box 8-4).[17] The description indicates that this form of rehabilitation is effective for a variety of conditions, in addition to maintaining health and fitness in well individuals.

The beneficial effects of aquatic therapy depend largely on the fundamental principles of physics, such as the buoyancy, viscosity, and hydrostatic pressure of water. Both physiologic and psychological benefits are derived from aquatic physical therapy. The physiologic benefits include improved cardiovascular status, increased muscle strength and flexibility, decreased pain, and improved balance without the impact that occurs with exercises on land. Psychological benefits include general relaxation from the warmth of the water, the socialization process

BOX 8-4

Description of Aquatic Therapy

Aquatic physical therapy is the evidence-based and skilled practice of physical therapy in an aquatic environment by a physical therapist or by a physical therapist assistant under the supervision of a physical therapist. Aquatic physical therapy includes, but is not limited to, treatment, rehabilitation, prevention, health, wellness, and fitness of patient/client populations in an aquatic environment with or without the use of assistive, adaptive, orthotic, protective, or supportive devices and equipment. The unique properties of the aquatic environment enhance interventions for patients/clients across the age span with musculoskeletal, neuromuscular, cardiovascular-pulmonary, and integumentary diseases, disorders, or conditions. Aquatic physical therapy interventions are designed to improve or maintain function, aerobic capacity and endurance conditioning, balance, coordination and agility, body mechanics and postural stabilization, flexibility, gait and locomotion, relaxation, and muscle strength, power, and endurance. Interventions used in aquatic physical therapy include, but are not limited to, therapeutic exercise, functional training, manual therapy, breathing strategies, electrotherapeutic modalities, physical agents, and mechanical modalities using the properties of water and techniques unique to the aquatic environment.

From American Physical Therapy Association (APTA): APTA Aquatic Physical Therapy Section, Alexandria, VA, 2010, APTA. Available at: www.aquaticpt.org.

8

BOX 8-5

Precautions and Contraindications for Aquatic Therapy

- Fevers, infections, rashes.
- Cardiac history.
- Incontinence without protection.
- Open wounds without appropriate dressings.
- Fear of water.
- Limited lung capacity.
- Unstable cardiac condition.

Modified from Hall CM, Brody LT: *Therapeutic exercise: movement towards function*, ed 2, Baltimore, 2005, Lippincott Williams and Wilkins.

that may be associated with group sessions in a pool, and the increased patient confidence and level of satisfaction that accompany patient performance.

Certain contraindications and precautions must be considered when planning and implementing any aquatic therapy session (Box 8-5). These contraindications and precautions must be carefully considered to ensure the safety of the individual.

HOME EXERCISE PROGRAMS

The use of therapeutic exercise in a rehabilitation program is an important component of the physical therapy plan of care. Aside from the physical benefits derived from exercise, it also encourages active participation in the rehabilitative process and allows patients to assume responsibility for their care. Home exercise programs are an important aspect of patient care. Performing exercises in the clinic two or three times per week is not usually adequate to achieve the desired long-lasting effects of rehabilitation, so home exercises given by the PT become an important component of physical therapy.

SUMMARY

This chapter has presented the role that PTs and PTAs perform in physical therapy for musculoskeletal conditions. Common conditions described were overuse and traumatic injuries and surgical and medical conditions. Components of the patient examination were presented. Interventions focused on patient/client instruction, biophysical agents, manual techniques, therapeutic exercise, and home programs. The emphasis in physical therapy for musculoskeletal conditions is on evaluating a patient's function and developing a plan of care that will assist the patient to return to optimal function in the environment, whether that be the athletic field, work site, home, or civic life.

CASE STUDIES

CASE STUDY
ONE

EXAMINATION

History

Jack, a 36-year-old male, is single and has an 8-year-old child. As an architect, he sits at a computer approximately 5 hours per day and drives 1 hour each way to work. His chief complaint is left-sided lower back pain that spreads into the buttock region and occasionally down the back of the thigh. Symptoms came on suddenly approximately 2 weeks ago after he bent down to pick up house keys; Jack had difficulty standing back up because of pain. He saw a physician, who recommended a course of muscle relaxants and physical therapy. Jack says that the pain has gradually improved since its onset and rates the pain level a 4 on a scale of 1 to 10. The pain worsens when he lifts his daughter from the floor and with prolonged periods of sitting. Symptoms improve with walking. Jack has no complaints of numbness or tingling in the lower extremity, but is currently unable to sit for more than 20 minutes without the onset of pain. His Oswestry score is 36% (higher scores represent greater disability). The Patient-Specific Functional Scale is scored as a 10 (sum of scores; goal is 30) with the following three activity limitations: decreased ability to don socks and pants, unable to go bike riding with daughter, and unable to transfer groceries from the cart to the car. Radiographs taken 1 week ago were "normal," according to Jack. He has a history of occasional low back discomfort after prolonged sitting, but no previous history of this type of pain. His medical-surgical history and family history are unremarkable. Jack is sedentary, but enjoys occasional weekend recreational activities.

Systems Review

Body type is endomorphic. Cardiovascular examination findings: blood pressure 136/88 mm Hg and resting heart rate 86 beats per minute. The patient's integumentary system is unremarkable, and he has full ROM of the lower extremity. Neuromuscular evaluation shows normal movement patterns of the lower extremities.

   Gait appears antalgic with decreased weight bearing on the left. In standing posture, Jack has a posterior pelvic tilt with a slight lateral shift to the right. Hip heights and iliac crest heights are symmetric. ROM testing demonstrates lumbar spine movements to be significantly limited in all directions; the chief complaint is exacerbated with flexion movements. Pain centralizes with lumbar extension in the prone position. In joint integrity and mobility testing, no swelling or temperature changes are noted over the lumbar erectors. Increased tone is palpated bilaterally in the spinal muscles. Muscle performance testing finds the lower extremity to be within normal limits; however, the trunk muscles were not tested because of pain. A straight leg raise reproduces the thigh pain at 40°, and there is a positive slump test. Sensation of the lower extremity is intact to light touch bilaterally. Testing of reflex integrity reveals symmetric deep tendon reflexes (DTRs) of 2 (range 0-4) in the lower extremity throughout.

EVALUATION

Based on Jack's signs and symptoms a diagnosis of lower back pain with radiating pain was made. His Oswestry score indicates a moderate level of disability. Impairments include increased muscle tone of the lumbar erectors, comparable pain with straight leg raise and slump test, poor posture, and decreased lumbar ROM. Activity limitations include a decreased ability to sit for prolonged periods. Participation restrictions include an inability to complete job tasks in a timely fashion because of a decreased ability to sit and an inability to participate in recreational activities.

8

Prognosis and Expected Range of Visits

Over the course of 4 to 8 weeks, Jack will return to his premorbid level of function with a minimal increase in symptoms. He is to be seen for 8 to 12 visits over the course of 3 months.

Short-Term Goals (2-4 Weeks)

The following short-term goals are set: (1) pain reduced to 1 to 2 (out of 10), (2) abolishment of lateral shift, (3) 50% increase in all lumbar movements, (4) independence in a home exercise program, and (5) ability to demonstrate proper sitting posture throughout the treatment session.

Long-Term Goals and Outcomes (6-8 Weeks)

For the long term, Jack's goals and outcomes are: (1) Oswestry score less than 10%, (2) PSFS score greater than 25, (3) secondary prevention—the risk of impairment, functional limitation, and disability is reduced through adherence to an independent exercise program, and Jack understands and demonstrates strategies to prevent the recurrence of symptoms, and (4) services provided by the PT are deemed acceptable by the patient.

Plan of Care and Intervention

Jack's home exercise program will begin with lateral shift and lumbar extension exercises and progress to flexion exercises. He will be educated on proper sitting posture and body mechanics, including lifting techniques. Manual techniques (joint and soft tissue mobilization) are to be used as appropriate for pain relief and to improve muscle tone. As pain resolves, exercises will increase to include functional movements, flexibility exercises, core strengthening exercises, and cardiovascular fitness training. The importance of adhering to the home exercise program will be explained. Work site analysis will be performed, followed by recommendations to improve Jack's computer workstation.

Outcomes and Patient Status at Discharge

After 6 weeks of physical therapy, Jack was free of symptoms and all goals had been met. He was discharged with a comprehensive home exercise program. A recommendation was made to initiate a general fitness program at the local health club.

CASE STUDY TWO

EXAMINATION

History

Alice, a 72-year-old widow and retired schoolteacher, lives alone. She is right hand dominant. Alice sustained a fractured right radius after slipping on ice 8 weeks ago. She was immobilized in a cast from her hand to midhumerus with her elbow positioned in 90° of flexion and her arm supported in a sling for comfort. The cast was removed yesterday. Her chief complaints are stiffness and weakness throughout the upper extremity and an inability to perform daily activities such as getting dressed and preparing meals. Her score on the PSFS is 56. Radiographs taken yesterday reveal "healing without complications." Alice has no past history of the current condition; her medical history includes osteoporosis, otherwise she is in generally good health. Her family history is unremarkable. Regarding social habits, Alice walks to miles a day and enjoys cooking, gardening, and the outdoors.

Systems Review
Cardiovasular: blood pressure of 140/90 mm Hg and a resting heart rate of 80 beats per minute. Integumentary: dry skin over the area covered by the cast. Musculo-skeletal: full ROM of left upper extremity movements and good range of strength in the left arm. See below for details of the right upper extremity. Neuromuscular: left upper extremity reveals normal movement patterns.

Tests and Measures
Observation reveals swelling over the dorsal aspect of the right wrist. Alice's stand-ing posture is with the head slightly forward and the shoulders rounded, and she holds her arm in a guarded position against her body. Muscle atrophy is noted throughout the right upper extremity. Joint integrity and mobility testing demon-strates limited and painful active movements of the right shoulder, elbow, and wrist. AROM of the right hand is within normal limits. PROM of the right upper extremity is as follows:

Shoulder:	Flexion=0-160°
	Abduction=0-60°
	External rotation=0-15°
	Internal rotation=0-70°
Elbow:	Unable to extend past 60° of flexion
Wrist:	Flexion=0-45°
	Extension=0-45°

Accessory motion is decreased at the right glenohumeral joint and distal radio-ulnar joint. In muscle performance testing, resisted tests reveal weakness in the fol-lowing muscle groups: right shoulder abductors and external rotators, elbow flexors and extensors, and wrist flexors and extensors. Manual muscle tests reveal the fol-lowing (see Table 8-1 for descriptions of grades; grades are based on a scale of 0-5):

Right biceps=4−/5	Left biceps=5/5
Right triceps=3+/5	Left triceps=5/5
Right hand grip=15 lb	Left hand grip=25 lb

Testing for pain reveals pain with movement of the right upper extremity. Sen-sory integrity testing reveals the upper extremity to be intact to light touch bilat-erally. In reflex integrity, Alice has upper extremity DTRs of 3 throughout (within a range of 0-4) and symmetric.

Evaluation
Alice has decreased ROM and strength secondary to immobilization after a radial fracture. Impairments include swelling, decreased upper extremity strength,

decreased upper extremity ROM, poor posture, and decreased accessory movement at the shoulder and wrist. Her activity limitations include a decreased ability to perform ADLs. Regarding participation restrictions, Alice is unable to participate in desired leisure activities, including cooking and gardening.

Prognosis and Expected Range of Visits

Over the course of 8 to 12 weeks, Alice will return to her premorbid level of function with minimal limitation. She is to be seen for 6 to 18 visits over the course of 3 months.

Short-Term Goals (2-4 Weeks)

Alice's short-term goals are as follows: (1) decrease swelling by 25%, (2) increase upper extremity strength to the next higher grade, (3) increase right grip strength to 18 lb, (4) increase ROM by 5 to 10° in all limited movements, (5) increase accessory motion to nearly full range, (6) be able to demonstrate proper cervical and shoulder posture, and (7) demonstrate independence in her home exercise program.

Long-Term Goals and Outcomes (10-12 Weeks)

Alice's long-term goals and outcomes include: (1) functional limitations and disabilities—Alice should be able to perform all ADLs independently and to return to all leisure activities, (2) patient satisfaction—services provided by the PT are deemed acceptable by Alice, and (3) secondary prevention—the risk of adhesive capsulitis and other upper extremity or postural pathology is reduced and risk of future falls is reduced through patient education and adherence to an independent exercise program.

Plan of Care and Intervention

Alice's home exercise program will progressively increase to enhance elbow and wrist ROM and strength. The program will include active assisted, active, and resisted exercises such as pendulum, pulley, and cane exercises (see Figure 8-13), in addition to balance training activities. Alice will be educated on proper posture and the relationship between proper posture and shoulder mechanics. Biophysical agents (superficial heat) and manual techniques (joint mobilization) will be used as appropriate. Proprioceptive neuromuscular facilitation patterns will be incorporated to improve functional movements. As strength and ROM increase, simulated ADLs will be added to the treatment program.

Outcomes and Patient Status at Discharge

After 9 weeks of physical therapy, Alice had functional use of her right upper extremity and was able to return to all activities with minimal limitation. She was discharged with a comprehensive exercise program.

CASE STUDY THREE

EXAMINATION

History

Megan is a 20-year-old female college student who was examined in the PT clinic through direct access with left (L) anterior knee pain. She states the pain has increased gradually over the past month and is aggravated by prolonged sitting in class, walking and running, and stair climbing. She has had to stop her recreational fitness workout of treadmill running and weight lifting because of the pain. She rates her pain as a 2 (scale of 0-10) during normal activities, but it can be 8 after climbing stairs to her dorm room or excessive walking. She denies any injury to the knee, but does report having similar symptoms 3 years ago during high school soccer season. At that time, she was referred to physical therapy and was instructed in quad-strengthening exercises that helped manage symptoms somewhat. Her past medical and family history is unremarkable with the exception of a recent 10 lb weight gain.

Systems Review
Blood pressure 115/75 mm Hg, resting heart rate 68; integumentary and neuromuscular examination of uninvolved extremities unremarkable; musculoskeletal: ht = 63 in., wt = 145 lbs, BMI = 25.7.

Tests and Measures
Standing posture examination reveals internally rotated position of (L) femur, and bilateral pes planus (flat feet). Demonstrates full AROM and PROM of both knees, but limited squat because of pain in (L) knee. Muscle performance testing is within normal limits (WNL) at both knees, with slight weakness noted in (L) hip abductors. Flexibility testing reveals + Straight Leg Raise and Ober's tests on (L). Patellar orientation reveals a lateral shift and glide both statically and dynamically on the (L). Functional testing with step-downs reveals poor pelvic control and reproduces pain. Score on Lower Extremity Functional Scale is 66/80.

Evaluation
(L) anterior knee pain caused by muscle imbalances and structural malalignment in the (L) lower extremity resulting in patellofemoral pain syndrome. Impairments include (L) knee pain, decreased flexibility of hamstrings and iliotibial band, weakness in hip abductors, and excessive foot pronation in standing. Activity limitations include difficulty sitting for prolonged periods of time and negotiating stairs because of pain; participation restrictions include inability to participate in desired fitness program of running and strength training.

Prognosis and Expected Range of Visits
Over the course of 6 to 8 weeks, this patient will be able to resume her desired level of activity, including running and strength training, with adequate pain management. She will be seen for 8 to 10 visits.

Short-Term Goals (2-4 Weeks)
(1) Decrease pain with walking and stair climbing to 2/10 or 3/10, (2) improve Lower Extremity Functional Scale score to 70/80, (3) become independent with hamstring and iliotibial band stretching exercises, (4) increase strength in hip abductors for improved pelvic control during step-down.

Long-Term Goals (6-8 Weeks)
(1) Improve lower extremity alignment, (2) improve score on Lower Extremity Functional Scale to 76/80, (3) resume desired level of fitness, including jogging and lower extremity strength training with manageable knee pain, (4) prevent further episodes of knee pain by adherence to an exercise program that addresses muscle imbalances, and (5) improve wellness by decreasing BMI to <25.

Plan of Care
Instruction in home exercise program, including cardiovascular training beginning with aquatic therapy and progressing to land-based training as tolerated, flexibility exercises, progressive hip and core strengthening, and functional exercises using weights and resisted bands and involving a variety of surfaces including exercise balls and foam rollers. Fit for custom orthotics to address overpronation.

Outcomes and Patient Status at Discharge
After nine visits, patient reported minimal symptoms and goals achieved. She was able to demonstrate good pelvic control while doing repeated step-downs without pain, and she reported tolerating a progressive running program with her orthotics. She was discharged with instructions to continue the prescribed home exercise program and progress running distance and weight with resistance training as tolerated.

REFERENCES

1. Magee DJ, Zachazewski JE, Quillen WS: *Scientific foundations and principles of practice in musculoskeletal rehabilitation,* St. Louis, 2007, Saunders Elsevier.
2. PTNow. http://ptnow.org/Default.aspx. Accessed October 14, 2014.
3. Guide to Physical Therapist Practice 3.0, American Physical Therapy Association. http://guidetoptpractice.apta.org/. Accessed October 14, 2014.
4. Boissonnalut WG: *Primary care for the physical therapist: examination and triage,* St. Louis, 2010, Elsevier Saunders.
5. Kendall FP, McCreary EK, Provance PG, et al.: *Muscles: testing and function,* ed 5, Baltimore, 2005, Lippincott Williams and Wilkins.
6. Sahrmann SA: *Movement system impairment syndromes of the extremities, cervical and thoracic spines,* St. Louis, 2011, Mosby, Inc.
7. Gray Institute Online Exercise Library. https://www.grayinstitute.com/educational_products.aspx?cat=7. Accessed October 14, 2014.
8. Teyhen DS, Shaffer SW, Lorenson CL, et al.: Clinical measures associated with dynamic balance and functional movement, *J Strength Cond Res* 28(5):1272–1283, 2014.
9. McKinnis LN: *Fundamental of musculoskeletal imaging,* ed 3, Philadelphia, 2010, FA Davis.
10. Michlovitz SL, Nolan TP: *Modalities for therapeutic intervention,* ed 5, Philadelphia, 2011, FA Davis.
11. Prentice WE: *Therapeutic modalities in rehabilitation,* ed 4, New York, 2011, McGraw-Hill Medical.
12. Robinson AJ, Snyder-Mackler L: *Clinical electrophysiology, electrotherapy and electrophysiologic testing,* ed 3, Baltimore, 2007, Williams and Wilkins.
13. Cyriax J: *Textbook of orthopedic medicine, vol 1, diagnosis of soft tissue lesions,* ed 8, London, 1982, Baillière Tindall.
14. Kostopoulos D, Rizopoulos K: *The manual of trigger point and myofascial therapy,* Thorofare, NJ, 2001, Slack.
15. Kisner C, Colby LA: *Therapeutic exercise: foundations and techniques,* ed 6, Philadelphia, 2012, FA Davis.
16. Wynn KE: Lily ponds, warm springs and fortunate accidents, *PT Mag Phys Ther* 2(12):44–45, 1994.
17. Mission statement, Aquatic Physical Therapy Section of the American Physical Therapy Association. http://www.aquaticpt.org/about.cfm. Accessed October 14, 2014.

ADDITIONAL RESOURCES

Andrade CK, Clifford P: *Outcome-based massage,* ed 3, Baltimore, 2013, Lippincott Williams and Wilkins. Provides theoretical background and comprehensive descriptions of a variety of manual techniques based on desired outcomes.
Andrews JR, Harrelson GL, Wilk KE: *Physical rehabilitation of the injured athlete,* ed 4, Philadelphia, 2012, Saunders. Offers a comprehensive, joint-by-joint approach to the management of athletic injuries. The book provides hundreds of illustrations of common exercises used in this population.

Brotzman SB, Wilk KE: *Clinical orthopedic rehabilitation,* ed 3, Philadelphia, 2011, Mosby. Thorough text on the examination techniques, differential diagnosis, treatment approaches, and intervention options for a variety of musculoskeletal disorders.

Cameron MH: *Physical agents in rehabilitation: from research to practice,* ed 4, St. Louis, 2012, Saunders. A comprehensive text on clinical decision making and the practical application of physical agents.

Cook C: *Orthopedic manual therapy: an evidence based approach,* ed 2, Upper Saddle River, NJ, 2012, Pearson Prentice Hall. This is a clinically applicable text that describes examination and manual therapy techniques of the extremities and spine.

Donatelli RA, Wooden MJ: *Orthopedic physical therapy,* ed 4, St. Louis, 2010, Churchill Livingstone, Elsevier. Includes fundamental principles of orthopedic physical therapy practice and specific examination and treatment approaches by anatomic region.

Dutton M: *Orthopedic examination evaluation and intervention,* ed 3, New York, 2012, McGraw Hill. A comprehensive text covering management of orthopedic injuries, including examination, evaluation, and intervention. An accompanying DVD demonstrates numerous manual techniques and therapeutic exercises.

Evans RC: *Illustrated orthopedic physical assessment,* ed 3, St. Louis, 2008, Mosby. Hundreds of tests can be used for making conservative care diagnoses of disorders of the nervous and orthopedic systems. This manual describes them in a clearly illustrated, sequential fashion. Organization of the text is by region and specifically by initial signs, symptoms, and indications.

Fetters L, Tilson J: *Evidence based physical therapy,* Philadelphia, 2012, FA Davis. A step by step approach to the five steps in the EBP process. Emphasis is on appraisal of diagnostic, prognostic, and intervention studies in additional to synthesized evidence and clinical practice guidelines. Also includes a chapter on technology used in EBP.

Hall CM, Brody LT: *Therapeutic exercises: moving toward function,* ed 3, Philadelphia, 2010, Lippincott Williams and Wilkins. Offers a comprehensive approach to therapeutic exercise, including separate chapters on aquatic physical therapy, proprioceptive neuromuscular functioning, and closed kinetic chain exercise.

Jewell DV: *Guide to evidence-based physical therapy practice,* ed 3, Boston, 2014, Jones and Bartlett. Designed to facilitate evidence-based practice in the clinic by describing what constitutes evidence, how to search and evaluate evidence found in the literature, and how to integrate evidence into clinical decision making. Also includes several chapters on research design and a review of inferential statistics.

Kolt GS, Snyder-Makler L: *Physical therapies in sport and exercise,* ed 2, London, 2007, Churchill Livingstone. A comprehensive text with an emphasis on the rehabilitation and prevention of injuries seen with exercise and sport. Several chapters devoted to special populations, such as children, female athletes, older adults, and athletes with disabilities.

Magee DJ: *Orthopedic physical assessment,* ed 6, Philadelphia, 2013, Saunders. An excellent text detailing the evaluation of joints, with good descriptions of special tests.

Magee DJ, Zachazweski JE, Quillen WS: *Scientific foundations and principles of practice in musculoskeletal rehabilitation,* St. Louis, 2007, Elsevier. A comprehensive text including the pathophysiology of tissue healing and repair and principles of practice grounded in scientific foundation.

8

REVIEW QUESTIONS

1. What is the difference between active and passive ROM?
2. Without looking at the text, how many questions can you come up with that may be helpful in a patient interview?
3. How would quantitative and qualitative measurements fit into the SOAP note?
4. Research some physical therapy books in your school's library to find examples of resisted tests and manual muscle testing. What, in your observation, is the main difference?

5. What is meant by an outcome measure? How does it differ from other tests and measures described in this chapter?
6. Try the following study technique: Photocopy Table 8-3 and block out the second column ("biophysical agents") with a folded strip of paper. Can you fill in the applicable agents? Repeat this exercise by filling out column 3 ("physiologic effects") or column 4 ("clinical indications"). Performing this exercise will reinforce the uses and effects of physical agents.
7. Describe the difference in purpose between exercising for muscular strength and muscular endurance.
8. Explain the difference between open and closed kinetic chain exercises.

A sense of history and an appreciation of why things happened can provide a perspective in understanding the present and in projecting the future.

Lucy Blair, PT

9 Physical Therapy for Neuromuscular Conditions

Katy Eichinger and Cynthia M. Zablotny

KEY TERMS

amyotrophic lateral sclerosis (ALS)
angiography
benign paroxysmal positional vertigo (BPPV)
bradykinesia
computerized tomography (CT)
constraint-induced movement therapy (CIMT)
electroencephalography (EEG)
electromyography (EMG)
exacerbation
expressive aphasia
Guillain-Barré syndrome (GBS)
hemiparesis
hypertonia
hypotonia

learned nonuse
lumbar puncture (LP)
magnetic resonance imaging (MRI)
motor control
motor learning
multiple sclerosis (MS)
muscle tone
nerve conduction velocity (NCV)
neuroplasticity
paraplegia
Parkinson's disease (PD)
perception
plaques
receptive aphasia
rigidity
sensation
spasticity
spinal cord injury (SCI)
stroke, or cerebrovascular accident (CVA)

tetraplegia
traumatic brain injury (TBI)
tremor
unilateral spatial neglect
vertigo

LEARNING OBJECTIVES

After reading this chapter, the reader will be able to:
1. Discuss the role of the physical therapist in the management of patients with neuromuscular disorders.
2. Describe some of the common neuromuscular conditions in which physical therapists play an essential role.
3. Compare the different roles a therapist may play, depending on the patient's condition and problems.

GENERAL DESCRIPTION

At the beginning of the last century, one could learn about the human nervous system from autopsy tissue samples only. Today, with new technologies, the brain can be seen in action in living human beings. The 1990s were declared the decade of the brain by the U.S. Congress. During this period, tremendous progress was made in the areas of neuroscience, clinical neurology, and genetics. Within the past 10 years, basic and clinical scientists involved in neurorehabilitation science have worked collaboratively to translate evidence addressing brain and nervous system function and repair following injury into clinical practice. As a result of this work, the knowledge base of physical therapists working in neurorehabilitation has expanded, enabling them to more accurately diagnose movement system problems, make predictions about future function, and select and design optimal interventions to promote recovery.

Patients with problems related to disorders of the neuromuscular system comprise a large proportion of individuals treated by physical therapists (PTs) and physical therapist assistants (PTAs) today. Disorders of the neuromuscular system can be inherited or acquired. Some examples of inherited disorders include Friedrich's ataxia or spinal muscular atrophy, which are both present from birth. Acquired disorders may impact individuals at any point in their lifetime. Some neurologic diseases, such as multiple sclerosis, Parkinson's disease, or Lou Gehrig's disease (amyotrophic lateral sclerosis—ALS) generally have their onset when individuals are within their thirties to sixties. Other acquired diseases, such as Alzheimer's disease, primarily affect older adults, while spinal cord injuries most frequently impact those in their teens to their thirties. The age of the patient at the time of disease onset serves as an important factor guiding physical therapy goal setting and interventions. When neurologic disease is diagnosed early in life, it may influence the motor, cognitive, or language development of the child. When an older adult acquires a neurologic condition, the prognosis for recovery will most certainly be influenced by the person's general health and the presence of other comorbidities and overall function prior to onset.

Primary neurologic disease may result from pathology of the vascular system, trauma, infection, toxic or metabolic disturbances, neoplasms (tumors), or degenerative disorders. The time course of onset of neuromuscular conditions varies, with some diseases having abrupt onsets, while others have signs and symptoms that develop across weeks, months, or even years. Depending on the cause of the disorder, the condition may be lifelong or temporary. It may be reversible, static, or progressive. The patient may go through periods of "plateaus" (i.e., relative stability) interspersed with progression. Because of the lengthy course of most neuromuscular disorders, PTs have extended contact with their patients and play a critical role in their care. PTs may provide services to these individuals within acute care, inpatient rehabilitation, outpatient, extended care, and home health settings. Each of these settings requires the physical therapist to develop a unique set of skills that go beyond basic care delivery. Depending on the condition, the stage of illness, and the setting of service delivery, the frequency of intervention will vary from daily sessions to monthly, quarterly, or yearly checkups for exercise prescription modifications, equipment assessment, and educational fine-tuning.

From the description just presented, it is apparent that PTs and PTAs who work with this population encounter diversity in their clients, their work settings, and the types of services they provide. Despite being prepared for autonomous practice through their education, physical therapists working in neurorehabilitation frequently function as part of a team of rehabilitation specialists who work collaboratively to coordinate patient care addressing all aspects of a person's needs. This team approach is optimal, as the majority of patients seen in neurorehabilitation present with impairments, activity limitations, or participation restrictions, which require expertise from the disciplines of occupational and speech therapy, neuropsychology, nursing, and medicine. As described in the patient/client management model, physical therapists are involved in examination, evaluation, diagnosis, prognosis, intervention, and outcomes in the clinical management of their patients/clients, such as those with neuromuscular disorders (see Chapter 2). The next section provides a brief overview of some common neuromuscular disorders and the role of physical therapy in the care and management of patients with these disorders.

9

COMMON CONDITIONS

STROKE

Stroke, or **cerebrovascular accident (CVA)**, is a leading cause of serious long-term disability in the United States and is one of the most common health conditions treated by neurorehabilitation therapists. Stroke refers to rapidly developing clinical signs that indicate a focal disturbance of cerebral function resulting from an interruption of blood flow.[1] This disruption may be caused by blockage from a clot that results in ischemia (decreased oxygen), or it may be caused by a blood vessel that bursts, creating a hemorrhage (bleeding). The range of resulting symptoms and their severity depend upon the area of brain tissue that is involved. The most common symptom is a complete paralysis or partial weakness on the side opposite the site involved (**hemiparesis**).[2] Depending on the site of the lesion, the paralysis may be accompanied by such symptoms as difficulty in speaking or understanding language, cognitive deficits, or neglect of the involved side. Poststroke depression affects more than a third of individuals who have survived a stroke.[3] If not diagnosed and managed appropriately, poststroke depression can impact functional recovery and social participation outcomes.

When a patient post stroke is seen emergently, a CT scan of the brain is performed to determine whether the etiology of the stroke is ischemic or hemorrhagic.[4] The result of this imaging will determine the medical course of action to be taken. If ischemia is the cause, and the person is being seen within the first 4 hours post stroke onset, the patient will be given a thrombolytic (clot busting) medication such as recombinant tissue plasminogen activator (rtPA) to reduce the blood clot and improve blood flow to the brain. In the case of a hemorrhagic stroke, the medical team will decide if surgery is necessary to remove excessive blood that may be putting pressure on the brain. Regardless of the cause of the stroke, acute medical management focuses on improving cerebral circulation and oxygenation, maintaining adequate blood pressure, and managing other systemic factors that may have contributed to the stroke, such as heart rhythm disturbances.

Neurologic and functional recovery from stroke occurs most rapidly during the first 3 months but may continue at a slower pace beyond this time. Initial stroke severity influences the time to reach maximal recovery.[5] Poststroke physical therapy interventions are designed to enhance recovery of task-related functions and resolve impairments so that individuals may optimally achieve the goals they have identified as being meaningful. Compensatory strategies, including equipment use, may augment training when deemed necessary because of the severity of residual stroke impairments and the task and environmental demands required for safe movement. Other essential components of a comprehensive rehabilitation program post stroke include (1) patient education to address stroke risk factors that may predispose the individual to recurrent stroke, which is common, and (2) assessment and management of fall risk factors to prevent future injury. Figure 9-1 illustrates gait training with an individual following a stroke affecting his left side.

TRAUMATIC BRAIN INJURY

Traumatic brain injury (TBI) is a significant cause of both death and disability in the United States. TBI is defined as an alteration in brain function, or other evidence of brain pathology, caused by an external force.[6] Evidence of a change in brain function includes a diminished or altered state of consciousness, posttraumatic amnesia, or the presence of a skull fracture, posttraumatic seizure, or an abnormal brain scan. Falls are the leading cause of TBI, and disproportionately affect children ages 0-4 and older adults (≥65 years of age). Unintentional blunt trauma, motor vehicle accidents, and assaults are also significant causes of TBI and frequently affect older adolescents and young adults.[7] Given the nature

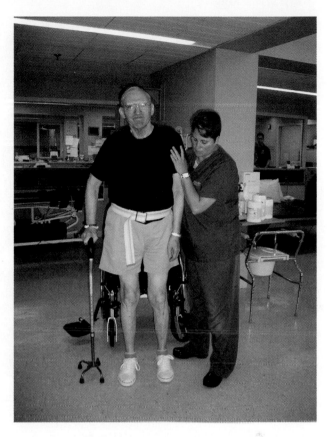

Figure 9-1 ■ Gait training for a patient following a stroke with left-side involvement.

of the causes of TBI, it is common to see numerous other systemic injuries, including fractures, dislocations, lacerations, and pulmonary complications, accompany the primary brain injury.[8]

Brain trauma is associated with both diffuse and focal insult to brain tissue that occurs at injury onset (primary injury). Injuries may range in severity from those considered mild, which may occur when someone sustains a concussion, to a severe injury, which results in a significantly altered level of consciousness. Initial acute care following TBI is focused on life preservation and minimizing the secondary mechanisms of injury, including events such as increased intracranial pressure and hypoxia, which further contribute to postinjury deficits. Impairments seen post-TBI are complex, impacting cognitive, physical, and emotional/behavioral domains. The cognitive deficits seen post-TBI may affect the individual's level of consciousness, memory storage and retrieval, attention, and information processing speed. Physical deficits may include paresis or paralysis, dyscoordination, and balance deficits, among others. Emotional/behavioral impairments are common and may include depression, lack of motivation, feeling anxious, and difficulty controlling emotions. Because of the variability and

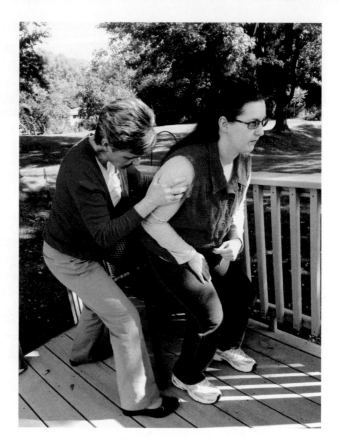

Figure 9-2 ■ Patient practicing sit to stand following a traumatic brain injury.

range of problems that can be encountered with each patient, management and intervention require an individualized plan and a multidisciplinary team approach in which each member plays a specific and significant role. Physical therapy intervention focuses on functional recovery and reinforces cognitive strategies appropriate to each individual's level.[8] Figure 9-2 provides an example of a functional training activity.

TBI results in

■ *Physical impairments*—Speech, vision, hearing, headaches, motor coordination, spasticity of muscles, paresis or paralysis, seizure disorders, balance, and fatigue.

■ *Cognitive impairments*—Short-term memory deficits, impaired concentration, slowness of thinking, limited attention span, impairments of perception, communication skills, planning, writing, reading, and judgment.

■ *Emotional impairments*—Mood swings, self-centeredness, anxiety, depression, lowered self-esteem, sexual dysfunction, restlessness, lack of motivation, and difficulty controlling emotions.

SPINAL CORD INJURY

Spinal cord injury (SCI) occurs when there is damage to the spinal cord or nerve roots, resulting in temporary or permanent loss of sensation and strength as well as body functions below the level of injury. Spinal cord injuries can result from motor vehicle accidents, falls, violence (especially gunshot wounds), and sports (diving and football). The age group most often affected is 16-30 years of age, and men are affected four times as often as women.[9] Spinal cord damage can also be precipitated by other diseases and conditions, and in these instances older patients are affected more commonly. Depending on the level of injury, all limbs may be affected (**tetraplegia**), or the lower part of the trunk and legs may be affected (**paraplegia**). If the lesion is complete, no residual sensory or motor function can be found below the level of the lesion ("-plegia"). The injury may also result in an incomplete lesion in which some distal motor and sensory functions may be preserved ("-paresis").

As with TBI, SCI may be accompanied by multiple injuries, and the early goal of management is preservation of life and prevention of further damage to neural tissue. Further damage is prevented through decompression and stabilization. Stabilization can be accomplished internally by fusing the vertebrae with bone grafts, rods, and wires, or externally with orthotic devices. Medications to control inflammation are often used to prevent further damage to neural tissue and enhance repair and recovery.

Acute physical therapy intervention focuses on maintaining flexibility and range of motion in the joints, strengthening unaffected muscles, and maintaining or improving cardiorespiratory capacity, and endurance. Once medical and orthopaedic clearance is obtained, more vigorous functional training is begun, often in a rehabilitation setting. Recent research provides evidence that the nervous system is able to recover from injury with time and applicable therapeutic interventions. Functional improvements, therefore, may be seen following the acute rehabilitation phase. The current health care climate has resulted in shortened rehabilitation stays, and despite the potential for recovery, individuals are often instructed in compensatory strategies to maximize functional independence as quickly as possible during the acute rehabilitation phase.[10]

In Figures 9-3 and 9-4, the patient is learning transfer and wheelchair manipulation skills. Physical therapists play a vital role in the identification of equipment requirements and environmental adaptations needed for each patient. For example, at discharge from a rehabilitation facility, most patients use a wheelchair as a primary means of mobility, and these must be custom ordered for each patient with specific size and adaptation requirements. The home will have to be made wheelchair accessible with ramps and other modifications. Thus the therapist plays a major role not only in the treatment but also in the rehabilitation of patients with SCI by providing family education and consultation on many related issues such as environmental modifications and assistive technology.

9

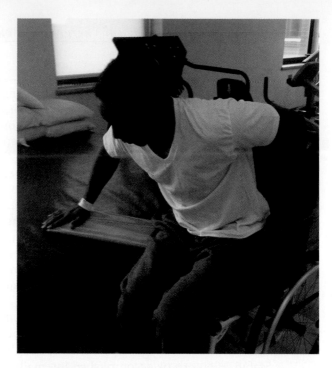

Figure 9-3 ■ Patient with a spinal cord injury transferring from the wheelchair to the mat table.

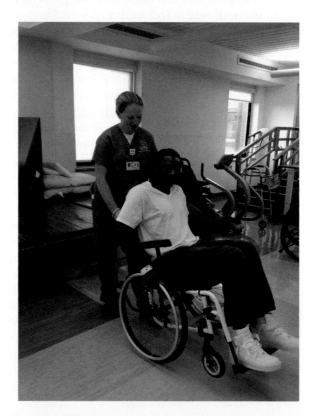

Figure 9-4 ■ Patient with a spinal cord injury working on wheelchair mobility skills.

VESTIBULAR DISORDERS

Dizziness is one of the most common presenting symptoms to primary care physicians, and it is also a common complaint heard by physical therapists working with individuals with primary neurologic health conditions. "Dizziness" is not a precise term; it is used by patients to describe sensations that may vary greatly and may include feelings of lightheadedness, unsteadiness, or spinning (**vertigo**). Vestibular dysfunction is a common cause of dizziness for many individuals.[11]

Understanding the anatomy and physiology of the vestibular system is essential to the correct diagnosis and management of pathologies affecting it. Vestibular dysfunction can result from involvement of the peripheral and/or central vestibular structures and pathways.[11] The peripheral vestibular apparatus includes the semicircular canals, which detect rotational movements, and the otolith organs, which detect linear movements and vertical orientation. These organs send their input via the vestibular nerve to the central nervous system vestibular structures, which include the vestibular nuclei, the cerebellum, and the central pathways connecting these structures. It is here that this information about motion, equilibrium, and spatial orientation is processed.

The physical therapy examination of an individual presenting with dizziness or other symptoms of vestibular pathology begins with a careful history to characterize the nature of the patient's symptoms (e.g., vertigo vs. feeling off-balance), the onset and timing of these symptoms (sudden vs. gradual onset; continuous vs. episodic) and the circumstances in which the symptoms are provoked (e.g., specific head movements or environments).[12] The physical therapist will then perform specific tests and measures to determine how well the eyes can coordinate their movements with one another and with movement of the head. This information helps in the diagnosis of the exact cause of the patient's symptoms, which is essential to setting up an optimal intervention program.

Peripheral vestibular injuries are most commonly the result of a disorder called **benign paroxysmal positional vertigo (BPPV)**, which occurs when calcium crystals that are normally part of the otolith organs break free and fall into the semicircular canals, causing a sensation of spinning when the head is moved in certain directions. Other causes of peripheral vestibular pathology include viral infections, tumors, toxicity from specific antibiotics, and genetics, as is the case with Meniere's disease. Central nervous system disorders, such as multiple sclerosis, stroke, and traumatic brain injury, can also lead to vestibular dysfunction.

Vestibular rehabilitation training programs are designed on an individualized basis to improve functional skills and participation by helping to enhance gaze stability, promote improved postural stability, and minimize symptoms of vertigo and feeling off-balance. These goals may be accomplished by prescribing specific eye and head movement exercises, engaging the patient in a balance retraining program, or, in the case of BPPV, having the physical therapist perform a "repositioning maneuver" of the head to move the calcium crystals back to their original location.[13]

9

MULTIPLE SCLEROSIS

Multiple sclerosis (MS) is a disease in which an abnormal immune-mediated process is triggered, attacking the myelin sheath that coats nerve fibers within the central nervous system. This results in areas of demyelination, also referred to as **plaques**, which lead to disturbances in the conduction of messages along the nerves. The nerve axons themselves may also be attacked. The condition is most often manifested from ages 15 to 45 years and affects women more often than men. There is a geographical pattern of MS prevalence worldwide, with the disease occurring more frequently in areas that are farther away from the equator. The specific cause remains unknown. MS can cause a variety of symptoms, depending on the location of the patches of nerve demyelination and axonal disruption. Common symptoms include visual deficits, sensory problems such as tingling and numbness, weakness, fatigue, problems with balance, dizziness and vertigo, and bladder dysfunction.[14] MS is considered to be a neurodegenerative disease, whose course varies for each individual. Many patients will experience a relapsing/remitting form of MS, which is characterized by periods of **exacerbations** (worsening of symptoms) followed by disease remission. Others may experience a more progressive form of MS, where symptom plateaus or remissions rarely occur. When initially diagnosed with this disease, it is not possible to discern what pattern of MS might evolve over time. This uncertainty is a significantly challenging aspect of this disease.

Physical therapists providing care for individuals with MS must direct their attention to managing primary disease impairments and functional limitations, as well as secondary impairments that may have arisen because of reduced function and immobility. Equipment assessment and home or work modifications may need to be addressed. Patient and caregiver education emphasizing safety in upright transitions and locomotion, energy conservation, and fatigue management are important elements of the care plan. Exercise prescription is now considered essential, as there is a growing body of evidence that patients with MS can benefit from a regular exercise program that includes both strengthening and endurance components.[15] These programs have been shown to provide physical, psychological, and social benefits to participants.

In current clinical practice, the majority of patients with MS seek physical therapy services whenever there is an increase in impairment or decline in functional abilities. Clinicians currently involved in MS care are advocating for a shift in the emphasis of physical therapy care toward a secondary prevention model, where health and wellness are optimized through sustained activity participation and exercise adherence across the lifespan.[16]

PARKINSON'S DISEASE

Parkinson's disease (PD) is a neurodegenerative condition that affects over 1 million individuals in North America. PD is commonly seen with advancing age and is characterized by a classic triad of symptoms including tremor, rigidity, and bradykinesia.[17] **Tremor**, alternating contractions of opposing muscle groups, is the presenting symptom in about 70% of individuals. It usually affects the hands and feet and tends to occur at rest. **Rigidity**, a disturbance in muscle tone, is manifested as resistance when the limbs are passively moved, regardless of movement speed. **Bradykinesia**, or slowness of movements, is the most common feature and is a major cause of disability in individuals with PD. Postural instability is often also considered a cardinal symptom of PD; however, it tends to occur later in the disease process.[18]

This condition results from a deficiency in dopamine, a neurotransmitter (chemical messenger) produced in a region of the brain called the *substantia nigra.* The specific cause of this depletion is unknown. Even though a cure does not yet exist, treatments including medications, surgery, and therapeutic interventions are used to manage the symptoms. Medications that restore neurochemical balance are available and can alleviate the motor symptoms. Unfortunately, the effectiveness of the medications diminishes over the years, and the symptoms continue to worsen. Deep brain stimulation of a specific area of the brain has been shown to be effective in improving motor symptoms in a select group of patients,[19] and neural cell transplantation is under investigation as an option for a more permanent treatment or cure.[20]

The tremor, rigidity, bradykinesia, and postural instability have a great impact on the patient's ability to perform functional activities such as rising from a chair, walking, climbing stairs, and reaching. Patients tend to demonstrate a stooped posture and walk with short, shuffling steps and decreased reciprocal arm movements. The PT can play a vital role in teaching patients with Parkinson's disease specific movement and/or compensatory strategies that allow them to move more easily.[21] These patients can also benefit from physical therapy interventions that target the secondary problems, such as weakness, decreased range of motion, and decreased aerobic capacity. Finally, it is important to assist the patient in developing a lifelong commitment to physical activity and to educate the patient on the importance of self-management skills to promote overall wellness.[16]

GUILLAIN-BARRÉ SYNDROME

Guillain-Barré syndrome (GBS) is an acquired neuromuscular condition that is a result of an inflammatory process affecting the peripheral nerve. It is considered a rare condition as it affects approximately 1-2 individuals per 100,000 per year.[22,23] GBS often presents following a viral infection and manifests with symmetric, progressive weakness, often beginning in the lower extremities. Weakness of the muscles involved in respiration, resulting in the need for ventilatory support, occurs in 10-30% of individuals. Symptoms usually progress rapidly over a period of 2 weeks, reaching a plateau after 4 weeks. Treatments using plasmapherisis or administration of intravenous immunoglobulin are often employed. Functional recovery occurs over weeks to months, with the majority of individuals regaining the ability to walk within a year after onset.[24]

Physical therapy intervention often begins in the hospital and there is evidence that multidisciplinary care is effective in the rehabilitation setting.[25]

9

Physical therapists often focus on functional training while facilitating proper limb positioning and posture. Strengthening exercises are also often part of the therapeutic intervention.[26]

AMYOTROPHIC LATERAL SCLEROSIS

Amyotrophic lateral sclerosis (**ALS**, also known as *Lou Gehrig's disease* after the famous baseball player), is a rapidly progressive neurologic disorder associated with the degeneration of motor nerve cells. Its cause is unknown. The median age at onset is in the fifties.[27] ALS is characterized by weakness, atrophy (loss of muscle bulk), fasciculations (muscle twitches), and spasticity. The weakness can be present in limb muscles and can cause difficulty with functional activities, or it can be present in the bulbar muscles (muscles involved in speech, swallowing, and breathing) and can cause difficulty with communication, feeding, and respiration. Progression of muscular symptoms results in decline of functional abilities, resulting in individuals requiring assistance with activities of daily living and use of powered mobility equipment. While advances in medical management and technology have greatly improved the quality of life for individuals with ALS, there is no cure for this disease. Survival time after diagnosis is between 3 and 5 years. Currently, there is one medication, riluzole (Rilutek), that has been shown to slow progression and can extend life by about 3 months.[28]

The role of physical therapy is to maximize functional abilities while minimizing secondary complications due to progressive weakness. Recommendations regarding exercise programs, bracing and orthotic needs, and adaptive and assistive equipment are necessary components of intervention. Patient and family education is also an essential piece of intervention for individuals with ALS.

PRINCIPLES OF EXAMINATION

The goal of physical therapy for individuals with neuromuscular conditions is to improve or maintain task-related functional movements and participation and promote optimal health and wellness. Functional movements include those required to complete basic self-care activities (e.g., dressing, eating, and bathing), transitional movements (e.g., bed mobility, transfers, and walking), and those necessary for educational, vocational, and recreational purposes. Through the examination process, the physical therapist determines which movement system components remain functional and which may need to be addressed through treatment.

HISTORY

Most patients with neurologic problems are referred to physical therapy after extensive evaluation by a neurologist, physiatrist, or both. The therapist begins the examination process with a thorough review of all pertinent medical records and data so that he or she can understand the patient's current medical condition, other comorbid conditions, and past health history, including relevant psychological, emotional, and social factors.

Therapists should be familiar with and understand the results and implications of special tests used by physicians to determine the patient's medical (etiologic or pathologic) diagnosis. Table 9-1 provides a summary of some of the more common medical tests used to diagnose neuromuscular conditions.[29]

Table 9-1
Medical Tests Used in the Diagnosis of Neuromuscular Conditions

Diagnostic Test	What It Measures	Why It Is Used
Computerized tomography (CT)	Uses X-rays and computer processing to measure the density of brain and spinal cord bony and soft tissues	■ Good for detecting bony abnormalities and fractures, hemorrhages, brain atrophy, and hydrocephalus ■ Quicker and cheaper than MRI
Magnetic resonance imaging (MRI)	Uses radio frequency waves and a magnetic field to measure the water content of different anatomic tissues within the nervous system	■ Provides high-contrast imaging and good anatomic detail for pathology in the brainstem and cerebellum, tumors in the brain and spinal cord, and plaques associated with multiple sclerosis
Angiography	Provides view of blood vessels and their connections; involves injection of radiopaque dye into blood vessels	■ Identifies areas of blood vessel narrowing, bulging, or malformations ■ Gives view of blood vessels supplying brain tumors
Lumbar puncture (LP)	Procedure used to collect fluid surrounding the brain and spinal cord (the cerebrospinal fluid—CSF) for analysis	■ Assists with measuring intracranial pressure ■ Used to collect CSF fluid for analysis to identify bacteria, viruses, and chemical/cellular content ■ Used to inject a radiopaque substance for a myelogram
Electroencephalography (EEG)	Records electrical potentials within the brain	■ Assists with diagnosis of seizures
Nerve conduction velocity (NCV)	Records the speed with which sensory and motor nerves conduct impulses	■ Identifies peripheral nerve pathology
Electromyography (EMG)	Records electrical activity of muscles	■ Identifies muscle pathology

9

Pertinent to the examination is an interview with the patient or a family member or caregiver. The interview gives the therapist an opportunity to hear firsthand the sequence of events that brought the patient to therapy. It allows the therapist to ask specific questions that will provide information about the patient's premorbid lifestyle and functional level, as well as assess the patient's cognitive and communicative capabilities. Most importantly, it provides insight into the societal roles and functional activities that are important to patients, giving them an opportunity to express their own goals and concerns to the therapist. It also offers a chance to ascertain the patients' understanding of their health condition and any contributing factors that may be associated with it.

SYSTEMS REVIEW

Since many neuromuscular conditions involve multiple body systems, it is important for the physical therapist to perform a systems review to screen for potential areas of concern. The systems review includes the cardiovascular/ pulmonary, integumentary, musculoskeletal, and neuromuscular systems. In addition, the patient's general levels of cognition, arousal, and attention are assessed. Patient data, such as weight, height, and vital signs, are collected. The purpose of the systems review is to examine the patient from a holistic perspective to (1) determine what body systems need further physical therapy assessment, (2) guide decision making regarding appropriate tests and measures that should be used with the patient, and (3) determine if a patient needs a referral to another health care provider to manage an issue outside of the scope of practice of the physical therapist.

MOVEMENT ANALYSIS OF FUNCTIONAL TASKS

When examining patients with neuromuscular conditions, therapists often rely on their movement analysis skills to determine the quality of the patient's movements (e.g., speed, smoothness, direction, and amplitude) and the amount of assistance that is needed for safe performance of certain tasks. The most common activities of daily living that might be assessed include bed mobility skills (moving or changing positions in bed), functional sitting balance, transitions in and out of bed, chairs, or other surfaces, sit-to-stand transitions, functional standing balance, walking and climbing stairs, and getting up from the floor. If a patient has identified additional functional tasks and goals that are meaningful to her, these may also be observed and assessed, as illustrated in Figure 9-5, which shows an individual with posttraumatic brain injury being assessed while descending a ramp at her home. When performing any movement analysis, the therapist needs to consider the prevailing environmental conditions in which the patient is moving, as these may influence his or her functional abilities. Movement analysis findings direct the therapist in the selection of relevant tests and measures to use when examining the patient.

COGNITION

Cognitive functions, such as level of consciousness, orientation, attention, long- and short-term memory, reasoning, and judgment can be impaired in disorders

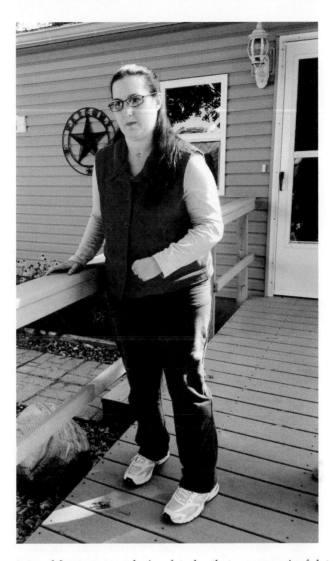

Figure 9-5 ■ Movement analysis of tasks that are meaningful to the patient, such as ramp negotiation, is an essential component of the examination process.

of the central nervous system. Impairments in this area may influence the patient's ability to follow commands and specific testing instructions while being examined by the physical therapist. Cognitive impairments will impact goal setting for the patient and will influence the structure and design of the therapeutic program. When working with patients with cognitive deficits, the neuropsychologist is a valuable resource for other team members regarding the optimal strategies that might be implemented to manage emotional and behavioral issues or assess changes in the level of cognitive functioning.

COMMUNICATION

Communication is another area that will have a major impact on how the therapist works with the patient. If the patient exhibits a diminished ability to receive and interpret verbal or written communication (**receptive aphasia**) or has an impaired ability to communicate his or her needs by speech (**expressive aphasia**), the therapist may have to use alternative communication strategies. For example, when working with patients with receptive aphasia, the therapist may need to demonstrate to the patient what is expected or required or use pictures to communicate basic concepts.

RANGE OF MOTION

Many individuals with neuromuscular conditions present with range of motion deficits that can affect the limbs, trunk, or neck. It is important for the therapist to document any range of motion impairments, as these will limit the movement options available to the patient. Movement restrictions are measured with the use of a goniometer. Deficits in range of motion can impact functional use of an extremity or create excessive energy costs during the execution of simple tasks.

MOTOR CONTROL

There are many different aspects of motor control that are addressed when examining an individual who has sustained some type of neurologic injury.[30] One of the first assessments is to observe whether the patient is capable of performing voluntary movement. If that is possible, the therapist can then determine whether the patient is able to isolate and control specific muscle actions in a coordinated manner, demonstrating smooth and accurate movement that is appropriately timed. Coordinated movement implies an ability to start, stop, reverse, change speed, change direction, and regulate force. Strength testing is an essential component of motor control testing, as weakness is a predominant problem in the majority of both central and peripheral nervous system conditions. In some cases, the therapist may notice the presence of some involuntary movements, such as a tremor, that might be seen either at rest or when the patient attempts to moves an extremity. Involuntary movements can sometimes interfere with functional limb use.

MUSCLE TONE

Muscle tone is generally defined as the inherent resistance that is felt when a muscle is passively stretched. Tone is considered to be a continuum from low (**hypotonia**) to high (**hypertonia**). Individuals who experience lower motor neuron disease tend to experience hypotonia, with a "floppy" feel to their muscles and joints. Individuals with central nervous system disorders are more apt to have **spasticity**, which is a velocity-dependent hypertonia. When muscle tone is altered from normal, a person's muscles may develop tightness, abnormal posturing, or reduced function. At times, hypertonia in certain muscle groups may be used by patients to assist with completing some functional tasks.

SENSATION AND PERCEPTION

Both sensation and perception are essential for normal coordinated movement. **Sensation** is the ability to receive sensory input from within and outside of the body and transmit it through the peripheral nerves and tracts in the spinal cord to the brain, where it is received and interpreted. Sensory information that is essential for movement comes through visual, vestibular, somatosensory, and auditory channels. **Perception** refers to the ability to integrate sensory information and interpret it in a meaningful manner. Perception is a cognitive function. An example of a perceptual deficit is a **unilateral spatial neglect**, which refers to an inability to integrate sensory information from one side of a person's body.

PRINCIPLES OF EVALUATION, DIAGNOSIS, AND PROGNOSIS

From the preceding brief descriptions, it is apparent that seemingly simple movements and activities are the result of complex and interconnected mechanisms. Sometimes therapists need several sessions to diagnose the movement disorders and functional limitations and identify the responsible components. Based on the findings of this detailed evaluation, a plan of care can be developed to meet goals of enhancing movement and function.

PRINCIPLES OF INTERVENTION

As procedural training unfolds in physical therapy, there are a number of general goals that are addressed, regardless of the etiology of the patient's neurologic deficits. The general goals of neurorehabilitation interventions include the following:

- Improve overall mobility and motor skill acquisition.
- Adapt functional mobility strategies to changing task and environmental conditions.
- Empower patients to solve their own motor problems when faced with novel situations.
- Resolve, reduce, and prevent impairments.
- Promote health and wellness.

Physical therapists use their patient assessment data to determine if the focus of their therapeutic interventions will be directed at recovery of function, compensation, or a blend of both.[31] Functional recovery implies that interventions will be designed to facilitate the patient's ability to successfully accomplish a task in the same manner it was performed prior to neurologic injury. Interventions that are designed to focus on compensation direct the patient's efforts at successful task completion using alternative methods or substitutions. For example, training a patient to complete a normally bimanual task using just one hand is an example of a compensatory technique. Oftentimes, procedural interventions may include a blend of both recovery and compensatory strategies. An example of a blended interventional strategy would be to encourage a patient to walk in therapy without an assistive device while simultaneously requiring him or her to use a cane for safe ambulation outside of therapy.

MOTOR CONTROL THEORIES AND APPROACHES

The field of **motor control**, which addresses how movement is organized and coordinated, provides the theoretical basis for the design and progression of task-oriented procedural interventions for neuromuscular conditions. Motor control theories have changed significantly across the years as our understanding of movement science has evolved. In response to this evolution, different interventions and training techniques have been developed and used clinically across the years.

From a historical perspective, early approaches to managing the movement deficits seen following upper motor neuron lesions were based on the work of several famous neurophysiologists who studied animals with different nervous system lesions.[32] These scientists addressed the contribution of reflex activity to movement and theorized relationships among different movement control centers located in the brain and the spinal cord. Their work supported a view of the central nervous system as having a reactive role in movement control. From the 1940s to the 1970s, several key physical therapists applied this work and the motor control theories that developed from it to their observations of individuals with upper motor neuron dysfunction, creating "traditional" treatment approaches such as proprioceptive neuromuscular facilitation (PNF), the Brunnstrom approach to hemiplegia, and neurodevelopmental treatment (NDT). Although the theory upon which many components of these approaches was based is no longer supported with current research evidence, each of these approaches made contributions to our understanding of movement following nervous system injury. For example, the PNF approach focused on the contribution of sensation to the movement system and emphasized the interaction of multijoint extremity muscle activity and proximal control to normal human movement. Both of these topics continue to be relevant today. The Brunnstrom approach, which was based on qualitative observations of poststroke motor recovery, continues to influence outcome measures used to assess the effectiveness of physical therapy interventions. At its inception, the NDT approach strongly emphasized the inhibition of abnormal movement patterns and abnormal muscle tone so that normal movement could occur. This approach also emphasized the importance of trunk control and posture to overall human movement, which is a concept that continues to influence current practice.[31] To date, many physical therapists continue to use modified elements of these traditional approaches to help them solve their patients' movement problems, although the rationale underlying their choice has been reframed to better align with current theories of motor control.

The traditional motor control theories and approaches were each somewhat distinct in their management of activity and impairment-based problems. Today, the predominant theories and approaches are a bit more congruent with one another and tend to be heavily influenced by the science of motor learning, which refers to one's ability to acquire motor skills and modify movement with practice. Currently, there are several theories of motor control influencing neurorehabilitation. Some of these are directed at an understanding of movement from an integrated perspective, taking into account the contribution of multiple body systems, including the nervous, musculoskeletal, cardiovascular, and cognitive/psychological systems. These theories suggest a more active role of the nervous system in movement control, rather than a reactive, passive role. Current theories also emphasize how movement emerges from an interaction of the person, the task he or she is attempting to perform, and the environment in which he or she is working.[30]

NEUROPLASTICITY AND INTERVENTION DESIGN

An understanding of **neuroplasticity**, which refers to the brain and spinal cord's ability to adapt and remodel themselves as they learn new behaviors and skills, has had a significant impact on the clinical decision making associated with selecting physical therapy interventions for individuals with neurologic disorders.[33] The current emphasis on task-specific training has evolved as a result of this body of work. Studies addressing neuroplasticity show that neurons within the brain are able to alter their function or anatomic structure in response to both internal and external circumstances surrounding injury and postinjury experiences. Through the work of basic and clinical scientists, we have learned some key factors that govern a patient's ability to acquire new motor skills. For example, there is ample evidence that when confronted with a movement goal such as reaching for and grasping an object following a neurologic injury, patients learn by trial and error that they can be quicker and more efficient with task completion if they use their lesser involved upper extremity, rather than their weaker extremity. Over time, this **learned nonuse** of the involved extremity, which is the phenomenon illustrated by this example, results in a reduction in brain activation and support for these actions. Kleim and Jones[33] refer to this concept as the principle of "use it or lose it." These researchers also emphasize principles such as the importance of task repetition, specificity of action, training intensity, and meaningful goal-directed movement. Each of these principles, when used in a positive manner, is capable of creating neuroplastic changes that may enhance movement and functional recovery. The opposite is true as well—brain activation in specific anatomic regions can be negatively impacted when motor skill acquisition training does not emphasize these concepts. These findings from basic science and clinical research hold important and exciting implications for physical therapists. They support the concept that whether postneurologic injury recovery is enhanced or inhibited depends, in part, on the design of the training experiences and the interventions that are selected by the physical therapist.

MOTOR LEARNING

Principles of motor learning serve as additional factors that influence the structure of therapy sessions in neurologic clinical practice. Clinicians strive to create therapeutic situations that will enhance **motor learning**, which implies that there has been a relatively permanent change in a patient's ability to perform some type of skill. Motor learning occurs in stages, where the learner first learns what to do (cognitive stage), then refines his movements (the associative stage), and finally develops skill (autonomous stage).[31] At each stage, the action of the therapist will change so that the patient's motor learning can be optimized.

Studies addressing motor skill acquisition point to the importance of practice for successful motor skill acquisition. As patients practice performing different tasks, the physical therapist is charged with the task of creating the most appropriate training environment to optimize motor learning. Different motor learning variables can be manipulated by the physical therapist during training, depending upon the task being practiced, the patient's stage of motor learning, the response of the patient, the environmental conditions, and the desired therapeutic goal associated with the training. Some examples of motor learning variables that can be modified include those addressing the practice conditions and the feedback that is provided to the patient.[30]

Practice condition variables include:

■ Blocked practice: Practice of one task for a block of trials.
■ Random practice: Practice of several different tasks in a random order.
■ Whole versus part task training: Refers to practice of either a complete continuous task versus breaking down a task into its component parts and having the patient learn these first before tackling the entire task.

Feedback variables include:

■ Intrinsic feedback: Refers to sensory input about the movement process that the patient receives from his own sensory organs.
■ Extrinsic feedback: This refers to movement information that comes from sources outside of the patient's internal sensory systems (e.g., auditory or tactile cuing provided by the therapist).
■ Feedback schedule: Frequency and timing of feedback.
■ Type of feedback: Positive feedback (movement success) versus negative feedback (movement errors).
■ Focus of attention: Directing the learner's attention to himself (internal focus) versus attending to movement variables outside of himself.

ACTIVITY-BASED TRAINING PARADIGMS

Several different activity-based motor skill training paradigms have been used to improve both upper and lower extremity function following neurologic injury. **Constraint-induced movement therapy (CIMT)**, which was developed by Dr. Edward Taub, focuses on regaining the use of a more involved upper extremity. It has been most widely used as a functional training technique for those who have some active wrist and finger movement following stroke.[34] This paradigm involves constraining use of the patient's lesser involved arm while engaging the involved arm in intensive training and practice of specific tasks. This enables the patient to overcome the phenomenon of learned nonuse. Locomotor training with body weight support is a technique that focuses on facilitating trunk and lower limb alignment and movement for walking. The patient dons a harness that provides some trunk and pelvic support, with straps that attach to an overhead suspension system for support (Figure 9-6). Training can be performed on a treadmill with the therapist facilitating limb and trunk movements and postures as needed. The body weight support system can also be used for overground walking. This technique has been used for locomotor training in individuals who have sustained a stroke, spinal cord injury, or who have Parkinson's disease.[35]

MANAGEMENT OF IMPAIRMENTS

In addition to activity-based procedural training for motor skill acquisition, physical therapists treating individuals with neurologic involvement frequently

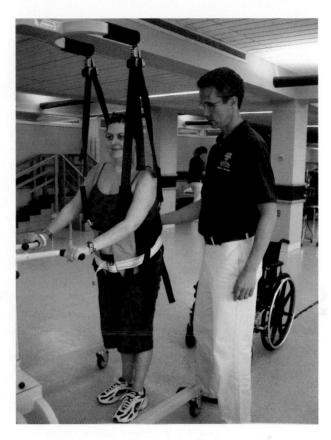

Figure 9-6 ■ Patient gait training using a body weight support system.

prescribe interventions that target body structure/function impairments.[31] Stretching and strengthening exercise programs are frequently needed to improve flexibility and strengthen key muscle groups. Figure 9-7 illustrates an individual following a spinal cord injury working on upper body strengthening. Neuromuscular electrical stimulation (NMES) or functional electrical stimulation (FES) are sometimes used as adjunct treatments to facilitate motor control or the timing of a muscle contraction, assist in maintaining range of motion, or provide an orthotic assist to an extremity joint. Assistive devices and bracing options may need to be used as compensatory techniques to assist with balance, safety, and function. The therapist may also recommend environmental modifications to help the patient function more effectively.

PATIENT-RELATED INSTRUCTION

A large part of neurorehabilitation is devoted to educating patients about their disease and its sequela. Many neurologic diseases are associated with other comorbidities, so educational efforts may need to address these issues as well. Since the majority of neurologic health conditions are chronic in nature, patients

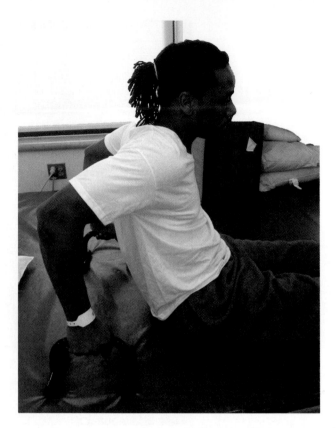

Figure 9-7 ■ Patient with a spinal cord injury working on upper body strengthening.

and their families require health-related instruction to enable them to optimize health and wellness and prevent future adverse health events or emergencies.

SUMMARY

The goal of neuromuscular physical therapy is to evaluate movement and activity limitations resulting from damage to the nervous system and to design therapeutic interventions that enable a patient to acquire the necessary motor skills to recover function. If the problems are untreatable and progressive, the goal is to teach the patient and caregivers to accommodate and compensate for the problems and prevent secondary complications. The therapist—in conjunction with the patient, family, and other caregivers—will draw up a plan of care with appropriate short- and long-term goals and specific strategies, which may include hands-on interventions using some of the approaches described earlier, as well as education of the patient and family members regarding exercises and activities the patient or family can perform to meet these goals. An ongoing process of examination, evaluation, and intervention modification will occur to assure that the patient's goals are met. The ultimate objective is to help rehabilitate the patient to function at the highest level attainable within the constraints of the health condition.

CASE STUDY Jim is an 18-year-old man who sustained a gunshot wound to his thoracic spine. The bullet shattered his vertebra and caused damage to the spinal cord that resulted paraplegia. He also sustained abdominal injuries that required surgery. Jim is now medically stable and has been referred to therapy to begin the long process of rehabilitation.

The first task of the team members (which include a physiatrist, nurse, psychologist, social worker, and physical and occupational therapists) is to complete a thorough evaluation. After all evaluations are complete, a team meeting is scheduled to discuss the plan of care including short- and long-term goals. A family meeting may also be scheduled during the rehabilitation stay in order to discuss discharge plans. Early in the rehabilitation stage, it is often difficult to tell how extensive and permanent the neurologic damage is—it usually takes several months to make a definitive prognosis, and hence these goals will probably need periodic review and adjustment.

Even as team members were conducting their evaluations, the PT had already started treatment and management to maintain mobility, increase strength in the uninvolved muscles, and educate the patient about problems arising from loss of sensation. The nurses had initiated a program to manage bowel and bladder function. The psychologist had begun helping Jim cope with the trauma of this unexpected event and the loss of body image and body functions. The social worker was starting to determine Jim's needs at discharge and whether these needs could be met by his family and in the current home environment.

During the next several weeks the team will continue to reevaluate Jim thoroughly for any changes in sensory or motor recovery, which will help determine the prognosis. The team members will start making discharge and placement plans based on Jim's recovery, his functional abilities, the family's needs in being able to care for him at home, their insurance coverage for necessary services, and so on. Team members will continue to work with Jim to teach the new skills necessary to function as independently as possible. The PT will play a major role in teaching Jim mobility skills such as moving around in bed and getting in and out of the wheelchair. The therapist will also be involved in making recommendations for equipment, such as the appropriate wheelchair and cushion, to meet the needs of his lifestyle. The therapist will also educate Jim and his family regarding home accessibility needs such as a ramped entrance, widened doorways, and bathroom adaptations. The family may be able to get some financial help for home modifications or may end up bearing the complete financial burden themselves.

Not only is Jim dealing with many physical and psychological challenges, but the family is also dealing with many emotional issues. As the therapist works with Jim and his family, they will frequently be very open during these sessions and voice their fears and concerns. The therapist's role is to provide not only technical support for the physical needs but also psychological and emotional support for both the patient and the family.

9

REFERENCES

1. Sacco RL, Kasner SE, Broderick JP, et al.: An updated definition of stroke for the 21st century: a statement for healthcare professionals from the American Heart Association/American Stroke Association, *Stroke* 44(7):2064–2089, 2013.
2. O'Sullivan SB: Stroke. In O'Sullivan SB, Schmitz TJ, Fulk GD, editors: *Physical rehabilitation*, ed 6, Philadelphia, PA, 2014, FA Davis Co., pp 645–720.
3. Ostir GV, Berges IM, Ottenbacher A, et al.: Patterns of change in depression after stroke, *J Am Geriatr Soc* 59(2):314–320, 2011.
4. Jauch EC, Saver JL, Adams HP, et al.: Guidelines for the early management of patients with acute ischemic stroke: a guideline for healthcare professionals from the American Heart Association/American Stroke Association. http://stroke.ahajournals.org/content/early/2013/01/31/STR. 0b013e318284056a.full. Accessed October 1, 2014.
5. Teasell R, Hussein N: Background concepts in stroke rehabilitation, Evidence-Based Review of Stroke Rehabilitation (EBRSR) website. Update November 2013. http://www.ebrsr.com/sites/default/files/Chapter3_Background-Concepts_FINAL_16ed.pdf. Accessed October 1, 2014 (chapter 3).
6. About brain injury, Brain Injury Association of America website. http://www.biausa.org/about-brain-injury.htm#definitions. Accessed October 1, 2014.
7. Traumatic brain injury in the United States: fact sheet, Centers for Disease Control and Prevention website. http://www.cdc.gov/traumaticbraininjury/get_the_facts.html. Accessed October 1, 2014.
8. Fulk GD, Nirider CD: Traumatic brain injury. In O'Sullivan SB, Schmitz TJ, Fulk GD, editors: *Physical rehabilitation*, ed 6, Philadelphia, PA, 2014, FA Davis Co., pp 859–888.
9. Fulk GD, Behrman AL, Schmitz TJ: Traumatic spinal cord injury. In O'Sullivan SB, Schmitz TJ, Fulk GD, editors: *Physical rehabilitation*, ed 6, Philadelphia, PA, 2014, FA Davis Co., pp 889–964.
10. Field-Fote EC: *Spinal cord injury rehabilitation,* Philadelphia, PA, 2009, FA Davis Co.
11. Schubert MC: Vestibular disorders. In O'Sullivan SB, Schmitz TJ, Fulk GD, editors: *Physical rehabilitation*, ed 6, Philadelphia, PA, 2014, FA Davis Co., pp 965–999.
12. Tusa RJ: Bedside assessment of the dizzy patient, *Neurol Clin* 23(3):655–673, 2005.
13. Furman JM, Cass SP: Benign paroxysmal positional vertigo, *N Engl J Med* 341:1590–1596, 1999.
14. O'Sullivan SB: Multiple sclerosis. In O'Sullivan SB, Schmitz TJ, Fulk GD, editors: *Physical rehabilitation*, ed 6, Philadelphia, PA, 2014, FA Davis Co., pp 721–768.
15. Latimer-Cheung AE, Martin Ginis KA, Hicks AL, et al.: Development of evidence-informed physical activity guidelines for adults with multiple sclerosis, *Arch Phys Med Rehabil* 94:1829–1836, 2013.
16. Ellis T, Motl RW: Activity behavior change in persons with neurologic disorders: overview and examples from Parkinson disease and multiple sclerosis, *J Neurol Phys Ther* 37:85–89, 2013.
17. O'Sullivan SB, Bezkor EW: Parkinson's disease. In O'Sullivan SB, Schmitz TJ, Fulk GD, editors: *Physical rehabilitation*, ed 6, Philadelphia, PA, 2014, FA Davis Co., pp 807–858.
18. Gelb DJ, Oliver E, Gilman S: Diagnostic criteria for Parkinson disease, *Arch Neurol* 56(1):33–39, 1999. http://dx.doi.org/10.1001/archneur.56.1.33.
19. Foltynie T, Hariz MI: Surgical management of Parkinson's disease, *Expert Rev Neurother* 10 (6):903–914, 2010.
20. Urbaniak HK, Yarbrough C, Ciacci J: Gene- and cell-based approaches for neurodegenerative disease, *Adv Exp Med Biol* 671:117–130, 2010.
21. Morris ME, Martin CL, Schenkman ML: Striding out with Parkinson disease: evidence-based physical therapy for gait disorders, *Phys Ther* 90:280–288, 2010.
22. Cosi V, Versino M: Guillain-Barré syndrome, *Neurol Sci* 27(Suppl 1):S47–S51, 2006.
23. Office of Rare Diseases, National Institute of Health. http://rarediseases.info.nih.gov. Accessed October 2, 2014.
24. El Mhandi L, Calmels P, Camdessanché JP, et al.: Muscle strength recovery in treated Guillain-Barré syndrome: a prospective study for the first 18 months after onset, *Am J Phys Med Rehabil* 86:716–724, 2007.
25. Khan F, Amatya B: Rehabilitation interventions in patients with acute demyelinating inflammatory polyneuropathy: a systemic review, *Eur J Phys Rehabil Med* 48:507–522, 2012.
26. Orsini M, de Freitas MRG, Presto B, et al.: Guideline for neuromuscular rehabilitation in Guillain-Barré syndrome: what can we do? *Rev Neurosci* 18(4):572–580, 2010.

27. Brooke M: Diseases of the motor neurons. In Brooke M, editor: *A clinician's view of neuromuscular diseases*, Baltimore, MD, 1986, Williams and Wilkins.
28. Miller RG, Mitchell JD, Lyon M, et al.: Riluzole for amyotrophic lateral sclerosis (ALS)/motor neuron disease (MND), *Cochrane Database Syst Rev* 2:CD001447, 2002.
29. Blumenthal H: Introduction to clinical neuroradiology. In Blumenthal H, editor: *Neuroanatomy through clinical cases*, Sunderland, MA, 2010, Sinauer Associates, Inc., pp 86–123.
30. Shumway-Cook A, Woollacott MH: *Motor control: translating research into clinical practice, theory and practical applications*, ed 3, Philadelphia, PA, 2007, Lippincott Williams & Wilkins.
31. O'Sullivan SB: Strategies for improving motor function. In O'Sullivan SB, Schmitz TJ, Fulk GD, editors: *Physical rehabilitation*, ed 6, Philadelphia, PA, 2014, FA Davis Co., pp 393–443.
32. Pinkston D: Evolution of the practice of physical therapy in the United States. In Scully RM, Barnes MR, editors: *Physical therapy*, Philadelphia, PA, 1989, JB Lippincott.
33. Kleim JA, Jones TA: Principles of experience-dependent neural plasticity: implications for rehabilitation after brain damage, *J Speech Lang Hear Res* 51:S225–S239, 2008.
34. Wolf S, Winstein C, Miller J, et al.: Effect of constraint-induced movement therapy on upper extremity function 3 to 9 months after stroke: the EXCITE randomized clinical trial, *JAMA* 296 (17):2095–2104, 2006.
35. Fulk GD, Schmitz TJ: Locomotor training. In O'Sullivan SB, Schmitz TJ, Fulk GD, editors: *Physical rehabilitation*, ed 6, Philadelphia, PA, 2014, FA Davis Co., pp 444–484.

ADDITIONAL RESOURCES

The following is a list of websites providing the most up-to-date information regarding the cause, prevention, treatment, and management of various neuromuscular conditions. Several of the lay organizations provide a wealth of educational materials for patients and families, and some also provide links to support groups.

http://www.ninds.nih.gov/—National Institute of Neurological Disorders and Stroke (NINDS).
www.cdc.gov—Centers for Disease Control (CDC) and Prevention.
www.neuropt.org—Neurology Section of the American Physical Therapy Association.
www.strokeassociation.org—American Stroke Association.
www.spinalcord.org—National Spinal Cord Injury Association.
http://www.apdaparkinson.org/—American Parkinson Disease Association.
www.nmss.org—National Multiple Sclerosis Society.
www.vestibular.org—Vestibular Disorders Association.
mdausa.org—Muscular Dystrophy Association.

9

REVIEW QUESTIONS

1. Why might the physical therapy plan of care change several times for a patient recovering from a stroke?
2. List the kinds of information you might hope to gain from interviewing the patient and family. What other insights does the interview provide?
3. Why is movement analysis an important part of the examination process in a patient with a neuromuscular condition?
4. Describe the purposes of at least three diagnostic tests for neuromuscular disorders.
5. What purpose do braces, assistive devices, and environmental modifications serve in neuromuscular rehabilitation?

Those aspects of physical therapy commonly referred to as cardiovascular/pulmonary physical therapy are fully recognized as fundamental components of the knowledge and practice base for all entry-level physical therapists.

E.A. Hillegass, PT, and H.S. Sadowsky, PT

10

Physical Therapy in Cardiovascular and Pulmonary Conditions

Tiffany Hilton

KEYWORDS

angina
arteriosclerosis
blood gas analysis
cardiac catheterization
cardiac muscle dysfunction
cardiac pacemaker
chronic obstructive pulmonary disease (COPD)
conducting airways
congestive heart failure (CHF)
coronary artery bypass graft (CABG)
coronary heart disease (CHD)
dyspnea
echocardiography
electrocardiogram (ECG)

embolus
exercise stress testing
expiration
FITT principle of exercise prescription
heart failure
inspiration
ischemia
myocardial infarction (MI)
obstructive lung disease
percutaneous coronary intervention (PCI)
postural drainage
pulmonary function test
respiration
restrictive lung disease
spirometer
tachypnea
target heart rate (THR)
training zone
ventilation

LEARNING OBJECTIVES

After reading this chapter, the reader will be able to:

- Describe the normal anatomy and physiology of the cardiovascular and pulmonary systems.
- Define and describe the effects of common diseases that alter normal function of the cardiovascular and pulmonary systems.
- Outline how the functions of the cardiovascular and pulmonary systems are evaluated both normally and when disease is present.
- Discuss how physical therapists examine, evaluate, and provide interventions to individuals who have cardiovascular or pulmonary disease.

GENERAL DESCRIPTION

PREVALENCE

Physical therapists (PTs) and physical therapist assistants (PTAs) promote heath and wellness and the prevention and management of cardiovascular and pulmonary conditions. Regardless of the clinical setting, PTs and PTAs may treat patients with cardiac and pulmonary conditions as primary or secondary diagnoses. Significant advances in the diagnosis and treatment of cardiovascular and pulmonary conditions during the past 30 years, coupled with positive changes in modifiable risk factors, have resulted in a decline in the number of deaths. As individuals with these conditions are living longer lives, PTs and PTAs play a major role in improving functional performance, enhancing quality of life, and increasing the chances of living an independent life after disease. Despite the remarkable progress, cardiovascular and pulmonary conditions remain leading causes of morbidity and mortality.

Cardiovascular disease (CVD) remains the number one cause of death for men and women in the United States, claiming approximately 600,000 lives in 2010 (last full data set available).[1] This represents 24% of the more than 2.4 million people who died that year (Figure 10-1).[2] The economic impact and prevalence of this disease are extensive. Estimated direct and indirect costs for 2010 were $485.6 billion for the 81.1 million American adults who had CVD. A policy statement from the American Heart Association indicates that 40.5% of the U.S. population is projected to have CVD by 2030.[3] Total direct medical costs of CVD are projected to triple and total indirect costs are projected to increase 60% between 2010 and 2030. These substantial increases in CVD prevalence and costs demonstrate that effective strategies for prevention are essential.[3] Data from 2007 to 2010 indicate that 33% of U.S. adults have hypertension, ~14% of U.S. adults have high cholesterol, and 8.3% of the population have diagnosed diabetes

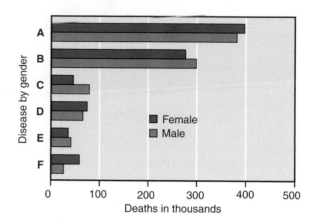

Figure 10-1 ■ Leading causes of death in the United States, 2010. **A**, Total cardiovascular disease. **B**, Cancer. **C**, Accidents. **D**, Chronic lower respiratory disease. **E**, Diabetes mellitus. **F**, Alzheimer's disease. (Modified from Go AS, Mozaffarian D, Roger VL, et al: Heart disease and stroke statistics 2014 update: A report from the American Heart Association, *Circulation*, 129(3):e28–e292, 2014.)

mellitus.[2] In 2011, 18% of high school students reported cigarette smoking.[2] The U.S. Department of Health and Human Services launched Million Hearts® in 2011 to focus clinical attention on the prevention of heart attack and stroke. Strategies to reduce the prevalence of leading CVD risk factors such as hypertension, high cholesterol, and smoking are emphasized by the campaign to reduce CVD.[4] Coronary heart disease (CHD), disease specifically of the heart and its vascular supply, is responsible for 48% of all the deaths caused by CVD (Figure 10-2).[2] This represents 1 of every 6 deaths in the United States in 2010. Approximately every 34 seconds an American undergoes a coronary event, and about every 1 minute 23 seconds, an American dies of a cardiac event. For 2010, an estimated 785,000 Americans had a new heart attack (myocardial infarction [MI]) and 470,000 had recurrent attacks.[2]

Besides attempts to alter the lifestyle of a person who is at risk for heart disease to decrease the risk factors, direct intervention is commonly used to manage heart disease. In 2010, an estimated 492,000 **percutaneous coronary interventions (PCI)** were performed. The most common PCI procedure requires inserting a tube into a coronary vessel and inflating a balloon on the end of the tube to open up a blockage in the vessel to restore normal blood flow. Nearly 397,000 coronary artery bypass procedures were performed, 370,000, pacemaker procedures were completed, and 2378 heart transplantations were performed in 2012.[2]

Chronic obstructive pulmonary disease (COPD) comprises a group of lung diseases that are characterized by obstruction of airflow through the bronchial system and in some cases destruction of lung parenchyma. Emphysema and chronic bronchitis are the two most common COPD conditions and are often found together in the same patient. Asthma is not included in this definition of COPD.

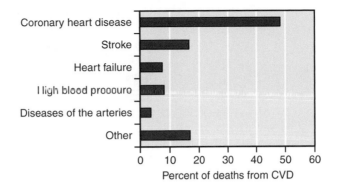

Figure 10-2 ■ Percentage breakdown of deaths attributable to cardio-vascular diseases in the United States, 2010. (Modified from Go AS, Mozaffarian D, Roger VL, et al: Heart disease and stroke statistics 2014 update: A report from the American Heart Association, *Circulation*, 129(3):e28–e292, 2014.)

In 2011 (last full data set available), 12.7 million people in the United States aged 18 or over had a diagnosis of COPD.[5] COPD is the third leading cause of death in the United States, and for the past 11 years more women than men have died of COPD. As in CVD, gender, race, and age affect the population in which COPD develops. Women are two times as likely to have chronic bron-chitis compared to men. In 2011, 6.8 million women and 3.3 million men were diagnosed with chronic bronchitis. In 2011, chronic bronchitis prevalence was greatest in non-Hispanic blacks. Historically, men have had higher prevalence rates of emphysema than women. However, this trend appears to be changing as the prevalence rate of emphysema among women increased greater than 60% in women and decreased 6% in men. In 2011, 2.5 million women were diagnosed with emphysema compared to 21.1 million men. In 2010, the projected annual cost of COPD to the nation was $49.9 billion. This included $29.5 billion in direct health care costs, $8 billion in indirect morbidity costs, and $12.4 billion in indi-rect mortality costs.[5]

Physical therapists must have a thorough understanding of the normal anat-omy and physiology of the cardiac and pulmonary systems. With this knowl-edge, the therapist can evaluate these systems, determine if the patient is appropriate to treat, and develop optimal rehabilitation programs.

CARDIOVASCULAR SYSTEM

HEART

The heart is positioned left of center in the chest cavity (mediastinum), with the base located superiorly and the apex inferiorly and left of center. A fibrous tissue known as the *pericardial sac* surrounds the heart. The major portion of the heart is made up of muscle tissue referred to as the *myocardium*. This tissue is cross-striated with layers of muscle fibers arranged in multiple directions.[6]

The heart has two pairs of matched chambers. The two atria are thin-walled chambers, whereas the two ventricles have much thicker muscular walls

10

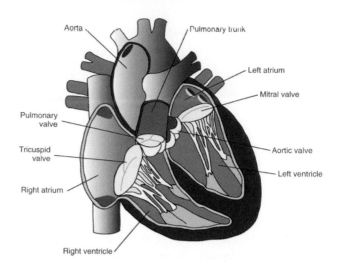

Figure 10-3 ■ Schematic view of the heart and the heart chambers and valves. (From Workman ML, LaCharity L, Kruchco S: *Understanding pharmacology*. Saunders, St. Louis, 2011.)

(Figure 10-3).[7] These chambers are separated by valves that direct the blood through the chambers in a specific pattern.

The right atrium receives venous blood from the body through the superior and inferior venae cavae. With atrial contraction (atrial systole) the blood then passes through the tricuspid valve into the right ventricle (Figure 10-4, *A*).[7] The left atrium receives oxygenated blood through the pulmonary veins coming from the lungs. During atrial systole, this oxygenated blood passes through the bicuspid (mitral) valve into the left ventricle (Figure 10-4, *B*).[7]

Once the right and left ventricles have received blood from their respective atria, ventricular contraction (ventricular systole) occurs. This contraction results in an increase in pressure in the ventricular chambers, which causes the tricuspid and bicuspid valves to close tightly and prevents blood from passing back into the atria. As ventricular contraction continues, venous blood leaves the right ventricle through the pulmonic or semilunar valve and flows into the lungs to be reoxygenated. Oxygenated blood leaves the left ventricle through the aortic valve into the aorta to be transported to the body through the systemic circulation.

It is significant that the ventricles have thicker muscular walls than the atria. This greater muscle mass, especially in the left ventricle, must provide enough force to overcome the resistance to flow that blood encounters as it moves through the peripheral arteries.[8]

CONDUCTION

The myocardium contains special types of tissue responsible for conducting the electrical impulse that causes the myocardium to contract in a synchronized pattern. The synchronized depolarization and repolarization of cardiac muscle

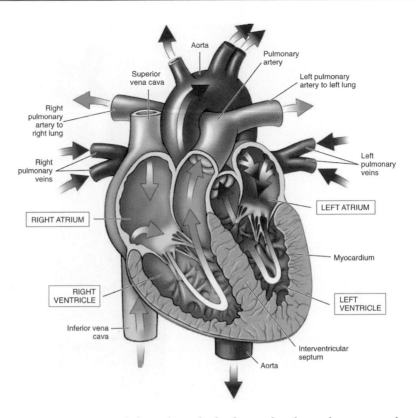

Figure 10-4 ■ Blood flow through the heart chambers: deoxygenated blood flow (blue) from the right atrium to the right ventricle to the lung through the pulmonary artery; oxygenated blood (red) returning to the left atrium from the lungs via the pulmonary veins, moving into the left ventricle, and exiting through the aorta. (From Herlihy B: *The human body in health and illness.* ed 5, Saunders, St. Louis, 2014.)

result in efficient movement of blood through the chambers of the heart and through the coronary and peripheral vessels.

The specialized tissues are called *nodal* and *Purkinje fibers* (Figure 10-5).[7] The sinoatrial (SA) node initiates the impulse (sinus rhythm) and is referred to as the *pacemaker* of the heart. Once a signal is initiated by the SA node, it travels quickly through the walls of the atria on special tracts to the atrioventricular (AV) node. The impulse also travels to the muscle fibers of the atria and causes them to contract. The AV node transports the signal to the bundle of His, which is where the Purkinje fibers start to spread out into the muscle fibers of the ventricles. For every heartbeat or contraction, the depolarization signal that causes the myocardium to contract must travel through this conduction system of the heart.

Both the SA and AV nodes receive autonomic nerve fibers via the sympathetic and parasympathetic systems. These nerve fibers release special neurotransmitters that influence the rate of contraction and myocardial contractility. The ability

10

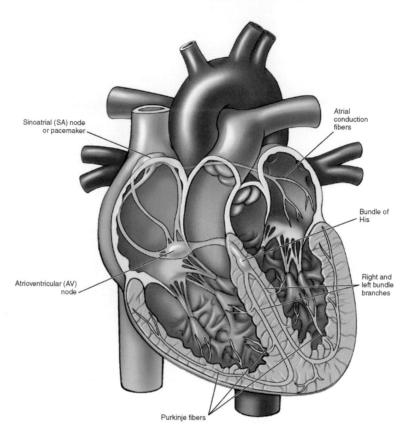

Figure 10-5 ■ Conduction system of the heart, illustrating the location of the sinoatrial (SA) and atrioventricular (AV) nodes. (From Herlihy B: *The human body in health and illness.* ed 5, Saunders, St. Louis, 2014.)

to influence the heart's rate and contractility is extremely important because this mechanism allows the central nervous system to tell the heart how to respond to increases in demand, such as those made during exercise.[8]

CORONARY ARTERIES

The myocardium receives its blood supply from two major vessels: the right and left coronary arteries (Figure 10-6).[9] These arteries arise from the ascending aorta, which is the major artery leaving the left ventricle and carrying blood to the body (see Figure 10-3). In general, the right and left coronary vessels supply the right and left sides of the heart, respectively; however, this arrangement can vary a great deal among individuals. If something occurs that causes blockage of a coronary vessel, it is important to determine exactly how that blockage alters blood flow to the individual's myocardium. A blockage that prevents oxygen supply to the heart, causing permanent damage to the heart cells, is known as an MI or heart attack.

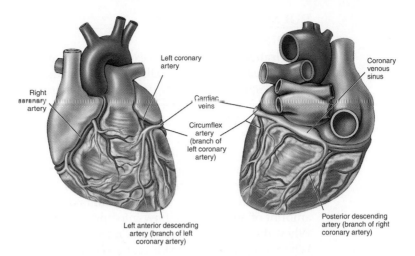

Figure 10-6 ■ Blood is supplied to the tissues of the heart by the right and left coronary arteries. The left coronary artery branches into the left anterior descending artery and the circumflex artery. The coronary veins collect blood and empty it into the coronary sinus, which eventually empties into the right atrium. (From Edmunds M: *Introduction to clinical pharmacology.* ed 7, Mosby, St. Louis, 2013.)

PERIPHERAL CIRCULATION

The blood vessels that comprise the peripheral circulation are arteries, capillaries, and veins, and disorders in these vessels can result in cardiovascular and pulmonary dysfunction. PTs and PTAs work with a variety of patients who have disabilities caused by pathologic changes in the peripheral circulation.

The arteries, of which the aorta has the largest diameter, and the arterioles have elastic fibers and smooth muscle in their walls. If the smooth muscle contracts, the diameter of the vessel is decreased, which causes an increase in the resistance to blood flow through the vessels. Arterioles are often referred to as "resistance vessels." Changes in resistance to blood flow in the peripheral circulation directly affect how hard the heart has to work to pump blood through the body. A disease called **arteriosclerosis**, which is often referred to as "hardening of the arteries," occurs when the walls of the arteries become thick and stiff. Arteriosclerosis decreases the elasticity of the vessel resulting in higher resistance to blood flow, subsequently restricting blood flow to the tissues and organs.

Capillaries are the smallest vessels in the peripheral circulation. They connect arteries to veins and can be so small that they allow only one red blood cell to pass through at a time. Their walls are only one cell thick, which permits efficient exchange of oxygen and carbon dioxide. Nutrients and waste products also pass through the wall. Capillaries are often referred to as "exchange vessels."

The veins, which return blood to the heart from the body, have much less elastic fiber and smooth muscle in their walls. The larger veins can act as a blood reservoir and are often called "capacitance vessels."

PULMONARY SYSTEM

RESPIRATION

Respiration is the process of exchanging oxygen and carbon dioxide between the air we breathe and blood cells that pass through the lungs. **Ventilation** is the process of exchanging air between the atmosphere and the lungs through inspiration and expiration.[10] The mechanics of inspiration and expiration depend on many factors, including the structure of the lungs, chest, and muscles. **Inspiration** occurs when the muscles of ventilation, the most important being the diaphragm, contract to cause an increase in the space within the thoracic cavity. This expansion causes air pressure to drop inside the lungs, which causes air to move into the lungs. **Expiration** is the reverse of this process.

If the body needs increased amounts of oxygen, such as during exercise, the amount of air that must flow into and out of the lungs must markedly increase. When this situation occurs, the muscles of ventilation must work extensively. When disease affects the lungs, the results can be the same. In this case, however, the body is not requiring more oxygen. The ability of air to move normally into and out of the lungs is compromised because of blockage of the tubes that conduct the air. This obstruction results in high resistance to airflow and increased work for the muscles of ventilation.[11]

CONDUCTING AIRWAYS AND LUNGS

Conducting airways are the passageways and tubes that transport air into and out of the lungs. The upper conducting airway includes the nose, pharynx, and larynx. This component of the air transport system cleans and humidifies the air and terminates at the beginning of the trachea. The lower conducting airway is made up of the trachea and bronchiole system (Figure 10-7).[11] The bronchiole system consists of tubes branching from the main bronchus out to the terminal bronchioles. This is where the conduction system ends, air enters into the alveolus, and where gas exchange takes place. The alveoli are surrounded by capillaries that contain deoxygenated blood coming from the right ventricle of the heart. It is at this junction that oxygen and carbon dioxide are exchanged, with the reoxygenated blood returning to the left atrium. The lungs are compartmentalized into a system of lobes, which are present because of the structure of the bronchial airway system (see Figure 10-7). A special membrane, the pleura, covers the outer surface of the lungs and the inner surface of the chest wall. The pleura is extremely important to the process of ventilation and maintenance of the continuity of the lungs.[6]

CARDIOVASCULAR AND PULMONARY SYSTEM INTEGRATION

The importance of interaction between the cardiovascular and pulmonary systems is clear: when disease affects one system, eventually the other system will also be affected. For example, if arteriosclerosis develops in the coronary vessels, the amount of oxygen going to the heart muscle will be decreased. With time the heart muscle begins to fail and will not pump blood to the lungs and body efficiently. Eventually, this insufficiency results in an increase in blood volume and

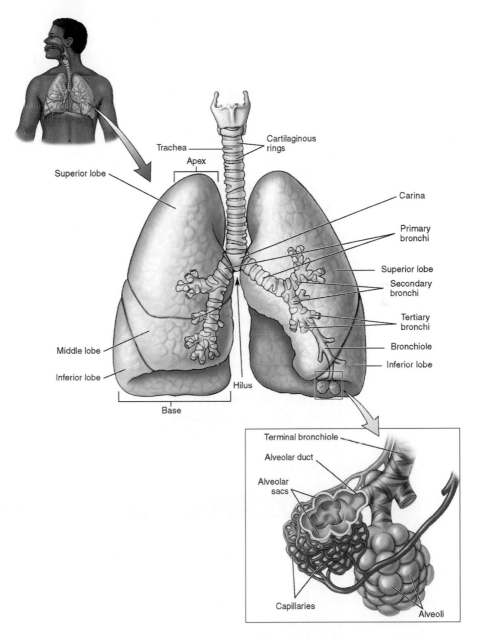

Trachea

Cartilaginous rings

Apex

Superior lobe

Carina

Primary bronchi

Superior lobe

Secondary bronchi

Tertiary bronchi

Bronchiole

Inferior lobe

Middle lobe

Inferior lobe

Hilus

Base

Terminal bronchiole

Alveolar duct

Alveolar sacs

Capillaries

Alveoli

Figure 10-7 ■ Anterior view of the lower airway showing the bronchial tree, alveoli, and pulmonary circulation. (From Herlihy B: *The human body in health and illness.* ed 5, Saunders, St. Louis, 2014.)

pressure in the lungs, which in turn causes a decrease in lung efficiency and, finally, permanent damage.

The degree of success that PTs or PTAs have in establishing appropriate examination and intervention procedures for individuals with cardiovascular or pulmonary disease depends in part on how well they understand how each system functions and interacts. The following section briefly describes common cardiovascular and lung diseases that are treated with physical therapy.

CARDIOVASCULAR DISEASES

Two major categories of disease processes influence the myocardium: ischemic conditions and cardiac muscle dysfunction.[12]

ISCHEMIC CONDITIONS

Ischemia occurs in the presence of insufficient blood flow and results in inadequate oxygenation of tissues because of a blocked blood vessel. In CVD, arteriosclerosis affects the coronary vessels and is commonly called **coronary heart disease**. **Angina** is the condition in which chest pain occurs from ischemia of the heart muscle.

The cause of arteriosclerosis, which can affect all vessels of the body, is not completely understood. It is clear, however, that the severity of the arteriosclerotic process can be influenced by many risk factors (Box 10-1).[13] Some of these factors cannot be changed, such as having a family history of CHD. However, most of these risk factors can be modified or eliminated completely by changes in behavior. PTs and PTAs promote a healthy lifestyle and help patients with cardiac dysfunction to alter their behavior as they progress through the rehabilitation process.

CARDIAC MUSCLE DYSFUNCTION

Cardiac muscle dysfunction refers to various pathologic conditions associated with heart failure.[12] **Heart failure** occurs when a disease process or congenital defect either directly or indirectly causes a decrease in the pumping capability of the heart muscle. These disease processes can occur either acutely or gradually.

BOX 10-1

Risk Factors That Promote the Development of Cardiovascular Disease

Positive Risk Factors
- Age
- Family history
- Cigarette smoking
- Sedentary lifestyle
- Obesity
- Hypertension
- Elevated cholesterol (low-density lipoprotein, total cholesterol)
- Prediabetes

Negative Risk Factor
- High-density lipoprotein cholesterol

(Data from *American College of Sports Medicine's Guidelines for Exercise Testing and Prescription.* ed 9, 2014.)

An example of an acute change in the heart's pumping capability is the occurrence of an MI. In this case, one of the coronary arteries suddenly becomes blocked by an **embolus** (clot). When embolism occurs, blood flow to heart muscle beyond the embolus stops, and the part of the heart muscle no longer receiving blood dies. If this embolus causes an interruption in blood flow to a large amount of heart muscle, death can result.

If an individual survives a heart attack, other symptoms may develop that further complicate the condition. One of the major complications after infarction is an abnormal rhythm in the sequence of heart muscle contraction (abnormal conduction). This problem makes the heart contraction inefficient. If the left ventricle is seriously damaged from the infarct, it may not contract strongly enough to move the blood through the body appropriately. This deficiency can cause the blood to back up into the lungs, or it may seriously limit function, such as the heart's ability to respond to an increase in physical activity.

When the heart muscle is compromised to the point that it cannot move blood volume effectively, **congestive heart failure (CHF)** will develop. This disorder can occur acutely or chronically. When CHF is present, the ventricles are not adequately pumping the appropriate volume from their chambers. When the right ventricle is not contracting efficiently, blood volume backs into the venous system and fluid collects in the liver, abdominal cavity, and legs. If the left ventricle does not contract appropriately, an abnormal amount of blood volume remains in the lungs, which results in fluid collection. The right ventricle then has to work harder because it must try to push blood into the lungs against increased resistance. This increased workload eventually leads to compromised function of the right ventricle (see Figure 10-4, *A*).

A person with CHF has many clinical problems. If fluid collects in the lungs, breathing becomes more difficult and the blood is not oxygenated appropriately. If fluid has collected in the legs, walking becomes more difficult. Because of increasing difficulty in performing activities, the patient would have to expend more energy to accomplish simple tasks. With increased energy expenditure, the heart would have to work harder to support simple functional activities. To develop an appropriate treatment program for a patient with problems of this type, a PT must have a thorough understanding of how these disease processes compromise function.

LUNG DISEASES

Diseases of the lung are generally classified as being obstructive or restrictive. If pathologic changes in the lung cause an abnormality in airflow through the bronchial tubes, the process is defined as **obstructive lung disease**, whereas if pathologic changes cause the volume of air in the lungs to be reduced, the process is defined as **restrictive lung disease.**[12] How lung diseases are classified is controversial. What is most important is that the common diseases that change lung function eventually demonstrate both obstructive and restrictive characteristics.[14]

CHRONIC OBSTRUCTIVE PULMONARY DISEASE

COPD is a group of disorders that produce certain specific physical symptoms. These symptoms include chronic productive cough, excessive mucus production, changes in the sound produced when air passes through the bronchial tubes, and **dyspnea** (shortness of breath). The specific disorders that can produce these changes include chronic bronchitis (inflammation of the bronchi), emphysema (trapping of air in the alveoli), and peripheral airway disease (collapse of terminal bronchioles). Other disorders sometimes included in this disease group include bronchial asthma (spasm like contraction of bronchi, resulting in air trapping) and cystic fibrosis (dysfunction of mucous glands, causing blockage of bronchi).[14] Differences between these obstructive diseases include their cause, pathology (what tissues are affected and how they are changed), and management. However, all of them cause similar symptoms in varying degrees.

The signs and symptoms that develop as COPD progresses include bronchial wall abnormalities that cause a decrease in lumen size and alveolar destruction. This process results in trapping of air in the lungs, which causes the lungs to become hyperinflated, and in a decrease in gas exchange in the alveoli, which results in hypoxemia (below-normal oxygenation of blood). Hypoxemia occurs when the lungs cannot adequately supply oxygen to or retrieve carbon dioxide from the red blood cells as the cells pass by the alveoli.

As resistance to airflow increases because of the decreasing lumen size of the bronchioles, the thorax enlarges as a result of air trapping. This enlargement of the thorax causes the respiratory muscles to work harder. With time, the effectiveness of the respiratory muscles decreases. With chronic hypoxemia, changes begin to occur in the function of the heart, in blood pressure, and in the thickness of the blood. All of these changes can lead to respiratory failure.[12,14]

RESTRICTIVE LUNG DISEASES
Restrictive lung diseases cause a decrease in the ability of the lungs to expand, which results in a decrease in the volume of air that can move into and out of the lungs. This disease process that affects lung tissue directly is most commonly of idiopathic, or unknown, origin. Known causes include chronic inhalation of air pollutants such as coal dust, silicon, or asbestos. Infections such as pneumonia, cancer of the lung, and changes in heart function (causing chronic fluid collection in the lungs) can also result in restrictive changes. Diseases or trauma to the nerve supply to the muscles of ventilation or disease of the muscles themselves can also result in decreased movement of the chest wall. Thus, many disease groups and structural changes in the chest wall can cause restrictive changes.

The signs and symptoms that develop as restrictive disease progresses include some of the same changes seen in COPD, such as shortness of breath and chronic cough. In the case of restrictive lung disease, however, the cough is nonproductive (does not bring mucus out of the lungs). Other changes include **tachypnea**, or an increase in the rate of breathing, which results in a marked increase in the amount of energy expended on breathing. This increased energy cost can be so severe that it results in weight loss and an emaciated appearance. Patients with restrictive lung disease are also subject to the problems associated with hypoxemia.[12,14]

PRINCIPLES OF EXAMINATION   The examination performed by PTs and PTAs is an inclusive process that involves not only the patient, but also the family and other caregivers who are participating in the overall care of the patient. It includes a review of the patient's past medical and social history, review of the body systems, and tests and measures to gather data about the patient's condition. Areas reviewed include not only physical parameters, but also functional, psychological, social, and employment conditions. The tests and measures that are selected to examine a patient/client depend on various parameters, including the age of the patient/client; severity of the problem; stage of recovery (acute, subacute, or chronic); phase of rehabilitation (early, intermediate, late, or return to activity); and home, community, and work status.[15] Table 10-1 describes tests and measures commonly performed in the examination of patients with cardiovascular and pulmonary conditions.[15]

Table 10-1
Description of Common Tests and Measures for Patients with Cardiovascular and Pulmonary Conditions

Function or Characteristic	Description
Work Life	Analyses to determine whether the patient/client can assume or resume a role in work settings
Balance	Ability to maintain the body in equilibrium
Circulation (arterial, venous, lymphatic)	Analysis of blood and lymph movement to determine adequacy of cardiovascular pump, circulation, oxygen delivery, and lymphatic drainage
Community, Social, and Civic Life	Ability to engage in social activity outside of the home
Self-care and Domestic Life	Analysis of activities necessary for independent living at home
Ergonomics and Body Mechanics	Determination of the dynamic capabilities required of the patient to safely perform within various environments (e.g., home, work, school, and leisure)
Aerobic Capacity/Endurance	Ability to use the body's O_2 uptake and delivery system
Ventilation and Respiration	Assessment of movement of air into and out of the lungs and exchange of gases to perform activities of daily living and exercises
Anthropometric Characteristics	Body dimensions and fat composition
Muscle Performance (Including Strength, Power, Endurance, and Length)	Capacity of a muscle or group of muscles to generate force
Posture	Analysis of body alignment and positioning
Range of Motion	Amount of active and passive movement at a joint

10

Adapted from *Guide to physical therapist practice*, 3.0, Alexandria, VA, 2014. Available at: http://guidetoptpractice.apta.org/. Accessed August 20, 2015.

Other diagnostic tests of the cardiovascular and pulmonary systems beyond the scope of the PT are useful for determining the diagnosis and prognosis of the disease. It is essential that PTs understand the results of these tests so that they can identify contraindications for treatment, establish an appropriate plan of care, and be aware of potential complications during treatment sessions. Diagnostic tests can be invasive or noninvasive and generally place the patient at a certain amount of risk.

CARDIOVASCULAR DIAGNOSTIC TESTS AND PROCEDURES

INVASIVE PROCEDURES

Various pieces of equipment can be used to assess how the heart is functioning or how adequately blood is flowing through an artery. Invasive procedures used to evaluate heart function require that some type of instrument be placed in the body or dye be injected into the blood. One of the most common invasive procedures used to assess heart function is **cardiac catheterization**. The procedure requires passing a catheter (a flexible tube) into an artery in the leg until it reaches the heart. The catheter can then be placed in the left chambers of the heart or in the coronary arteries or pulmonary veins. The catheter can have a special sensory device on the tip to measure pressure; thus, its use allows assessment of how much pressure is being generated in chambers of the heart. This measure in turn evaluates the strength of myocardial contraction. Dye can be released directly into the coronary arteries from the catheter, and a special type of imaging technique can then record how well blood flows through the vessels and demonstrate where blockage has occurred. The catheter could also have a small camera in the tip to allow viewing of the heart chamber valves and the inside of the coronary vessels. Other types of invasive procedures may also be performed, all of which require highly trained personnel and sophisticated equipment. These procedures are expensive and generally involve some risk to the patient.[7]

NONINVASIVE PROCEDURES

Noninvasive procedures are also used to assess heart function. Some of the more common procedures include echocardiography, electrocardiography, and exercise testing. **Echocardiography** ("cardiac echo") is the use of high-frequency ultrasound to assess the size of the heart chambers, the thickness of the chamber walls, and the pumping ability and motion of the chamber walls and heart valves. Generally, the transducer (device that produces the ultrasound and records the returning echo) is placed directly on the chest. In cases of pulmonary disease, obesity, and chest wall abnormalities, it may be difficult to view the heart using the traditional cardiac echo. Transesophageal echocardiography is an alternative method that provides a better view of the heart. With the patient under conscious sedation, the transducer is placed in the esophagus by having the patient swallow the catheter to improve the accuracy of its recording and allow assessment of the posterior aspect of the heart.[7]

One of the most common and inexpensive methods of noninvasive evaluation of heart function is the **electrocardiogram (ECG)**. In the hospital setting, a patient who is at risk of abnormal heart activity may be continuously monitored via telemetry (a system that sends the electrocardiographic signal to a distant receiver). PTs who work with individuals being monitored by electrocardiography must be able to interpret normal ECG readings and recognize abnormal rhythms that could be life threatening. This ability requires a basic understanding of the anatomy and conduction system of the heart (see Figure 10-5).

As previously discussed, the conduction system is responsible for initiating depolarization or contraction of the heart muscle. When the conduction and muscle tissues depolarize, a change in electrical potential occurs across the individual cell membranes. This minute electrical change is detected by special electrodes placed on the skin of the anterior chest wall, and the "signal" can be recorded. The output of the ECG is a graph (Figure 10-8).[12]

The ECG allows assessment of the heart's rate and rhythm (Figure 10-9).[16] When the heart is functioning normally, it produces a consistent ECG pattern. As seen in Figure 10-9, different components of the waveform are assigned names and represent specific events in the heart cycle. For example, the P wave represents atrial depolarization, and the QRS complex represents ventricular depolarization (contraction). If the heart does not depolarize in a normal way or if part of the heart muscle is not functioning correctly, characteristic changes will be observed in the ECG. Other heart problems that can be assessed by ECG include heart muscle hypertrophy and the presence of MI.[13]

Exercise stress testing is a noninvasive method of determining how the cardiovascular and pulmonary systems respond to controlled increases in activity. The most common activities are treadmill walking and cycling. This assessment technique is most frequently used to diagnose suspected or established CVD. However, it is also valuable in other applications, such as assessing a patient's performance after MI, coronary artery bypass surgery, or heart valve replacement. Exercise stress tests are often used to assess someone's functional status, to evaluate the effectiveness of treatment, and to help prescribe limitations for

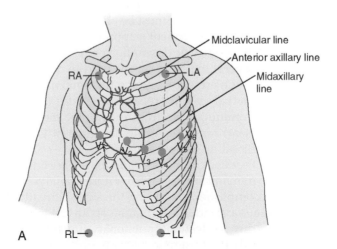

Figure 10-8 ■ Electrode placement for electrocardiographic monitoring. (From Black J, Hawks J: *Medical-surgical nursing*. ed 8, Saunders, St. Louis, 2009.)

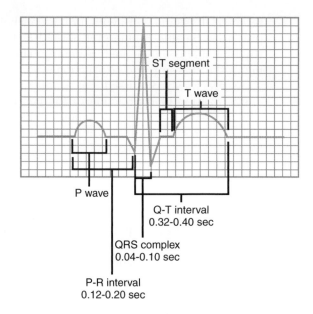

Figure 10-9 ■ Normal electrocardiogram tracing during a single heart-cycle. From Paz JC, West MP: *Acute care handbook for physical therapists*, ed 4, St. Louis, 2014, Saunders.

occupational activities. The results from an exercise stress test can be used to guide exercise prescription.[13]

A PT can be involved in administering an exercise stress test. Generally, the therapist is required to have training in the techniques of testing, especially if the testing protocol requires the patient to exercise at maximum capability. At a minimum, the PT must be able to interpret the data recorded during a stress test to establish a patient's appropriate level of exercise prescription, which should include a specific description of exercise intensity, duration, frequency, and mode.

Several methods can be used to administer an exercise stress test; the most common are walking on a treadmill and riding a bicycle ergometer. Generally, the actual testing procedure includes the following:

■ Continuous electrocardiographic monitoring.
■ Heart rate monitoring (from the ECG).
■ Blood pressure monitoring.
■ Feedback from the patient by reporting symptoms.

In many stress test laboratories, analysis of expired gas (air) from the lungs is accomplished by having the subject breathe into a collection device. This technique provides information about the amount of oxygen the patient consumes during the test and pulmonary function.[12,13]

When an exercise test is performed on a treadmill or bicycle ergometer, the exercise intensity or "protocol" used is very specific and has been tested in many laboratories. The Bruce protocol is one of the most common treadmill tests (Table 10-2).[17] The advantage of following a protocol is that the results of the test

Table 10-2 Bruce Treadmill Protocol			
Stage of Exercise	Time of Each Stage (min)	Speed of Treadmill (mph)	Grade of Treadmill (%)
I	3	1.7	10
II	3	2.5	12
III	3	3.4	14
IV	3	4.2	16

Modified from *American College of Sports Medicine Guidelines for Exercise Testing and Prescription*, ed 9, Philadelphia, 2014, Lippincott Williams & Wilkins.

can be compared with established results from other patients. This comparison helps determine the status of the patient.

PULMONARY DIAGNOSTIC TESTS AND PROCEDURES

As with cardiovascular diagnostic testing, both invasive and noninvasive procedures have been developed to assess lung function and the severity of pulmonary disease. PTs are not generally involved in performing these assessments; however, the information that is provided must be used by PTs so that appropriate evaluation and treatment procedures are established.

CHEST IMAGING

Chest imaging is the most common noninvasive method of assessing the lungs, chest wall, and heart. Baseline images can provide information about the presence of fluid in the lungs, air spaces, rib fractures, heart size, diaphragm shape and position, and nodules in the lungs. Subsequent images may be used to track the progression of pulmonary disease and the effectiveness of treatment.

Radiographs ("X-rays"), computed tomography (CT), and magnetic resonance imaging (MRI) are different techniques used to image the chest. Radiography uses ionizing radiation to generate a picture of the chest. Dense tissues, such as bone, appear white on the radiograph because they absorb the most radiation, whereas air spaces appear black on the radiograph. CT is a technique by which X-rays are used to take pictures of small slices of the chest and lungs and then a computer is used to put these individual images into a single picture. MRI uses the same principle as the CT scan except that the energy source used to take the picture is not X-rays, but magnetic waves.[18]

The ventilation-perfusion (V/Q) scan and CT pulmonary angiography (CTPA) are two diagnostic tests to diagnose a pulmonary embolus. For the V/Q scan, radioactive isotopes are inhaled into the lungs and injected into the bloodstream. V/Q scans are performed to locate the isotopes and to determine if there is a "mismatch" between the ventilation and perfusion of the lungs. CTPA uses CT to image the pulmonary arteries after injection of a radiocontrast agent.[7]

10

Even though highly technical equipment can provide a great deal of information concerning the condition of the lungs, the standard chest radiograph is often the first diagnostic test used. A PT must be competent in interpreting a standard chest radiograph. To assess the result of this common diagnostic procedure, the therapist must have a thorough understanding of normal anatomy and disease processes that affect the lungs.

BRONCHOSCOPY

A flexible fiber-optic tube is used for diagnosis and treatment. The tube is placed in the bronchial tree to permit visualization of the structures and suctioning of any secretions that have accumulated.[7]

PULMONARY FUNCTION TESTS

A **pulmonary function test** is an assessment of the effectiveness of the respiratory musculature and the integrity of the airways and lung tissue. The testing procedure can help classify the lung disease pattern as obstructive or restrictive by assessing the following:

- Lung volumes.
- Lung capacities.
- Gas distribution.
- Gas diffusion.
- Gas flow rate.

Generally, in a pulmonary function test the patient blows as hard as possible with the biggest breath into a machine called a **spirometer**. This device measures the various volumes and airflow rates, which are then compared with a normal scale. The degree of change from normal helps assess the seriousness of the obstructive or restrictive disease.[19]

BLOOD GAS ANALYSIS

Blood gas analysis involves assessing arterial blood to determine the concentration of oxygen and carbon dioxide. This measure helps determine how well the lungs are being ventilated or whether the patient has any deficits in respiration. Another parameter that is assessed is the acid balance of the blood. If the lungs are having difficulty in maintaining appropriate levels of oxygen and carbon dioxide, the blood generally becomes more acidic. In humans, blood must be maintained at a very specific acid level. Small changes in this acid level can result in severe reactions, possibly even death.[20]

PRINCIPLES OF EVALUATION, DIAGNOSIS, AND PROGNOSIS

The evaluation process results in establishment of a diagnosis and prognosis. A diagnosis is a description of a specific disease obtained by assessing the clinical signs, symptoms, or syndromes resulting from various pathologic conditions. Prognosis estimates the maximum level of improvement the patient will experience while progressing through the treatment process.[10] During the process of establishing a diagnosis and prognosis the PT also develops a plan of care. This plan establishes the specific outcomes the patient should be able to demonstrate at the end of the treatment process. It also includes an estimate of how long and how frequently the treatment process will have to be administered to reach the established goals and outcomes, as well as the criteria for discharge.

As a team member, the PT will be treating a patient in conjunction with several other medical personnel (e.g., doctors, nurses, nutritionists, psychologists, occupational therapists, social workers, and exercise physiologists). Each of these specialists will be applying specific management procedures. Therefore, the PT must be aware of all the treatments the patient is receiving and develop the treatment plan accordingly.

MEDICAL MANAGEMENT

One of the major forms of treating heart and lung disease is medical or pharmacologic management. Each year new pharmacologic agents become available to treat specific components of the complex symptoms that develop in individuals with cardiovascular and pulmonary disease. Generally, drugs used to treat cardiovascular and pulmonary disease relieve or improve symptoms, but do not eradicate the disease.

Understanding the effects of drugs used to treat specific heart diseases is extremely important. Many of these drugs can alter the heart's ability to respond to exercise. For example, drugs that alter how the sympathetic nervous system influences the heart can result in a decreased heart rate and prevent the rate from increasing in response to exercise. Other drugs used to treat the heart can help control the rhythm of contraction, increase or decrease the rate, and increase or decrease the strength of myocardial contraction. They can also improve coronary blood flow or help decrease the resistance to blood flow, thereby decreasing the work the heart must perform. Medical management of symptoms caused by cardiac disease focuses primarily on reducing oxygen demand and increasing oxygen supply.[21]

Medical management of symptoms caused by pulmonary disease focuses primarily on promoting bronchodilation and decreasing inflammation. Drugs producing bronchodilation improve airflow through the bronchial tubes, which helps oxygen reach the alveolus and thereby decreases the work of breathing. Anti-inflammatory agents help control the results of infection or inflammation. As in the case of cardiac drugs, pulmonary drugs can have adverse effects, including alteration of heart function, gastrointestinal distress, nervousness, muscle tremor, headache, anxiety, sweating, and insomnia.[21]

SURGICAL MANAGEMENT

Like pharmacologic management, surgical management of cardiovascular and pulmonary disease does not generally alter the disease process, but does improve the quality of life by relieving symptoms. In the case of CHD the arteriosclerotic process is not stopped, but coronary artery blood flow can be improved through surgery, which in turn enhances heart performance.

Two methods are commonly used to improve coronary blood flow to the heart: PCI and **coronary artery bypass graft (CABG).** PCI, which is the process of mechanically dilating the coronary artery, does not require surgically opening the chest. A catheter is placed through an artery in the leg and then positioned in the coronary vessel blocked by arteriosclerotic plaque. A balloon is then inflated (known as *percutaneous transluminal coronary angioplasty*), or a procedure using

10

laser light (known as *coronary laser angioplasty*) or a blade (known as *directional coronary atherectomy*) is used to destroy the plaque. A stent, or mesh tube, can be implanted to help the vessel remain open.[22]

CABG requires surgically opening the chest wall and grafting a small artery or a leg vein from the aorta to a point beyond the blockage or plaque. This technique bypasses the blockage and thereby reestablishes blood flow to the heart through the previously blocked vessel. Several vessels may be bypassed during the same surgery.[23]

Valve dysfunction most commonly occurs because of degenerative changes as a result of aging. The valves can become stenotic (narrowed) or insufficient, causing a regurgitation (leaking of the valve). Valve surgery can involve a repair or complete replacement, and the surgical approach varies according to the valve that is involved and the procedure.[24]

Surgical intervention is also required for inserting a pacemaker. A **cardiac pacemaker** is an electronic device that produces a pulse to control heart depolarization. In other words, it replaces the function of the SA node. This intervention is generally done to control severe cardiac arrhythmias. The electrodes can be inserted through a vein in the arm up to the heart and placed on the inner surface of the heart. The generator is then placed below the skin on the anterior chest wall and sutured in place. When a pacemaker is present in a patient, the PT and PTA must monitor the patient closely during exercise. Most pacemakers produce variable rates in response to exercise; however, if maximum-intensity exercise is performed, careful monitoring is mandatory.[25]

Surgical management is not as frequently used for common lung diseases as it is in the management of cardiac diseases. Resection of lung disease generally applies to removal of malignant and benign tumors, fungal infections, cysts, tuberculosis, fistulas, or bronchiectasis. As with heart transplantation, lung transplantation is performed only for end-stage lung disease. A multidisciplinary team evaluates the patient and determines if the patient is an appropriate candidate for the transplant. Pathologic changes that occur from obstructive or restrictive diseases generally do not necessitate surgery. When surgery on the heart or lungs is performed, however, the PT and PTA play a major role in pre- and postoperative care.

When the chest wall is opened, the patient generally must be connected to a machine that breathes for the patient and, in the case of heart surgery, a machine that pumps the blood because the heart is stopped. This very serious interruption of the normal function of the heart and lungs results in certain changes that will have to be managed no matter what surgical procedure is performed.[26] Box 10-2 identifies some of the problems a patient will have pre- and postoperatively that must be managed by a PT.[27]

PHYSICAL THERAPY CARDIAC REHABILITATION PROCEDURES

The PT is responsible for establishing an appropriate level of intensity, duration, frequency, and type of exercise for an individual with cardiac disease, which means monitoring the patient's cardiovascular response to the exercise to ensure the patient's safety. In addition, the therapist must review all the medical data

BOX 10-2

Factors Influencing Recovery after Chest Surgery

Preoperative Factors
- Risk factor profile
- Underlying pulmonary or heart disease
- Other medical problems

Factors during Operation
- Pulmonary collapse and hypoxemia
- Direct trauma to heart or lungs
- Heart arrhythmias
- Danger of emboli (clots) in lungs
- Damage to the mucous membrane of the lungs
- Poor humidity to lungs
- Reaction of lungs to anesthesia
- Drying of pleura

Postoperative Factors
- Atelectasis (collapse of alveoli)
- Narcotics to suppress pain
- Incisional pain preventing deep breathing
- Inactivity promoting shallow breathing
- Inability to clear lung secretions because of decreased coughing
- Pain
- Weakness

Modified from Howell S, Hill J: Acute respiratory care in open heart surgery, *Phys Ther* 52:253–260, 1972.

obtained from invasive and noninvasive testing procedures to select an appropriate level of activity for the patient's program.

After cardiothoracic surgery, upper extremity lifting and range of motion exercises should be restricted for 5 to 8 weeks. Unilateral upper extremity exercises are avoided until there is no evidence of sternal instability. In addition, patients are advised to cough with splinting and to limit range of motion at the onset of pain or pulling on the incision.[13]

To help the PT develop the plan of care, individuals with cardiac disease are classified according to the severity of the condition. Table 10-3 presents a functional classification system and four stages of heart failure that are used to determine the patient's basic condition and the type of activity in which the individual might engage. These scores are used to document the patient's symptoms and can be used to determine the response to treatment and the progression of the disease.[28,29]

Other guidelines used by the PT to help establish appropriate cardiac rehabilitation activities include phases of recovery. Cardiac rehabilitation is typically divided into inpatient and outpatient stages. As the length of inpatient hospital stays decrease, outpatient cardiac rehabilitation programs have an increasingly

10

Table 10-3
Functional Classifications of Patients with Diseases of the Heart and Stages of Heart Failure (HF)

FUNCTIONAL CLASSIFICATION		STAGES OF HEART FAILURE	
Class	Description	Stage	Description
I	Patients with cardiac disease but without resulting limitations of physical activity. Ordinary physical capacity does not cause undue fatigue, palpitation, dyspnea, or anginal pain.	A	Patients at high risk of developing HF because of the presence of conditions that are strongly associated with the development of HF. Such patients have no identified structural or functional abnormalities of the pericardium, myocardium, or cardiac valves and have never shown signs or symptoms of HF.
II	Patients with cardiac disease resulting in slight limitation of physical activity. Patients are comfortable at rest. Ordinary physical activity results in fatigue, palpitation, dyspnea, or pain.	B	Patients who have developed structural heart disease that is strongly associated with the development of HF but who have never shown signs or symptoms of HF.
III	Patients with cardiac disease resulting in marked limitation of physical activity. Patients are comfortable at rest. Less than ordinary physical activity causes fatigue, palpitation, dyspnea, or anginal pain.	C	Patients who have current or prior symptoms of HF associated with underlying structural heart disease.
IV	Patients with cardiac disease resulting in an inability to carry out any physical activity without discomfort. Symptoms of cardiac insufficiency or anginal syndrome may be present even at rest. If any physical activity is undertaken, discomfort is increased.	D	Patients with advanced structural heart disease and marked symptoms of HF at rest despite maximal medical therapy and who require specialized interventions.

Data from New York Heart Association Functional Classification, 1994, and the American College of Cardiology/American Heart Association Guidelines, 2005.

important role. The inpatient stage is often referred to as Phase I (acute), whereas the outpatient stage is generally broken down into Phase II (subacute), Phase III (intensive rehabilitation), and Phase IV (ongoing rehabilitation).[12,22,30] This classification system varies a great deal and often remains specific to a program. For instance, Phase IV is frequently combined with Phase III.

Rehabilitation during the early recovery period will be dependent on the cardiac event, complications, and contraindications. A baseline assessment should be performed on all patients. Inpatient activities include self-care activities, arm and leg range of motion, postural/position changes, and walking short distances.[13] Inpatient rehabilitation recommendations follow the "Frequency, Intensity, Time, and Type of Exercise," or **FITT principle of exercise prescription** and

Table 10-4
FITT Recommendations for Inpatient Programs

Frequency	Mobilization 2 to 4 times per day for the first 3 days of the hospital stay
Intensity	Seated or standing resting heart rate (HR_{rest}) + 20 beats/min^{-1} for patients with an MI and + 30 beats/min^{-1} for patients recovering from heart surgery; with an upper limit ≤ 120 beats/min^{-1} that corresponds to a rate of perceived exertion ≤ 13 on a scale of 6 to 20
Time	Intermittent walking bouts lasting 3 to 5 min as tolerated with exercise bouts of progressively increasing duration. The rest period may be a slower walk (or complete rest) that is shorter than the duration of the exercise bout. Goal is to achieve a 2:1 exercise/rest ratio
Type	Walking
Progression	When continuous exercise duration reaches 10 to 15 min, increase intensity as tolerated within the recommended rate of perceived exertion and HR limits

Data from *American College of Sports Medicine Guidelines for Exercise Testing and Prescription*, ed 9, Philadelphia, 2014, Lippincott Williams & Wilkins.

progression.[13] Table 10-4 lists FITT recommendations for inpatient programs.[13] The therapist or assistant must monitor the ECG, heart rate, blood pressure, and other physiologic parameters to ensure that the patient stays within the predetermined safety range. It is important to note that the patient is involved in educational activities, including risk factor modification, understanding of the medications prescribed, and discharge planning.

After discharge, the individual participates in the outpatient phases of the cardiac rehabilitation program. These phases focus on exercises that will gradually and safely increase the individual's functional capacity. The early stages of outpatient rehabilitation (Phase II) are performed under supervision and monitored closely. Generally, patients attend outpatient cardiac rehabilitation programs that have representatives of the entire rehabilitation team (e.g., occupational therapy, physical therapy, and nutrition). During Phase II, close physician management is always available. Depending on the severity of the problem, the patient will attend supervised training sessions three or four times a week for 10 to 12 weeks. If recovery has continued well, a stress test will be performed to help determine whether the patient has improved or responded to the exercise program.

Progression to Phases III and IV involves more independent and aggressive activities. To proceed to these levels, the individual must (1) be able to self-monitor the exercise program, (2) have no contraindications to exercise, and (3) be emotionally stable.[20] These phases include a gradual increase in exercise intensity. Periodic checkups by the professional team occur most frequently in Phase III. Once Phase IV has been attained, the patient should be functioning at the maximum safe capacity.

During the outpatient phases of the cardiac rehabilitation program, the exercises emphasize aerobic training that includes rhythmic activity of large muscle

10

masses. Appropriate aerobic training involves a warm up period, a peak period, and a cool-down period. The length of time for these periods may vary with the status of the patient, but generally the warm up and cool-down phases should be at least 5 to 10 minutes each. The peak period should last 20 to 60 minutes. It is during the peak period that the patient must reach and maintain the prescribed exercise intensity.[12,14] Table 10-5 lists FITT recommendations for outpatient programs.[13] There are several techniques for quantifying exercise intensity including heart rate reserve, **ratings of perceived exertion (RPE),** percent age-predicted heart rate, percent oxygen uptake, and metabolic equivalents (METs). RPE is a subjective report from the patient that indicates how hard he/she feels their body is working. Exercise intensity should be prescribed using the exercise stress test results when that information is available. In the heart rate reserve method, a **target heart rate (THR)** is calculated by subtracting the heart rate at rest from the maximum heart rate, multiplying that value by the intensity desired, and adding the product to the heart rate at rest.[13]

Table 10-5 FITT Recommendations for Outpatient Programs	
Frequency	Exercise should be performed at least 3 days, but preferably on most days of the week. Frequency of exercise depends on several factors including baseline exercise tolerance, exercise intensity, fitness and other health goals, and types of exercise that are incorporated into the overall program. For patients with very limited exercise capacities, multiple short (1-10 min) daily sessions may be prescribed. Patients should be encouraged to perform some of these exercise sessions independently (i.e., without direct supervision)
Intensity	Exercise intensity may be prescribed using one or more of the following methods: • Based on results from the baseline exercise test, 40% to 80% of exercise capacity using the HR reserve (HRR), oxygen uptake reserve ($\dot{V}O_2R$), or peak oxygen uptake ($\dot{V}O_{2peak}$) methods • RPE of 11 to 16 on a RPE scale of 6 to 20
Time	Warm-up and cool-down activities of 5 to 10 min, including static stretching, ROM, and light-intensity (i.e., $<40\%$ $\dot{V}O_2R$, $<64\%$ peak heart rate [HR_{peak}], or <11 RPE) aerobic activities, should be a component of each exercise session and precede and follow the conditioning phase. The goal for the duration of the aerobic conditioning phase is generally 20 to 60 min per session. After a cardiac-related event, patients may begin with as little as 5 to 10 min of aerobic conditioning with a gradual increase in aerobic exercise time of 1 to 5 min per session or an increase in time per session of 10% to 20% per week
Type	The aerobic exercise portion of the session should include rhythmic, large muscle group activities with an emphasis on increased caloric expenditure for maintenance of a healthy body weight and its many other associated health benefits. To promote whole body physical fitness, conditioning that includes the upper and lower extremities and multiple forms of aerobic activities and exercise equipment should be incorporated into the exercise program. The different types of exercise equipment may include the following:

Table 10-5
FITT Recommendations for Outpatient Programs—cont'd

- Arm ergometer
- Combination of upper or lower (dual action) extremity cycle ergometer
- Upright and recumbent cycle ergometer
- Recumbent stepper
- Rower
- Elliptical
- Stair climber
- Treadmill for walking

Aerobic interval training (AIT) involves alternating 3 to 4 min periods of exercise at high intensity (90%-95% HR_{peak}) with exercise at moderate intensity (60%-70% HR_{peak}). Such training for approximately 40 min, three times per week has been shown to yield a greater improvement in $\dot{V}O_{2peak}$ in patients with heart failure and greater long-term improvements in $\dot{V}O_{2peak}$ in patients after CABG compared to standard continuous, moderate-intensity exercise. Although AIT has routinely been used in athletes, its use in patients with CVD appears to have potential but cannot yet be universally recommended until further data regarding safety and efficacy are available

Progression   There is no standard format for the rate of progression in exercise session duration. Thus, progression should be individualized to patient tolerance. Factors to consider in this regard include initial physical fitness level, patient motivation and goals, symptoms, and musculoskeletal limitations. Exercise sessions may include continuous or intermittent exercise depending on the capability of the patient

Data from *American College of Sports Medicine Guidelines for Exercise Testing and Prescription*, ed 9, Philadelphia, 2014, Lippincott Williams & Wilkins.

$$THR = ([HR\,max - HR\,rest] \times Intensity\ desired) + HR\,rest$$

The maximum heart rate is most accurately measured by a maximum stress test. However, it is commonly estimated by subtracting one's age from 220. The 220 − age formula is the most simple method to predict maximum HR, but often will underestimate or overestimate measured maximum HRs.[13] The THR is used to establish a person's **training zone**, or the minimum and maximum heart rates that must be achieved to produce an aerobic training effect. The percentage of intensity desired depends on the individual's level of fitness, symptoms, and ECG findings. If the person has cardiac disease, 40% to 80% heart rate reserve may be indicated.[13] By contrast, a training zone for a young athlete may fall between THRs of 60% and 85% of that person's maximum heart rate capacity. To produce a "training effect" or a change in aerobic capacity, this individual would have to reach a heart rate in the established training zone. The important thing to remember is that as aerobic capacity improves, the amount of work the heart has to perform at a specific exercise intensity decreases. This improvement in aerobic capacity in turn improves the patient's functional capacity without causing the heart to be overworked.

10

Besides the intensity of exercise (how hard a patient works during a single exercise period) and the duration of exercise (the length of time each exercise period should last), factors to consider in the planning of an aerobic training program include the type of exercise (what the patient does, such as walking, jogging, and bicycle riding) and the frequency of exercise (how many times a day or week the patient exercises).[13] The type of exercise must allow for aerobic performance, which includes rhythmic contraction of large muscle groups over several minutes (20-60 minutes). Walking, upper or lower cycle ergometer, and elliptical training all promote this type of activity. An individual with cardiac disease, however, may not be able to sustain 20 minutes of exercise at one time; therefore, several periods of exercise throughout the day would be more appropriate. The frequency of exercise may also be determined by the patient's condition. Normally, in the latter phases of their program, individuals with cardiac disease must generally perform a minimum of 20 minutes of exercise three to five times per week to promote or maintain aerobic training.[9]

The PT and PTA must continuously monitor the patient during all phases of the exercise program. Appropriate monitoring includes assessing heart rate, blood pressure, and respiratory rate responses to the specific exercise intensity. This monitoring is important, especially in the early phases of rehabilitation, to ensure that the patient does not exercise at an unsafe level. As the patient progresses, the therapist must teach self-monitoring for safe participation in activities, thus moving the patient one step closer to independent activity. When the patient can function independently at maximum functional capability, the therapist's responsibilities have been met.

PHYSICAL THERAPY PULMONARY REHABILITATION PROCEDURES

As with patients who have cardiac dysfunction, the PT is responsible for establishing an appropriate level of exercise programming for individuals with pulmonary disease. The intensity and duration of the program must be at an appropriate level to promote a training effort that will enhance the patient's ability to perform daily functions aerobically. Aerobic performance occurs when the active muscles receive all the oxygen they need to perform their task. To select the appropriate intensity and duration of exercise, the PT must review the results of all examination procedures performed on the patient. From these data and the physical therapy evaluation, the appropriate exercise program can be established. It is important to remember that during aerobic exercise the PT and PTA must monitor the patient's cardiovascular response to the exercise, such as the heart rate, blood pressure, and breathing rate and depth, as well as eliciting feedback on how the patient feels. In this way, excessive exercise that could put the patient at risk is prevented.

Other components of physical therapy treatment for patients with pulmonary disease include techniques for secretion removal, respiratory muscle training and breathing, and energy conservation. Secretion removal techniques are performed in patients who produce excessive mucus in the bronchi of the lungs as occurs in obstructive pulmonary disease. The technique applied to promote mucus removal is called **postural drainage**. The patient is placed in a certain position ("posture") to passively drain fluid from a specific portion of the lung. The therapist applies percussion (or clapping), vibration, and shaking to specific areas of the chest wall overlying specific lobes of the lung (Figure 10-10).[31] Percussion promotes movement of mucus through the bronchial tubes. Having the patient assume the Trendelenburg (inverted) position and cough immediately after the percussion or vibration procedure also helps move mucus out of the different sections of the lungs.

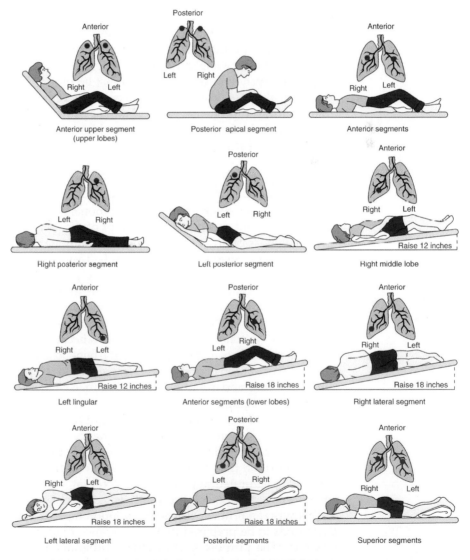

Figure 10-10 ■ Positions for performing postural drainage to remove secretions from the lungs. (Modified from Potter PA, Perry AG: Fundamentals of nursing: concepts, process and practice. ed 4, St Louis, 1997, Mosby. In Wilkins RL. *Egan's fundamentals of respiratory care*. ed 9. St. Louis, 2009, Mosby.)

Producing a good cough is essential for maintaining normal lung function in everyone. If the respiratory muscles are weakened or do not work properly, the efficiency of the cough mechanism is reduced. This reduced cough efficiency can occur in both the obstructive and restrictive disease patterns. It also occurs in patients who have experienced trauma, such as an individual with quadriplegia after spinal cord injury or patients who have had thoracic surgery.

The PT can help the patient enhance coughing in three ways: by strengthening both the primary and secondary muscles of ventilation, by changing the breathing pattern, and by teaching the patient how to use different devices to support the chest wall so that the expiration force generated during coughing is enhanced.[26]

The PT and PTA engage in direct intervention during pulmonary rehabilitation. They also participate in helping to modify the patient's risk factor profile, such as promoting weight management, good nutrition, smoking cessation, and a positive psychological state. They must be prepared to monitor the activities of other health care professionals and ensure that their treatment program is integrated into a comprehensive care plan. The primary goal for pulmonary rehabilitation is to help the patient achieve the highest functional level allowed by the pulmonary impairment.

THE "WELL" INDIVIDUAL

A discussion of cardiovascular and pulmonary physical therapy would not be complete without reviewing the concept of the "well" individual (person without a diagnosis of any cardiovascular or pulmonary disease). Even though the emphasis of physical therapy tends to be restorative care, preventative care is included in the scope of physical therapy practice. Prevention strategies can be implemented in susceptible populations to prevent disease.[32]

PTs have a responsibility to implement prevention strategies, to promote a healthy lifestyle, and to act as role models for their patients. The goals of the Million Hearts® initiative are relevant to PTs because they can have a significant impact on behaviors and can promote the beneficial effects of a healthy lifestyle.[4] The implementation of prevention strategies and the promotion of a healthy lifestyle in young and middle-aged individuals will result in more individuals "successfully aging."

Proper nutrition, regular exercise, weight control, blood pressure control, cholesterol management, and smoking avoidance are all modifiable risk factors that can significantly reduce mortality rates. PTs can provide information about proper nutrition that includes eating a diet high in fiber, fruits, and vegetables and low in saturated fat, cholesterol, total fat, and sodium. PTs can encourage smoking cessation and physical activity to prevent overweight and obesity. Physical activity is a primary disease prevention measure for all age groups. A PT or PTA needs to be prepared to offer guidance to individuals starting an exercise program. The purpose of an exercise program may include stress reduction, weight management, improvement in body composition (percentage of body fat), alteration of cardiac risk factors, or enhancement of functional capacity.[12,33]

The aging population represents a large group of "well" individuals who can benefit from exercise, but have a tendency to be sedentary. Specific cardiovascular and pulmonary changes occur with aging, one of the most specific being a decrease in the safe maximum heart rate. It is well established that the heart rate is inversely related to age. As a person grows older, the maximum heart rate declines. At the same time, the pulmonary system demonstrates a decline in both static and dynamic measurements. Although endurance training in the elderly cannot reduce cardiac changes, it can reduce pulmonary changes.[9]

Just as an individual with cardiac or pulmonary disease needs an examination, so does the "well" individual. This examination should include reviewing the risk factor profile, including smoking and family history. The PT should examine the functional status of the musculoskeletal system. The performance results of an exercise stress test, body composition, strength, and flexibility should also be reviewed. Any preexisting conditions, such as orthopaedic abnormalities, must also be considered. An important aspect of the examination is to determine the individual's specific interests. Does he or she like to swim, run, or ride a bicycle? Understanding the person's interests could help the therapist design a program more likely to induce compliance with the exercise routine.

Box 10-3 presents a summary of benefits gained from aerobic and strength training programs.[12] This type of information can be used to encourage a sedentary person to engage in a regular exercise program. Appropriate assessment and monitoring, however, must accompany any regular exercise.

SUMMARY

Cardiovascular and pulmonary physical therapy has, over the past three decades, become an integral part of the knowledge and practice base of the PT. This chapter has presented the prevalence of the cardiovascular and pulmonary impairments, a fundamental review of the structure and function of the related systems, common conditions, a description of invasive and noninvasive diagnostic tests, principles of medical and rehabilitation procedures, and the physical therapy approach to the "well" individual. A thorough understanding of the anatomy, physiology, and function of the cardiovascular and pulmonary system is essential to develop the skills necessary to make appropriate clinical decisions for proper examination, management, and progression of patients with cardiovascular and pulmonary diseases. It is also essential for PTs and PTAs to remember that no matter what the diagnosis, when exercise is applied as an intervention, the cardiovascular and pulmonary response to that exercise must always be monitored.

PTs working with individuals who have cardiovascular or pulmonary disease must also be acutely aware of their role as team members. Whether guiding a PTA in applying appropriate exercise intensity or discussing maximum exercise intensity levels with a cardiologist, the PT must take into account the total management program the patient with cardiovascular or pulmonary disease is experiencing.

10

BOX 10-3	*Benefits of Aerobic Exercise and Strength-Training Programs*

Benefits of an Aerobic Exercise Program

■ Improvement in aerobic capacity
■ Increased efficiency to extract oxygen in trained muscles
■ Increase in stroke volume
■ Decrease in resting heart rate
■ Decrease in submaximal heart rates
■ Change in body composition (loss of fat)
■ Decreased clotting factors in blood
■ Decrease in resting blood pressure in hypertensive individuals
■ Altered method of cholesterol transport
■ Increase in high-density lipoproteins (HDLs)
■ Slight decrease in low-density lipoproteins (LDLs)
■ Decrease in various fats produced by the body
■ Increase in using carbohydrates as an energy source
■ Improvement in psychological well-being
■ Improved response to stress
■ Decrease in physiologic responsiveness to stimuli
■ Improved self-image
■ Decrease in risk of developing heart disease as a result of elimination of a number of the risk factors

Benefits of a Strength-Training Program

■ Increase in strength of trained muscles
■ Increase in use of anaerobic metabolism
■ Improved ease in performing many activities of daily living, especially with upper body strength training
■ Increase in bone mass
■ Increase in size, endurance, or both, of trained muscles
■ Improvement of body image and self-esteem

Modified from Hillegass EA, Sadowsky HS: *Essentials of cardiopulmonary physical therapy*, ed 2, Philadelphia, 2001, Saunders.

CASE STUDIES

CASE STUDY ONE

CLINICAL HISTORY

Joe is a 60-year-old man who retired after 30 years as a high school math teacher. He had not experienced any previous symptoms of heart disease, such as chest pain or shortness of breath, but had been taking medicine over the previous 3 years for mild high blood pressure, which was well controlled. His risk factor profile included the following:

■ Family history—mother (age 82) and older brother (age 55) died of heart disease.
■ Smoking—between the ages of 16 and 40, one pack per day.

- Sedentary—has not engaged in any regular exercise program since the age of 50.
- Obesity—states he has "been carrying" an extra 30 lb since his mid-40s.

One week ago he was admitted to the emergency room after 1 hour of severe chest pain. The ECG demonstrated severe abnormalities indicating a change in the function of the anterolateral part of his heart. He was rushed to the operating room, where cardiac catheterization revealed a complete blockage of his left coronary artery. Coronary artery bypass grafting was performed.

CARDIAC REHABILITATION

After surgery, Joe was admitted to the cardiac care unit. He was prescribed medications that helped control his heart rate, improve the strength of the heart's contractions, and prevent arrhythmias. The PT assessed the patient's status and, after conferring with the cardiologist and nurse, initiated the activities outlined in Table 10-4. The PT reported the following results at the end of the exercise period:

1. Resting heart rate (beats per minute): 86 while lying in bed, 98 while sitting, 105 while standing, and 135 while performing activities of daily living such as brushing teeth at the bedside.
2. Blood pressure: 130/90 while lying in bed, 110/80 while sitting, 110/65 while standing, and 100/60 while performing daily activities.

ECG: no indication of any change in pattern except when performing daily activities. This change demonstrated possible mild ischemia.

On the third day of the exercise program, Joe demonstrated appropriate physiologic responses to walking and to the exercises. The patient was discharged on the fifth day after surgery.

Joe had an understanding that the medicine he took was to help prevent arrhythmias. He had learned how to take his own pulse and was instructed to not engage in any activities that caused his heart rate to exceed 135 beats per minute. At the time of discharge, he was instructed to move his bed to the first floor of his home to avoid a flight of stairs.

OUTPATIENT PROGRAM

Joe returned to the outpatient cardiac rehabilitation program conducted in the physical therapy department 3 days after discharge. He reported that he had not had any difficulty at home; however, further inquiry revealed that he did not engage in any activity other than activities of daily living and walking around the house.

The PT initiated Phase II of cardiac rehabilitation by determining how long Joe could walk on a treadmill at his preferred rate before reaching the THR of 120 to 135 beats per minute. This rate was established by the cardiologist at the time of discharge as the maximum exercise heart rate that Joe could reach. Over the next three outpatient visits (1 week), the PT established the following exercise routine to be performed at home twice daily:

1. Fifteen minutes of warm up and stretching.
2. Twenty minutes of stationary bicycle riding.
3. Fifteen minutes of cool-down exercises.

10

Joe remained on this exercise program for 3 more weeks. During that time he came to the cardiac rehabilitation program to meet with a nutritionist and a psychologist. He then underwent an exercise stress test on a treadmill, which revealed that he could safely reach a maximum heart rate of 146 beats per minute before incurring serious changes in heart function. Phase III cardiac rehabilitation was then initiated and included bicycle riding and fast walking with increasing intensity, duration, and frequency. At the end of 6 weeks of monitored Phase III activities, another stress test revealed that Joe could reach a safe maximum heart rate of 160 beats per minute. His resting heart rate and blood pressure were now within normal limits, he lost 20 lb, and his diet was cholesterol free. He was no longer taking any cardiac medication. The cardiologist approved Joe's transfer into Phase IV cardiac rehabilitation with 3-month checkups by the PT and another stress test in 1 year.

CASE STUDY TWO

CLINICAL HISTORY

Martha is a 58-year-old homemaker with a history of shortness of breath on exertion. She admits to a 25-year history of smoking, but stopped 5 years ago. She states that she has a productive cough in the morning. Recently, she was admitted to the hospital with a temperature of 102° F and a productive cough. Severe upper respiratory tract infection was the diagnosis. This was Martha's third such admission in the past year. After discharge, the physician requested a full pulmonary examination and initiation of rehabilitation to reduce the frequency of hospitalization.

The results of pulmonary testing revealed that her ability to forcefully expire a normal volume of air in 1 second was markedly decreased even though the total volume of air in her lungs remained near normal. The carbon dioxide concentration in her blood was elevated, and the amount of oxygen was below normal. A chest radiograph demonstrated mild inflammation of the bronchial tubes.

EXAMINATION

Physical therapy examination of her chest revealed that her breathing pattern depended mostly on the diaphragm with little chest wall motion. The angle between her ribs and sternum has increased, which indicates that her lower chest wall has permanently expanded beyond normal. There is evidence that her accessory muscles of ventilation around the neck and shoulders contract during quiet inspiration. When Martha was placed on a treadmill and asked to walk at 3 mph with no grade, she demonstrated a further drop in the oxygen saturation of her blood, shortness of breath, and mild wheezing.

PULMONARY REHABILITATION

The results of the examination led to a diagnosis of moderate obstructive lung disease accompanied by physical deconditioning. The primary goals for Martha's rehabilitation program would be to achieve a daily walk or jog of 30 continuous minutes without shortness of breath, improve her functional capacity, and perform pulmonary hygiene to assist with clearing of her lungs each morning.

The PT instructed Martha in the appropriate postural drainage positions that she will use for 10 minutes on each side of the chest before getting out of bed in the morning. She was taught breathing exercises that will help mobilize her lower chest wall, increase the strength of her diaphragm and intercostal muscles, and improve her ability to perform a forceful cough. Martha must also learn specific diet modifications and how to monitor for symptoms that might occur if her blood oxygen concentration were to drop too severely.

Martha's exercise program includes progressive walking. The heart rate achieved when shortness of breath requires her to stop will be used as the maximum heart rate. Warm up and cool-down periods will occur before and after the continuous walking period. The duration, intensity, and frequency of the exercise program will be increased until she can achieve 30 continuous minutes of walking without shortness of breath. In conjunction with the exercise program, the PT must educate the patient on how she will monitor herself safely and perform the exercise routine independently.

REFERENCES

1. Heron M: Deaths: Leading Causes for 2010, *Natl Vital Stat Rep* 62(6):1–97, 2013. 2013 Dec 20, http://www.cdc.gov/nchs/data/nvsr/nvsr62/nvsr62_06.pdf. Accessed July 9, 2014.
2. Go AS, Mozaffarian D, Roger VL, et al: Heart disease and stroke statistics—2014 update. A report from the American Heart Association, *Circulation* 129(3):e28–e292, 2014.
3. Heidenreich PA, Trogdon JG, Khavjou OA, et al: Forecasting the future of cardiovascular disease in the United States. A policy statement from the American Heart Association, *Circulation* 123 (8):933–944, 2011.
4. Centers for Disease Control and Prevention: Million Hearts: strategies to reduce the prevalence of leading cardiovascular disease risk factors—United States, *MMWR* 60(36):1248–1251, 2011. http://www.cdc.gov/mmwr, September 16, 2011, Accessed August 8, 2014.
5. Trends in COPD (chronic bronchitis and emphysema): morbidity and mortality. New York, American Lung Association. http://www.lungusa.org/finding-cures/our-research/trend-reports/copd-trend-report.pdf. Accessed July 31, 2014.
6. Standring S: *Gray's anatomy: the anatomical basis of clinical practice*, ed 40, Philadelphia, 2009, Elsevier.
7. Frownfelter D, Dean E: *Cardiovascular and pulmonary physical therapy evidence to practice*, ed 5, St Louis, 2012, Mosby, Inc., an affiliate of Elsevier, Inc.
8. Moore KL, Dalley AF, Agur AM: *Clinically oriented anatomy*, ed 6, Philadelphia, 2010, Lippincott Williams and Wilkins.
9. McArdle WD, Katch FI, Katch VL: *Exercise physiology: energy, nutrition and human performance*, ed 7, Philadelphia, 2009, Lippincott Williams and Wilkins.
10. Dorland WAN: *Dorland's illustrated medical dictionary*, ed 32, Philadelphia, 2011, Saunders.
11. Van De Graaff KM, Fox SI: *Concepts of human anatomy and physiology*, ed 5, Dubuque, Iowa, 1998, WC Brown.
12. Hillegass EA: *Essentials of cardiopulmonary physical therapy*, ed 3, St Louis, 2010, Saunders.
13. Pescatello Linda S: *American college of sports medicine guidelines for exercise testing and prescription*, ed 9, Philadelphia, 2014, Lippincott Williams & Wilkins.
14. Brannon FJ, Foley MW, Starr JA, Sand LM: *Cardiopulmonary rehabilitation: basic theory and application*, ed 3, Philadelphia, 1998, FA Davis.
15. *Guide to Physical Therapist Practice* 3.0. American Physical Therapy Association. http://guidetoptpractice.apta.org/. Accessed November 24, 2014.
16. Paz JC, West MP: *Acute care handbook for physical therapists*, ed 4, St. Louis, 2014, Saunders.
17. Pescatello Linda S: *American college of sports medicine guidelines for exercise testing and prescription*, ed 9, Philadelphia, 2014, Lippincott Williams & Wilkins.
18. Minter RA: *Chest imaging: an integrated approach*, Baltimore, 1981, Williams and Wilkins.
19. Cohen S: *Pulmonary function tests in patient care*, New York, 1980, American Journal of Nursing Company.
20. Cohen S: *Blood gas and acid base concepts in respiratory care*, New York, 1976, American Journal of Nursing Company.
21. Ciccone CD: *Pharmacology in rehabilitation*, ed 4, Philadelphia, 2007, FA Davis.

10

22. Wenger NK, Hellerstein HK: *Rehabilitation of the coronary patient,* ed 3, New York, 1992, Churchill Livingstone.
23. Heart Transplants: Statistics The American Heart Association, Dallas, Texas. www.americanheart.org/presenter.Jhtml?identifier=4588. Accessed June 1, 2010.
24. Malone DJ, Lindsay KLB: *Physical therapy in acute care: a clinician's guide,* Thorofare, NJ, 2006, Slack.
25. Reul GJ: Implantation of a permanent cardiac pacemaker. In Cooley DA, editor: Techniques in Cardiac Surgery, ed 2, Philadelphia, 1984, Saunders.
26. Frownfelter DL: *Chest physical therapy and pulmonary rehabilitation: an interdisciplinary approach,* ed 2, Chicago, 1987, Year Book.
27. Howell S, Hill J: Acute respiratory care in open heart surgery, *Phys Ther* 52:253–260, 1972.
28. ACC/AHA: Guideline Update for the Diagnosis and Management of Chronic Heart Failure in the Adult, *Circulation* 112(12):E154–E235, 2005.
29. The Criteria Committee of the New York Heart Association: *Nomenclature and criteria for diagnosis of diseases of the heart and great vessels,* ed 9, Boston, 1994, Little, Brown and Co, 253–256.
30. Irwin S, Tecklin JS: *Cardiopulmonary physical therapy,* ed 4, St Louis, 2005, Mosby.
31. Rothstein JM, Roy SH, Wolf SL, Scalzitti D: *The rehabilitation specialist's handbook,* ed 3, Philadelphia, 2005, FA Davis, 31.
32. Fair SE: *Wellness and physical therapy,* Sudbury, 2011, Jones and Bartlett Publishers.
33. Centers for Disease Control and Prevention and National Institutes of Health: Healthy People 2010, Heart Disease and Stroke. www.healthypeople.gov/document/html/volume1/12heart.htm. Accessed May 25, 2010.

REVIEW QUESTIONS

1. Explain how the cardiovascular and pulmonary systems function together.
2. Describe how pulmonary dysfunction can lead to cardiac dysfunction and how cardiac dysfunction can lead to pulmonary dysfunction.
3. Describe the movement of blood as it returns from the periphery through the heart to the pulmonary circulation.
4. Create a diagram that illustrates the processes of respiration and ventilation.
5. Explain the risk factors for CVD.
6. Research the use of at least one of the cardiovascular or pulmonary diagnostic tools discussed in this chapter.
7. Describe a patient in need of cardiac rehabilitation. (A paragraph is long enough.) Then create a flow chart of the typical therapy process and the changes made as the patient progresses.
8. Repeat the steps assigned in question 7, but this time apply it to a patient in pulmonary rehabilitation.

11

Physical Therapy for Integumentary Conditions

R. Scott Ward

KEY TERMS

arterial insufficiency
chronic inflammation
collagen
dermatitis
dermis
epidermis
ground substance
hypertrophic scar
inflammatory phase
inflammatory skin diseases
integument
keloid scar
maturation phase
neoplastic skin diseases
neuropathic (neurotropic) ulcer
pressure ulcer
proliferative phase
scar contraction
scar contracture
total body surface area (TBSA)
Vancouver Burn Scar Scale
venous insufficiency

LEARNING OBJECTIVES

After reading this chapter, the reader will be able to:

- Discuss the structure and function of the skin.
- Discuss the process of wound healing, including the three major phases—inflammation, proliferation, and maturation.
- Describe common problems associated with the integument (including vascular

compromise, trauma, and disease) and the basic examination principles related to those conditions.
- Describe basic intervention principles and strategies necessary in complete patient care (including prevention, management, and education).

Various types of integumentary (skin) wounds or impairments in skin integrity, the consequences of these wounds, and any associated effects of the wound such as inflammation, pain, edema, and scar formation can lead to significant functional limitations and disability. Physical therapists (PTs) and physical therapist assistants (PTAs) must be aware of the importance of the integumentary system in normal human function. They should be able to provide programs or interventions to prevent loss of skin integrity. Appropriate management of patients with various impairments of the skin is a critical part of physical therapy practice.

GENERAL DESCRIPTION

INTEGUMENT

The **integument**, the largest organ of the body, ranges from about 1 to 4 mm in thickness and consists of two layers—the epidermis and the dermis. Beneath the dermis lies a layer of subcutaneous tissue. The integument is basically a protective organ, but it also plays a role in temperature control and provides important sensory information regarding the environment. Figure 11-1 illustrates the structure of the skin and its appendages.

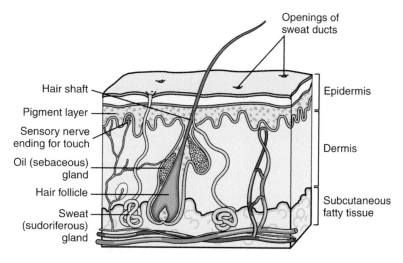

Figure 11-1 ■ Structure of the integument and its appendages. (From Sorrentino S: Mosby's Textbook for Long-term Care Nursing Assistants, ed 6, Mosby, St. Louis, 2011.)

EPIDERMIS

The **epidermis** is very thin in comparison with the overall thickness of the skin. The thickness of the epidermis generally ranges from about 0.06 to 0.1 mm. It is thicker only on the soles of the feet and the palms of the hands, where the most superficial layer of the epidermis, the stratum corneum, may increase the thickness to 0.6 mm. This thicker stratum corneum is often referred to as *callus.* The preponderant cells in the epidermis are keratinocytes produced in the basal cell layer. The basal cell layer is also where the epidermis is anchored to the dermis. Keratinocytes take a minimum of 28 days to differentiate through their epidermal phases until they are finally sloughed off the most external surface of the stratum corneum. It is the stratum corneum that restricts the loss of fluids from internal tissue and separates this same internal tissue from the external environment.

Other cells that make up the epithelium are Langerhans cells, Merkel cells, and melanocytes. Langerhans cells play a role in the immune response in skin. Merkel cells are acknowledged as sensory receptor cells that provide information about tactile stimuli. Melanocytes (located in the basal cell layer) synthesize melanin, which is a pigment that principally serves as primary protection against harmful ultraviolet radiation. Once produced, melanin is transferred from melanocytes to keratinocytes. Melanocytes are also present in the dermis and hair follicles (as well as other sites, such as the retina).

Other components of the epidermis that penetrate into the dermis are hair follicles, sebaceous glands, apocrine glands, and sweat (eccrine) glands. The basal cell layer surrounds each of these structures because of their connection with the epidermis. Hair is formed at the follicle by a process of keratinization that produces three layers of cells. The hair follicle is an invagination of the epidermis. Hair type and amount depend on several factors, including hormonal influence, age, and heredity. Sebaceous glands produce a fatty secretion and are found in association with every hair follicle (pilosebaceous glands). Some sebaceous glands not associated with hair follicles are also found in a general distribution over the body with the exception of the soles of the feet, the palms of the hands, and the lower lip. The main function of the sebaceous glands is to keep the skin "moisturized" and pliant and to prevent it from drying and cracking. The apocrine glands begin to secrete a commonly colorless and odorless oily sweat at the onset of puberty. These glands are localized in the anogenital and axillary areas. The odor associated with perspiration in these areas results from bacterial decomposition of the secretions. Sweat is a hypotonic solution that is delivered to the skin surface by sweat glands. Normal function of the sweat glands is critical in temperature regulation.

DERMIS

The **dermis** consists of fibrous and elastic connective tissue encompassed by a ground substance. The dermis varies from 1 to 4 mm in thickness and has two subdivisions—the papillary and the reticular dermis. The papillary dermis, which is composed of a loosely organized collagen matrix and is highly vascular, forms in reflection to the basal cell layer of the epidermis. The junction between these two layers of skin is far from flat. The ridges formed at the dermal-epidermal

11

junction (dermal papillae and epidermal ridges, respectively) provide protection against potentially damaging perturbations such as shearing and deepen the dispersion of the epidermal basal cell layer. The reticular dermis is composed of more densely bundled collagen fibers and less ground substance than the papillary dermis. The ground substance of the dermis is made up of various proteoglycans, glycoproteins, hyaluronic acid, and water. This "gel" forms the interstitial environment that accommodates the composite of dermal elements—fibroblastic collagen, blood vessels, and nerves—along with the epidermal appendages. The fibrous collagen supplies fortification against mechanical stresses on the skin while still allowing the deformation necessary for movement. The elastic connective tissue restores the collagen network to its "resting" arrangement, and the ground substance acts as a "cushion" to protect against many detrimental compression forces.

Blood vessels and nerves are also found within the dermis. The vascular structure in the dermis is vast and allows typically efficient diffusion of gases and nutrients to promote healthy cell function. The vascular system of the dermis also participates in the inflammatory response, an important component of wound healing. Along with the sweat glands, the capillaries in the skin also contribute to human thermal regulation. An equally expansive and efficient lymphatic system is associated with the vascular system in the dermis. The dermal nervous network provides the central nervous system with essential sensory information about temperature, pain, and various tactile stimuli (light touch, deep touch, and vibration) singly or in combination to allow for recognition of objects and textures. Efferent nerves innervate the vessels, sweat glands, and arrector pili muscles of the hair follicles.

SUBCUTANEOUS TISSUE

The subcutaneous layer of tissue consists of loose connective tissue, often containing various amounts of adipose tissue. The loose connective tissue binds the skin to the organ immediately below it in a fashion that allows a reasonable amount of movement of the skin over the underlying organ without displacement or damage.

WOUND HEALING

Wound healing is commonly described in three phases: the inflammatory phase, the proliferative phase, and the remodeling phase.[1] Each of the phases, along with applicable interventions for each phase, are discussed briefly in this section. It is important that all the phases of wound repair occur simultaneously to some extent. For example, inflammation can occur while the proliferative process is in progress.

INFLAMMATORY PHASE

With any injury comes an **inflammatory phase** during which repair of the damaged tissue is initiated.[2] Local cellular and vascular reactions are included in this wound-healing phase.[3] Initial blood loss is decreased by the immediate vasoconstriction of vessels. The vasoconstrictive response may last about 5-10 min. This time frame also allows the accumulation of platelets and the formation of temporary "platelet clots" along the damaged endothelial lining of the vessels. Activation of the clotting cascade leading to the eventual formation of fibrin clots begins at this time.

The period of vasoconstriction is followed by an episode of vasodilatation and increased capillary permeability. Leukocytes, which are chemotactically recruited to the wound site, are delivered by the increased flow of blood with vasodilatation. Early battles against infection are waged at this point by neutrophils.[4,5,6,7] Macrophages also migrate to the wound site to phagocytose wound debris and spent cells. Macrophages release factors important in wound repair, such as cytokines, growth factors, and collagenases.[8] Lymphocytes also follow neutrophils into the wound site. They play an important role in the immune response because they release factors that stimulate macrophages and fibroblasts.[9] The increased capillary permeability during inflammation can lead to the formation of local edema. Edema hinders healing by reducing the local arterial, venous, and lymphatic circulation and increases the chance of infection for the same reasons. Edema may also restrict motion, which increases the possibility of tissue fibrosis.

Exposure of injured nerves and release of chemical mediators at the wound site can produce pain. Pain often causes a patient to restrict activity because the activity may increase the pain. Decreases in appropriate activity can lead to a reduction in motion and mobility.

The inflammatory phase of healing may normally last about 2 weeks. Longer periods of inflammation are referred to as **chronic inflammation**.

During this phase, appropriate physical therapy interventions might include wound care, edema management, positioning, splinting, cautious passive range-of-motion exercises, active range-of-motion exercises, ambulation, and functional activities such as activities of daily living.

PROLIFERATIVE PHASE

Fibroblasts start converging on the wound site during inflammation, and the **proliferative phase** of wound healing commences with the production of collagen by these cells. Fibroblasts produce a connective tissue scaffold made up of elastin, collagen, and glycosaminoglycans. This process contributes to one of the major events during the proliferative phase of healing—rebuilding and strengthening of the wound site. Elastin is an elastic fibrous protein that provides flexibility to the wound, but it makes up only a small percentage in comparison with collagen.

Collagen is the chief protein produced by fibroblasts.[10] Collagen fibrils formed by fibroblasts combine and form collagen fibers. Collagen fibers supply the preponderance of strength to the wound. The strength lies in the collagen fiber, not in the amount of collagen at the wound site,[11] so a patient does not need a big scar to have a strong and well-healed wound.

Ground substance (glycosaminoglycans, water, and salts) occupies the space among the elastin, collagen, vascular structures, and other cells in the healing wound.[12] The ground substance allows cell proliferation and migration and provides some cushion for the healing tissue.

11

Angiogenesis (the formation of new blood vessels) begins during the inflammatory phase of healing, but the majority of regrowth occurs during the proliferative healing phase.[13] Vascular genesis is important for the distribution of nutrients and oxygen to cells at the site of healing.

Wounds that are not deep enough to destroy the epidermal basal cell layer can heal through real epidermal regeneration. In epidermal regeneration, proliferation of both epithelial cells at the margin of a wound and epidermal cells from any existing basal cell (such as those in the dermis that encompass hair follicles or sweat glands) ultimately leads to wound coverage. Deeper wounds that do not have basal cells available may still achieve wound closure with epithelium that migrates from adjacent uninjured skin. This process generally occurs only in smaller wounds.

One other concern associated with the proliferative phase of healing is wound contraction. Wounds begin to contract slightly during inflammation; however, aggressive contraction at the wound commences during the proliferative phase. Fibroblasts, particularly myofibroblasts, have contractile capability.[14,15,16] It appears that the physiologic function of wound contraction is to decrease the surface area of the wound, but contraction takes place in wounds of all sizes. Although potentially beneficial in small wounds, contraction is more frequently the cause of decreased mobility and cosmetic change, particularly in wounds associated with joints.

Physical therapy interventions for the proliferative phase of healing may include wound care, edema management, positioning, splinting, cautious passive range-of-motion exercises, active range-of-motion exercises, ambulation, and functional activities such as activities of daily living, similar to interventions during the inflammatory phase. In addition, active assisted range-of-motion exercises, stretching, strengthening exercises, and endurance exercises may be appropriate. During this phase, wounds must be handled carefully because a wound will not be as strong as normal skin.[17]

MATURATION PHASE

The **maturation phase** of healing is also often referred to as the *remodeling phase.* During the maturation phase, collagen continues to be actively deposited while it is also going through active lysis. The balance between the amount of collagen deposition by fibroblasts and the magnitude of collagen lysis influences the ultimate appearance of the scar (if scar formation occurs). If deposition exceeds lysis, either a **hypertrophic scar** or a **keloid scar** forms.[18,19] Keloid scars differ from hypertrophic scars in that they extend beyond the original boundaries of the wound, they take longer to mature, and they are not associated with contracture. There may also be some biologic distinction between these types of scars.[20,21,22]

During the maturation phase, collagen fibers are deposited in an unorganized fashion. The arrangement of these fibers, however, is influenced by stresses placed on them. For example, stretching an actively forming scar will cause the collagen fibers to align themselves along the length of the stretch and, therefore, become oriented in an alignment that favors mobility over restriction of movement.

The maturation phase of wound healing may last for several months. While the phase is active—that is, while collagen is being produced—the wound continues to contract with varying degrees of vitality. As the phase nears its end, wound contraction tends to diminish. Contraction during this phase is often referred to as **scar contraction**. If scar contraction leads to either a permanent or a semifixed positional fault at a joint, it is referred to as a **scar contracture**. Race, family history, depth of the wound, size of the wound, patient age, and location of the wound all appear to be factors affecting scar formation.[22,23,24,25]

All therapeutic interventions listed for the previous two phases may be applied to the maturation phase of healing. However, the PT or PTA can generally be more aggressive with manipulation of the wound site. Depending on circumstances, the maturation phase may also be the phase when work-hardening and -conditioning exercises are energetically pursued. Moreover, depending on the size and location of the scar, techniques to control scar formation should be instituted.

ADDITIONAL CONSIDERATIONS

The variables of repair and patient response to skin wounds include depth of the damage, location of the injury, size of the wound, healing time, and cause of the disruption. The depth of injury probably has the greatest impact on repair and eventual healing of a wound. For example, superficial wounds that leave a majority of the epidermal basal cells intact often heal without complication. Deeper skin damage that destroys much if not all of the epidermal basal cell layer may take weeks to heal or require surgical intervention to hasten repair. Generally, the deeper the wound, the longer it takes to heal. Figure 11-2 illustrates depths of wounds and the integumentary structures involved at the varying depths.

The location of the injury can affect rehabilitation in many ways. For example, wounds on the feet can affect gait, wounds on hands can affect activities that

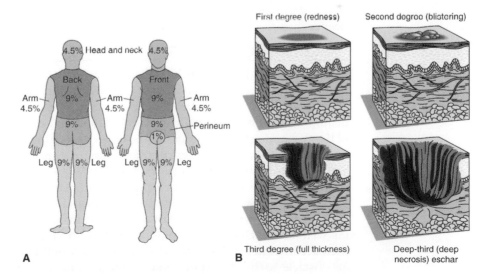

Figure 11-2 ■ Structures involved in varying depths of skin injury. (From Fordney M: Insurance Handbook for the Medical Office, ed 13, Saunders, St. Louis, 2014.)

require hand function, and wounds over any joint can lead to impairment in motion and, therefore, also lead to changes in strength and performance of activities of daily living. Furthermore, wounds at cosmetic sites such as the face and hands may offer psychological challenges for a patient to overcome.

The size of a wound, often measured as the percentage of **total body surface area (TBSA)** affected, has an effect on the extent of the physiologic response. A few of the physiologic responses that should be considered include the local inflammatory response, the basal metabolic rate, temperature control, cardiopulmonary stresses, hematopoietic reactions, and pain. For example, a large skin wound (such as an extensive burn injury) may dangerously decrease the ability of a patient to control body temperature. Also, a big wound will lead to an increased basal metabolic rate and impose extra nutritional demands on a patient that must be met to avert the protein catabolism that could lead to muscle loss. Infection is a potential problem with any open wound, and increased wound size may increase the risk of infection. As wound size increases, so does the magnitude of the physiologic response.

Wounds that require a long time to heal are associated with two primary problems. First, the risk of infection increases the longer that the wound is open. Second, a wound that takes longer than 2-3 weeks to heal is more likely to scar.

COMMON CONDITIONS

Damage to the integument most commonly results from vascular compromise or trauma. Vascular deficiencies such as local tissue ischemia (pressure ulcers and arterial disease) and venous insufficiency can create an unhealthy tissue environment that leads to skin breakdown. Wounds from various types of trauma may include cuts, abrasions, and burns.

The cause of a wound can provide insight into its prognosis. For example, patients with wounds caused by arterial disease usually require surgical intervention to improve arterial function and eventually improve healing of the associated skin wound. Electrical injuries should lead to the suspicion that tissue deeper than the skin has been damaged.

VASCULAR COMPROMISE

Wounds caused by **arterial insufficiency** are most commonly situated on the foot or ankle, but they also occur at other locations. These wounds are caused by primary loss of vascular flow to an anatomic site, which leads to tissue death.[26,27,28] **Venous insufficiency** (venous stasis) can also lead to ulceration of the skin and generally occurs on the lower part of the legs.[26,27,28] Venous stasis may result from venous hypertension, venous thrombosis, varicose (dilated) veins, or obstruction of a portion of the venous system. The precise cause of ulcers caused by venous stasis has not been determined. Various theories forwarded to explain venous stasis ulceration include the notion of "fibrin cuff formation" that occurs as a result of an increase in capillary leakage of fibrinogen (as well as other large molecules) secondary to venous hypertension.[26] Fibrin then accumulates in the interstitial space and around capillaries and produces an obstacle to the transportation of oxygen and nutrients to tissue. Another theory regarding venous stasis ulcers is referred to as "white cell trapping." Venous hypertension decreases capillary flow and the subsequent removal of leukocytes. The trapped cells then occlude capillaries, which leads to ischemic damage and may also release substances that may cause direct local tissue damage.[26,28,29,30,31,32]

Pressure on tissue causes ischemia, producing damage, tissue hypoxia and death, and a wound referred to as a **pressure ulcer**.[33] Only a few hours of pressure can cause severe tissue injury.[33,34,35] Pressure occurs most commonly over areas of bony prominence, such as the sacral or coccygeal area, ischial tuberosity, heel, lateral malleolus, and greater trochanter. Pressure may increase or decrease, depending on the patient's position.[36] Table 11-1 lists sites at risk for pressure ulcers by position. For example, simply being positioned incorrectly in bed can damage the skin.

Although most pressure ulcers occur at sites of bony prominence, they can develop at any location in which enough pressure is generated to cause ischemia. Inactivity and immobility increase the chance of development of pressure sores.[37,38] Shearing of the tissue at the site of pressure can further increase the tissue damage. Shearing may occur when a patient is moved from one surface to another or moves (slides) on the same surface. This activity causes friction damage to the skin. Friction can denude the epidermal covering and increase the likelihood for pressure ulcer formation. If the skin is exposed to moisture for a certain period, it may become macerated and more liable to break down. Common sources of moisture include sweat, urine, and feces. Poor nutrition increases the risk of pressure ulcers. Several age-related changes, such as a decrease in overall soft tissue mass that increases the protuberance of bony prominences, atrophy of the dermis, decreased vascularization, and impaired sensory perception, amplify the risk that pressure ulcers will develop.

Ischemic injury can occur as a result of loss of sensory feedback. An ulcer secondary to insensitivity is called a **neuropathic (neurotropic) ulcer**.[38] Decreased sensation limits a person from making appropriate adjustments to potentially damaging situations.[36,39] For example, a patient with sensory loss in the soles of the feet caused by diabetes mellitus may not notice a tiny pebble in the shoe.[40] Blood flow to the tissue compressed by the pebble decreases as the person continues to bear weight on the stone. Although not considered neuropathic ulcers, pressure ulcers may also occur with loss of sensory feedback, as in the case of a

Table 11-1 **Body Areas Commonly at Risk for Pressure Ulcer Development**	
Position	**Areas at Risk**
Supine	Occiput, elbows, scapulae, spinous processes, sacrum, coccyx, heels
Seated	Elbows, spinous processes, sacrum, coccyx, ischial tuberosities, greater trochanters, heels
Side-lying	Ear, shoulder, elbow, greater trochanters, medial and lateral aspects of knees, medial and lateral malleoli, heels
Prone	Forehead, nose, chin, anterior of shoulder, iliac crest, patella, dorsal surface of foot or toes

Data from Kosiak M: Etiology and pathology of ischemic ulcers, *Arch Phys Med Rehabil* 62:492–498, 1981.

11

patient with a spinal cord injury.[39] In the case of a spinal cord injury, if the patient does not perform frequent weight shifts, ischemia resulting from pressure will cause damage to the integument. Neuropathic ulcers may also form as a result of motor neuropathy, leading to anatomic deformity that causes pressure points that would not normally be present.

TRAUMA

Abrasions are integumentary wounds caused by scraping away skin through contact with a rough object or surface. Lacerations are cuts or tears of the integument and may be caused by sharp objects or surfaces. Injuries in which much if not all the skin and generally the subcutaneous tissue are separated from the underlying tissue are referred to as *avulsion injuries.* When an avulsion injury occurs to a hand or a foot, it may be called a *degloving injury.* A puncture wound is a hole in the skin created by a pointed, generally sharp object. Burn injuries include damage to skin from many possible causes, such as flame, chemicals, scalding, radiation, and electrical current.

As with some cases of ischemic skin damage, trauma can arise from loss of sensory feedback. Decreased sensation prevents a person from making appropriate adjustments to potentially damaging situations. For example, a patient with decreased sensation in the upper extremities because of edema resulting from surgical removal of axillary lymph nodes may not perceive the hazardous temperature of a dish when removing it from the oven or dangerously hot water, either of which could lead to a burn injury.

DISEASE

The skin can be affected by a number of disorders that may be either benign or life threatening. **Inflammatory skin diseases** are generally patchy sites of acute or chronic inflammation referred to as **dermatitis**. Dermatitis often includes associated symptoms of itching and some scaling of the epidermis. Certain viruses can lead to warts or rashes. Bacteria, foreign bodies, and plugged sebaceous glands are some of the causes that may lead to acne or other skin abscesses.

Neoplastic skin diseases (skin cancer) include basal cell carcinoma, squamous cell carcinoma, and malignant melanoma, which are the three most common types of cancers associated with the integument. Although other causes are possible, extensive exposure to sunlight is the most common cause of each of these cancers.

PRINCIPLES OF EXAMINATION

Examination of a wound should include a thorough history and physical assessment of the cause, depth, and size of the wound and signs of infection. Some variations in actual examination procedures may be applicable for different causes (see later). The skin adjacent to or otherwise associated with the wound should also be examined for any alteration from normal function (e.g., sensation, temperature, hair growth, mobility, and pliability) and appearance (e.g., texture and color [red for inflammation or bluish for cyanosis or poor perfusion]).

All ulcers, regardless of their cause, should be examined for size and depth. The size of a wound can be charted by several methods, some of which are tracing diagrams of the wound, TBSA estimates (see discussion of burns), and photography. The depth of a wound can be measured by injecting known volumes of saline into the wound cavity (the amount of saline left over is subtracted from the total to give a volume). Depth may also be measured by the use of a wound filler (such as dental alginate) that can be transferred to a volumeter to allow measurement of the depth of the wound via displacement of fluid from the volumeter. Depth can be further determined by observation of the exposed tissue. For example, a moist pink or red wound that is hypersensitive and on an even plane with adjacent, uninjured skin is probably a partial-thickness wound, whereas in deeper wounds subcutaneous adipose tissue or fascia can often be identified. In wounds that extend beyond defined subcutaneous tissue, muscle, tendon, ligament, bone, and other structures may be visible.

Besides assessing integrity of the integument, the PT should perform other tests and measures for a full evaluation of the patient. Assessment of the patient's ability to communicate and comprehend, joint mobility, muscle performance, gait (if applicable), ventilation, and circulation and sensory tests (including assessment of pain) should be part of the physical therapy examination.

VASCULAR COMPROMISE

ARTERIAL WOUNDS

Wounds caused by arterial insufficiency are commonly found on the lower part of the leg, including the feet and toes. Because of the poor circulation to the wound, minimal, if any, exudate is seen. The shape of these wounds is commonly irregular, and the wounds are often deep with a pale wound base. The diminished circulation contributes to poor wound healing. The pain associated with arterial wounds is severe and generally increases when the leg is elevated. Skin adjacent to these wounds is characterized by hair loss and pallor on elevation, is cool to the touch, and appears "thin" and shiny. Pulses associated with arterial wounds are weak or absent.

VENOUS ULCERS

Wounds caused by venous insufficiency are commonly found on the lower part of the leg. Exudate and edema are present, the shape of these wounds is commonly irregular, and the wounds are generally shallow with a red or pink wound base. Edema is a factor in poor wound healing. Some mild pain is associated with venous ulcers, and the pain can commonly be decreased when the leg is elevated. The skin adjacent to these wounds is characterized by inflammation, dilated veins, abnormal pigmentation, and induration (hardness) and may be dry or scaly. Pulses associated with venous ulcers are present.

NEUROPATHIC ULCERS

Neuropathic ulcers are usually located on the plantar surface of the foot at pressure points or bony prominences. The wound may bleed easily unless the condition is coupled with arterial insufficiency. The shape of these wounds is commonly circular, and the wounds are often deep. Because of the sensory neuropathy that led to the wound, these ulcers are normally painless. The skin adjacent to the wounds is characterized by sensory deficit, but might otherwise appear fairly normal.

11

PRESSURE ULCERS

Pressure ulcers may be located in diverse sites on the body but are generally found over bony prominences. Besides describing the location, the examiner should document the depth and size, which can vary. A well-accepted method for describing a pressure ulcer is to use a staging system provided by the National Pressure Ulcer Advisory Panel.[39] Staging of the ulcer is based on wound characteristics, mainly depth. Table 11-2 outlines the criteria for staging pressure ulcers. Once an ulcer is staged, the assigned stage should not change as the wound changes. For example, a Stage III ulcer that heals does not progress

Table 11-2
Criteria for Staging Pressure Ulcers

Ulcer Stage	Description of the Ulcer
I—Nonblanchable erythema	Intact skin with nonblanchable redness of a localized area usually over a bony prominence. Darkly pigmented skin may not have visible blanching; its color may differ from the surrounding area. The area may be painful, firm, soft, warmer or cooler as compared to adjacent tissue. Category I may be difficult to detect in individuals with dark skin tones. May indicate "at risk" persons.
II—Partial thickness	Partial thickness loss of dermis presenting as a shallow open ulcer with a red pink wound bed, without slough. May also present as an intact or open/ruptured serum-filled or sero-sangineous filled blister. Presents as a shiny or dry shallow ulcer without slough or bruising.* This category should not be used to describe skin tears, tape burns, incontinence associated dermatitis, maceration or excoriation. *Bruising indicates deep tissue injury
III—Full-thickness skin loss	Full-thickness tissue loss. Subcutaneous fat may be visible but bone, tendon or muscle are *not* exposed. Slough may be present but does not obscure the depth of tissue loss. *May* include undermining and tunneling. The depth of a Category/Stage III pressure ulcer varies by anatomic location. The bridge of the nose, ear, occiput and malleolus do not have (adipose) subcutaneous tissue and Category/Stage III ulcers can be shallow. In contrast, areas of significant adiposity can develop extremely deep Category/Stage III pressure ulcers. Bone/tendon is not visible or directly palpable.
IV—Full-thickness tissue loss	Full-thickness tissue loss with exposed bone, tendon or muscle. Slough or eschar may be present. Often includes undermining and tunneling. The depth of a Category/Stage IV pressure ulcer varies by anatomic location. The bridge of the nose, ear, occiput and malleolus do not have (adipose) subcutaneous tissue and these ulcers can be shallow. Category/Stage IV ulcers can extend into muscle and/or supporting structures (e.g., fascia, tendon, or joint capsule) making osteomyelitis or osteitis likely to occur. Exposed bone/muscle is visible or directly palpable.

From National Pressure Ulcer Advisory Panel and European Pressure Ulcer Advisory Panel. Pressure Ulcer Prevention and Treatment: Clinical Practice Guideline. Washington, DC: National Pressure Ulcer Advisory Panel, 2009. Used with permission of the National Pressure Ulcer Advisory Panel, August 18, 2015.

from a Stage III to a Stage II and then to a Stage I ulcer (referred to as *back staging*). Rather, healing of the wound is described in terms of changes in size, depth, and other characteristics and, when healed, the wound would be a healed Stage III ulcer.

TRAUMA

Any traumatic wound of concern should be initially referred for primary medical intervention. This recommendation would hold true for wounds such as abrasions, lacerations, puncture wounds, avulsion injuries, degloving injuries, and burn injuries, regardless of the cause of the wound.

Burn injuries include skin damage from one or more of the following sources: flame, chemicals, scalding, radiation, and electrical current. The severity of the burn injury depends on several factors, including percent TBSA affected, location of the burn, depth of the wound, presence of associated trauma (e.g., fracture, nerve injury), and smoke inhalation. Figure 11-3 provides a method for calculating percent TBSA and documenting the location and depth of injury. The size of the wound, as reported in percent TBSA affected, and the location of the

Area	1 year	1–4 years	5–9 years	10–14 years	15 years	Adult	Partial-thickness	Full-thickness	Total
Head	19	17	13	11	9	7			
Neck	2	2	2	2	2	2			
Ant. trunk	13	13	13	13	13	13			
Post. trunk	13	13	13	13	13	13			
Right buttock	2 1/2	2 1/2	2 1/2	2 1/2	2 1/2	2 1/2			
Left buttock	2 1/2	2 1/2	2 1/2	2 1/2	2 1/2	2 1/2			
Genitalia	1	1	1	1	1	1			
Right upper arm	4	4	4	4	4	4			
Left upper arm	4	4	4	4	4	4			
Right lower arm	3	3	3	3	3	3			
Left lower arm	3	3	3	3	3	3			
Right hand	2 1/2	2 1/2	2 1/2	2 1/2	2 1/2	2 1/2			
Left hand	2 1/2	2 1/2	2 1/2	2 1/2	2 1/2	2 1/2			
Right thigh	5 1/2	6 1/2	8	8 1/2	9	9 1/2			
Left thigh	5 1/2	6 1/2	8	8 1/2	9	9 1/2			
Right leg	5	5	5 1/2	6	6 1/2	7			
Left leg	5	5	5 1/2	6	6 1/2	7			
Right foot	3 1/2	3 1/2	3 1/2	3 1/2	3 1/2	3 1/2			
Left foot	3 1/2	3 1/2	3 1/2	3 1/2	3 1/2	3 1/2			
						Total			

Etiology of injury _____

Date of injury _____

Time of injury _____

Patient age _____

Patient sex _____

Patient weight _____

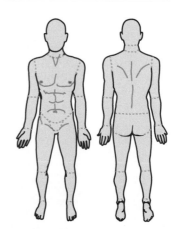

Figure 11-3 ■ Burn diagram used to calculate the size, location, and depth of a burn injury.

burns are important clues to the sites of potential impairment and functional loss. Impairments may be acute when related to pain or wound contraction in superficial, partial-thickness, and full-thickness burns, whereas wound and scar contracture at a burn site can lead to chronic problems of decreased function and potential disability. The location of the burn may also have cosmetic implications for long-term socialization of a patient with burns. The depth of a wound can be determined by the presence of certain clinical findings.[41] A superficial burn injury is painful and erythematous (like a sunburn), with the possibility of minor localized swelling. Partial-thickness injuries are typically painful, red, and weepy. The skin is normally pliable. Blistering is also commonly associated with a partial-thickness burn. A full-thickness burn is generally not painful when palpated, may be tan or yellowish brown, and has a leathery, nonpliable texture.

Associated trauma can increase the severity of a burn injury because of the increased impairment the patient will experience beyond that caused by the burns. Documentation of any associated trauma is critical to the establishment of a comprehensive plan of care. Smoke inhalation (inhalation injury) may lead to cardiopulmonary impairment. In the plan of care, the therapist may need to address impaired ventilation, gas exchange, aerobic capacity, and endurance related to inhalation injury.

DISEASE

A physician carries out the actual diagnosis and primary treatment of skin disease, but PTs and PTAs must be able to recognize the signs and symptoms of skin cancer so that they provide patients with an appropriate and prompt medical referral.[42] Key warning signs for skin cancer include a new skin growth, a sore that does not heal within 3 months, or a bump that is getting larger. Detection of possible melanoma is based on alterations in a growth on the skin or in a mole and may include changes in size, color, shape, elevation, surface appearance, or sensation.

SCAR TISSUE

As some wounds heal, scar tissue may form. Assessment of the scar tissue may be performed with the **Vancouver Burn Scar Scale.**[43] This scale rates characteristics of scars, including pigmentation, vascularity, pliability, and height (Table 11-3). A higher score on the Vancouver Burn Scar Scale correlates with more scarring. Scars are generally referred to as either *hypertrophic scars* or *keloid scars*. Both keloid and hypertrophic scars hypertrophy, but as keloid scars grow, they extend beyond the boundaries of the wound, whereas hypertrophic scars do not.[20] In addition to examination of the scar itself, the location of the scar should be assessed. Scars over or near joints may impede joint mobility, and scars in areas of cosmetic importance may have a detrimental effect on patient motivation and activity (Figure 11-4). Scar contraction, which can lead to contracture, is a major contributor to wound-related disability.

Table 11-3
Vancouver Burn Scar Scale

Score	Pigmentation	Vascularity	Pliability	Height
0	Normal pigmentation, close to the pigmentation of the rest of the body	Normal	Normal	Flat (normal)
1	Hypopigmentation	Pink	Flexible with minimal resistance	Raised <2 mm
2	Hyperpigmentation	Red	Gives way to pressure	Raised <5 mm
3		Purple	Firm, not easily moved	Raised >5 mm
4			Banding: raised tissue that blanches with stretching of the scar	
5			Contracture: permanent tightening that produces a deformity	

Adapted from Sullivan T, Smith J, Kermode J, et al.: Rating the burn scar, *J Burn Care Rehabil* 11(3):256–260, 1990.

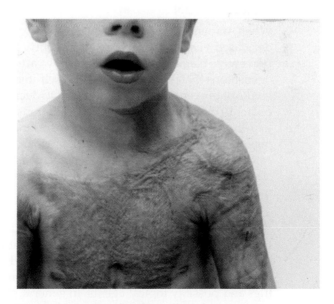

Figure 11-4 ■ Hypertrophic burn scar.

PRINICPLES OF EVALUATION, DIAGNOSIS, AND PROGNOSIS

Evaluation of a patient with a skin wound encompasses the extent of the condition, the identification of related impairments, the level of associated loss of function, the patient's basic health condition, and social factors affecting care. The decisions made through an evaluation render a diagnosis about the meaning of a patient's signs and symptoms.

The prognosis of a patient with integumentary involvement is related to the diagnosis and will be enhanced if the therapist ensures that the wound is stable, clean, and healing or healed. Some indication of the potential for scarring or the course of the scarring should be included in the prognosis because scarring clearly affects the time needed for treatment and follow-up. The prognosis of problems associated with wounds is influenced by the severity of the problems. For example, severe edema is associated with a poorer prognosis than mild edema. In addition, the presence of any comorbidity or infection, the chronicity of the problem, and any number of other physical, psychological, or social factors will affect the prognosis.

PRINCIPLES OF INTERVENTION

Proper attention by the PT and PTA to the integument ranges from preventing skin breakdown to promoting wound healing. Patients must also be educated about care of the wound, including management of the risks and signs of infection, wound care and dressing procedures, and management of scar tissue. Setting appropriate goals for interventions is imperative to minimize impairment and functional loss.

This section describes some basic elements of physical therapy intervention related to the integument. For details about integumentary management, the reader should refer to the Additional Resources at the end of the chapter and should continue to peruse current literature on the topic.

PREVENTION

When patients are at risk for ulcers (e.g., because of decreased sensation, decreased vascularity, decreased mobility, poor nutrition, or incontinence), the preventive element of physical therapy care is important. Positioning, supports, or cushions that reduce pressure and self-inspection of the skin are important elements of preventing ulcers secondary to decreased mobility, impaired sensation, or lack of circulation. Water-repellent lotions and absorbent products can be used to decrease the damaging effects of incontinence on the skin. Appropriate dressings and proper transfer techniques are important in preventing skin breakdown caused by shear and friction. When edema is associated with a wound, compression therapies such as intermittent compression pumps and compression garments may be beneficial.

WOUND MANAGEMENT

Depending on the depth of the wound and other complications, surgery such as grafting may be necessary to achieve wound closure. Many wounds, however, require short- or long-term conservative management with appropriate dressings and possibly topical agents. In general, the extent of physical therapy interventions is based on the depth of injury.

Conservative management of arterial wounds and neuropathic ulcers commonly consists of wound care, protection of the wound and surrounding tissue, and possibly bed rest. The wound should be cleansed when dressings are changed. Dressings that maintain or increase moisture at the wound site should be used because of the lack of exudate from the wound. Cushions or protective casting (total contact casting) may be useful in preventing further trauma to the wound as it heals. Bed rest may help to protect the wound, but it must be used with caution to avoid other impairments related to disuse.

Venous wounds should be managed by wound care and compression of the affected extremity.[44,45] Wound care should consist of cleansing the wound and applying a dressing. The dressing used depends on the amount of exudate at the wound site. The dressing of choice is usually a pliable semiabsorbent or gel-type dressing. If a dressing is to be worn during compression therapy, it should not be bulky. Compression of the extremity helps reduce swelling and venous hypertension in the limb. Activity such as ambulation, swimming, or cycling should be encouraged unless medically contraindicated.

Pressure ulcers require wound care and pressure relief.[36] Much like venous ulcers, pressure ulcers should be cleansed and dressed in a way that provides a moist healing environment but still manages excess exudate. Pressure-relieving devices might include any of the following options. Seat cushions should decrease the likelihood of shear and pressure while also protecting against heat and moisture. Wheelchairs should be appropriately aligned to minimize the chance of pressure ulcer formation. Foam that is either premanufactured for certain anatomic areas or custom cut by the therapist can be used to help position patients in bed. Air mattresses and other pressure relief mattresses help to decrease the buildup of pressure in any one location on the body. Turning schedules should be established and followed. In a typical turning schedule, the patient would be turned every 2 hours with equal time spent supine, prone, lying on the right side, and lying on the left side.

Treatment of burns is generally based on wound depth. Skin grafting is inevitable for full-thickness wounds of any consequential percent of TBSA. Wounds of any depth should be carefully cleansed. After cleansing, superficial burns require only a moisturizer, which may provide some pain relief, to help keep the skin moist. Partial-thickness burns are commonly covered with a topical agent, either an ointment such as Polysporin or a cream such as silver sulfadiazine. These wounds are then covered with nonadherent gauze and wrapped lightly with a gauze dressing. Full-thickness burns are characteristically treated with a topical silver sulfadiazine cream and wrapped in gauze dressing.

With any of these wounds, appropriate exercises and activities should be prescribed to decrease other impairments. Exercises should emphasize joint mobility, muscle performance, gait (if applicable), ventilation, and circulation.

SCAR MANAGEMENT

The major functional problem with scar tissue is the continuous contraction associated with it. Scar hypertrophy not only may contribute to loss of function but also may lead to cosmetic defects. Surgery to correct problems associated with scarring may be considered in an attempt to improve specific impairments or particular cosmetic deformities. Nonsurgical management of a scar is accomplished in a variety of ways. Positioning may be used to counterscar contraction by lengthening tissue for a maintained period. Generally, anticontracture positions are positions of extension at each affected joint region, such as elbow extension with supination or a neutral ankle position with no flexion of the toes. Splints may be used as static positioning devices to hold a joint in a certain position.[46] Serial splinting may also be used to progressively increase joint range of motion. Dynamic splints, which apply a gentle stretch to tissue, are used for mobilization or exercise purposes. Some prefabricated splints are available, but most clinicians fabricate custom splints from malleable thermoplastic material. Passive stretching may be used to gently elongate contracting tissue. Active exercise (including ambulation) is used for the same purpose as passive stretching but provides a way to involve patients in their own rehabilitation.[47] With any stretching, passive or active, the patient should feel the tissue stretch and try to "push the stretch" as much as possible (Figure 11-5). Effective stretching does not require induction of pain in the affected tissue during the stretch or exercise.

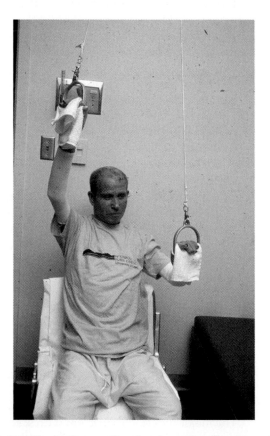

Figure 11-5 ■ Patient using overhead reciprocal pulleys to perform a self-stretch of scar tissue in the axillae and over the elbows. The patient is also wearing pressure garments to help control scar hypertrophy.

Pressure garments are used to decrease hypertrophy of the scar (see Figure 11-5). These supports also assist in conforming the scar to normal anatomic parameters. Typically, patients are prescribed pressure garments during the maturation phase of healing. The pressure garments can be custom ordered to fit a patient and can be made for any extremity, the face or head, the hands, the feet, and the torso.

PATIENT EDUCATION

The patient should be the most important member of the rehabilitation team. Those who will be assisting with care of the patient should also be included in all sessions preparing the patient for discharge. Obvious items that should be taught to the patient and other caregivers include skin care and wound management protocols, positioning techniques, exercise programs, and application and wearing of pressure garments (if needed). Demonstrating the technique and allowing the patient or caregiver to perform any of the protocols under observation should reinforce all these procedures. It is important to inform the patient about the reasons for the procedures being applied. If patients know what techniques or procedures they must perform, how to do them, and the reasons for the specific protocols assigned, they will be more apt to comply with their care.[45]

SUMMARY

This chapter has outlined the many components of integumentary care. The anatomy of the skin and the phases of wound healing are important elements to understand when interventions are being considered. Common conditions of skin breakdown arise as a result of problems with local circulation, decreased sensation, long-standing pressure, and trauma. Understanding the implications of wound depth, size, and location is critical in developing treatments. Beyond direct management of the wound, interventions that stress prevention of further skin breakdown and decrease impairments related to other systems have been discussed. Treatments that enhance wound healing and involve the patient directly as part of the rehabilitation team are most beneficial in generating optimum patient outcomes.

CASE STUDIES

CASE STUDY ONE

Mrs. George is a 53-year-old woman in whom venous insufficiency was diagnosed 5 years ago. She has managed it well until recently, when a small ulcer developed on the left lateral aspect of the lower part of her leg about 8 cm above her lateral malleolus. The ulcer is approximately 2 by 3 cm in size and is partial to deep partial thickness. A measurable amount of exudate is oozing from the wound. The limb is edematous (in comparison with the contralateral limb). Lower extremity pulses are palpable. The patient complains of mild pain at the wound site, but she is otherwise functionally independent in all activities.

GOALS

Management goals include a reduction in risk factors for infection, reduced wound size, attainment of wound healing, and a reduction in edema. The patient should understand these goals and the desired outcomes from intervention.

INTERVENTION

To decrease the risk of infection, the wound should be selectively debrided to remove nonviable tissue. Appropriate dressings should be applied, including (in this case) a semiabsorbent, nonbulky dressing that will maintain a moist wound environment but also absorb some of the exudate from the wound. Intermittent compression with an extremity lymphedema pump may be useful in decreasing edema. A graduated compression stocking should be fitted for the patient. She should be encouraged to ambulate and, if necessary, be prescribed a walking schedule. While seated, she should elevate the limb and perform ankle pumps. Standing for long periods should be discouraged. The patient should be educated and be able to demonstrate how to (1) perform dressing changes, (2) apply and operate the intermittent compression pump (one could be rented for home use), (3) apply and monitor the fit of the graduated compression stocking, and (4) describe the reasoning for the prescribed interventions and the importance of exercise and elevation in preventing further problems related to edema and venous stasis.

CASE STUDY TWO

Stan is 47 years old and was injured in a house fire. He incurred a 14% TBSA burn. Full-thickness injuries totaling 7% TBSA occurred on his right upper extremity and hand. The other 7% TBSA included the upper right portion of his chest and back. The patient is right hand dominant. He was previously healthy and sustained no associated injuries (e.g., smoke inhalation). Stan was employed as a worker in a warehouse and lives at home with his wife and three teenage children. Four days after his admission to the burn center, his right upper extremity and hand burns underwent skin grafting.

GOALS

Risk factors for infection need to be reduced to enhance partial-thickness wound healing and prepare full-thickness wounds for skin grafting. Joint mobility is to be maintained and soft tissue restriction (wound and scar contraction) reduced. The risk of impairment secondary to scar formation needs to be decreased. Independence in activities of daily living and the ability to perform tasks associated with Stan's work are goals to be regained. The patient should understand these goals and the desired outcomes from intervention.

INTERVENTION

When dealing with such a burn, the patient must be treated before any surgery to alleviate and prevent increased impairment and disability. The patient must continue with postsurgical treatment to achieve the final desired outcomes of therapy intervention.

PRESURGERY

The wounds should be cleansed and dressed twice a day to reduce the risk of infection and promote healing of the partial-thickness wounds and to prepare the full-thickness wounds for skin grafting. Active range-of-motion exercises for the upper extremity and hand will enhance joint mobility and decrease the soft tissue restriction associated with wound contraction. Positioning of the upper extremity will also help prevent decreases in mobility and increases in soft tissue restriction. The patient should also be encouraged to participate in his personal care (e.g., brushing teeth, combing hair, and personal hygiene), which will aid in future independence in activities of daily living.

POSTSURGERY

Any remaining partial-thickness wounds should be cleansed and dressed twice a day to reduce the risk of infection and promote healing. Active range-of-motion exercises and positioning that began presurgically should be continued after surgery. Passive range of motion or stretching of the upper extremity might be helpful in overcoming any relentless contraction of the scar tissue forming at the sites of skin grafting. The patient should be required to manage his personal care independently. Strengthening exercises and exercises specific to preparation for return to work should also be included as the patient can tolerate them. The patient's upper extremity should be measured for and fitted with a scar control compression garment (specifically, an arm sleeve and a glove). Scar control will help maintain anatomic contours and decrease the risk of soft tissue restriction caused by scar formation.

The patient should be educated about and be able to demonstrate (1) assisting with dressing changes, (2) performing any of the specifically prescribed exercises, and (3) applying and monitoring the fit of the scar control compression garments. The patient should also be able to describe the rationale behind each of the interventions.

REFERENCES

1. Baum CL, Arpey CJ: Normal cutaneous wound healing: clinical correlation with cellular and molecular events, *Dermatol Surg* 31(6):674–686, 2005.
2. Rankin JA: Biological mediators of acute inflammation, *AACN Clin Issues* 15:3–17, 2004.
3. Eming S, Krieg T, Davidson J: Inflammation in wound repair: molecular and cellular mechanisms, *J Invest Dermatol* 127:514–525, 2007.
4. Park J, Barbul A: Understanding the role of immune regulation in wound healing, *Am J Surg* 187:11S–16S, 2004.
5. Oberyszyn T: Inflammation and wound healing, *Front Biosci* 12:2993–2999, 2007.
6. Kennedy A, DeLeo F: Neutrophil apoptosis and the resolution of infection, *Immunol Res* 43:25–61, 2009.
7. Kolaczkowska E, Kubes P: Neutrophil recruitment and function in health and inflammation, *Nat Rev Immunol* 13:159–175, 2013.
8. Gordon S: The macrophage: past, present and future, *Eur J Immunol* 37:S9–S17, 2007.
9. Keen D: A review of research examining the regulatory role of lymphocytes in normal wound healing, *J Wound Care* 17:218–220, 2008.
10. Peacock E, editor: *Wound repair*, ed 6, Philadelphia, 1984, Saunders.
11. Hardy M: The biology of scar formation, *Phys Ther* 69:1014–1024, 1989.
12. Corr DT, Hart DA: Biomechanics of scar tissue and uninjured skin, *Adv Wound Care* 2:37–43, 2013.
13. Raines EW: The extracellular matrix can regulate vascular cell migration, proliferation, and survival: relationships to vascular disease, *Int J Exp Pathol* 81(3):173–182, 2000.

11

14. Eddy RJ, Petro JA, Tomasek JJ: Evidence for the nonmuscle nature of the "myofibroblast" of granulation tissue and hypertrophic scar. An immunofluorescence study, *Am J Pathol* 130 (2):252–260, 1988.

15. Li B, Wang JH: Fibroblasts and myofibroblasts in wound healing: force generation and measurement, *J Tissue Viability* 20:108–120, 2011.

16. Gurtner GC, Werner S, Barrandon Y, Longaker MT: Wound repair and regeneration, *Nature* 453 (7193):314–321, 2008.

17. Franz MG, Kuhn MA, Wright TE, et al.: Use of the wound healing trajectory as an outcome determinant for acute wound healing, *Wound Repair Regen* 8(6):511–516, 2000.

18. Ladin DA, Garner WL, Smith DJ Jr : Excessive scarring as a consequence of healing, *Wound Repair Regen* 3(1):6–14, 1995.

19. Armour A, Scott PG, Tredget EE: Cellular and molecular pathology of HTS: basis for treatment, *Wound Repair Regen* 15(Suppl 1):S6–S17, 2007.

20. Kose O, Waseem A: Keloids and hypertrophic scars: are they two different sides of the same coin? *Dermatol Surg* 34(3):336–346, 2008.

21. Slemp AE, Kirschner RE: Keloids and scars: a review of keloids and scars, their pathogenesis, risk factors, and management, *Curr Opin Pediatr* 18(4):396–402, 2006.

22. Burd A, Huang L: Hypertrophic response and keloid diathesis: two very different forms of scar, *Plast Reconstr Surg* 116(7):150e–157e, 2005.

23. Davies DM: Plastic and reconstructive surgery. Scars, hypertrophic scars, and keloids, *Br Med J (Clin Res Ed)* 290(6474):1056–1058, 1985.

24. Deitch EA, Wheelahan TM, Rose MP, et al.: Hypertrophic burn scars: analysis of variables, *J Trauma* 23(10):895–898, 1983.

25. van der Veer WM, Bloemen MC, Ulrich MM, et al.: Potential cellular and molecular causes of hypertrophic scar formation, *Burns* 35(1):15–29, 2009.

26. Grey JE, Harding KG: Venous and arterial leg ulcers, *BMJ* 332:347–350, 2006.

27. Paquette D, Falanga V: Leg ulcers, *Clin Geriatr Med* 18(1):77–88, 2002.

28. Rudolph DM: Pathophysiology and management of venous ulcers, *J Wound Ostomy Continence Nurs* 25(5):248–255, 1998.

29. Smith PC: The causes of skin damage and leg ulceration in chronic venous disease, *Int J Low Extrem Wounds* 5(3):160–168, 2006.

30. Raffetto JD: Dermal pathology, cellular biology, and inflammation in chronic venous disease, *Thromb Res* 123(Suppl 4):S66–S71, 2009.

31. Coleridge Smith PD: The microcirculation in venous hypertension, *Vasc Med* 2(3):203–213, 1997.

32. Stekelenburg A, Gawlitta D, Bader DL, Oomens CW: Deep tissue injury: how deep is our understanding? *Arch Phys Med Rehabil* 89(7):1410–1413, 2008.

33. Cushing CA, Phillips LG: Evidence-based medicine: pressure sores, *Plast Reconstr Surg* 132 (6):1720–1732, 2013.

34. Aronovitch SA: Intraoperatively acquired pressure ulcer prevalence: a national study, *J Wound Ostomy Continence Nurs* 26(3):130–136, 1999.

35. Krapfl L, Gray M: Does regular repositioning prevent pressure ulcers? *J Wound Ostomy Continence Nurs* 35:571–577, 2008.

36. Gillespis BM, Chaboyer WP, McInnes E, Kent B, Whitty JA, Thalib L: Repositioning for pressure ulcer prevention in adults, *Cochrane Database Syst Rev* 3(4):CD009958, 2014.

37. Allman RM: Pressure ulcers: using what we know to improve quality of care, *J Am Geriatr Soc* 49 (7):996–997, 2001.

38. Boulton AJ, Kirsner RS, Vileikyte L: Clinical practice. Neuropathic diabetic foot ulcers, *N Engl J Med* 351(1):48–55, 2004.

39. NPUAP: National Pressure Ulcer Advisory Panel. http://www.npuap.org/pr2.htm. Accessed September 15, 2014.

40. Connor H: Some historical aspects of diabetic foot disease, *Diabetes Metab Res Rev* 24 (Suppl): S7–S13, 2008.

41. Ward R: The rehabilitation of burn patients, *Crit Rev Phys Rehabil Med* 2:121–138, 1991.

42. Geller AC, Swetter SM, Brooks K, et al.: Screening, early detection, and trends for melanoma: current status (2000-2006) and future directions, *J Am Acad Dermatol* 57(4):555–572, 2007, quiz 573–576.

43. Sullivan T, Smith J, Kermode J, et al.: Rating the burn scar, *J Burn Care Rehabil* 11(3):256–260, 1990.

44. Amsler F, Willenberg T, Blattler W: In search of optimal compression therapy for venous leg ulcers: a meta-analysis of studies comparing diverse [corrected] bandages with specifically designed stockings, *J Vasc Surg* 50(3):668–674, 2009.

45. de Araujo T, Valencia I, Federman DG, Kirsner RS: Managing the patient with venous ulcers, *Ann Intern Med* 138(4):326–334, 2003.

46. Richard R, Ward RS: Splinting strategies and controversies, *J Burn Care Rehabil* 26(5):392–396, 2005.

47. Schnebly WA, Ward RS, Warden GD, Saffle JR: A nonsplinting approach to the care of the thermally injured patient, *J Burn Care Rehabil* 10(3):263–266, 1989.

ADDITIONAL RESOURCES

Sussman C, Bates-Jensen BM: *Wound care: a collaborative practice manual for physical therapists and nurses*, ed 4, Baltimore, MD, 2012, Lippincott Williams & Wilkins.

A well-written textbook that focuses on clinical examination and management of many common wounds.

Myers BA: *Wound management: principles and practice*, ed 3, Upper Saddle River, NJ, 2012, Pearson.

A very useful textbook that reviews wound healing and management of wounds.

REVIEW QUESTIONS

1. Describe the three phases of wound healing and develop a rationale for physical therapy involvement in each phase.
2. List the variables that should be identified during your examination of a patient to determine the cause and seriousness of the wound. How might these variables affect your intervention?
3. What characteristics differentiate a venous ulcer from an arterial ulcer, as well as these ulcers from a pressure ulcer?
4. Explain the differences involved in treating a superficial wound versus a deep wound.
5. How might an increased understanding of integumentary wounds and wound healing help you better understand injuries to tissues you cannot visualize (e.g., soft tissue injury, fracture, and tissue necrosis)?
6. Why is it important for PTs to be aware of scar formation?

The miracle of children is that we just don't know how they will change or who they will become.
Eileen Kennedy-Moore

12

Physical Therapy for Pediatric Conditions

Karen W. Nolan

KEY TERMS

anencephaly
autism
cerebral palsy (CP)
clubfoot
congenital muscular torticollis (CMT)
cystic fibrosis (CF)
developmental coordination disorder (DCD)
developmental delay
developmental dysplasia of the hip (DDH)
developmental milestone
disablement process
Down syndrome
Duchenne muscular dystrophy (DMD)
dynamical systems theory
eclectic approach
enablement process
family assessment
fetal alcohol syndrome (FAS)
goal-directed movement approach
hypotonia
Individualized Education Plan (IEP)
Individualized Family Service Plan (IFSP)
juvenile rheumatoid arthritis (JRA)
meningocele
meningomyelocele
neural tube defect
neurodevelopmental treatment (NDT)
norm referenced
normal developmental theory
osteogenesis imperfecta (OI)
pervasive developmental disorder (PDD)
plagiocephaly

prenatal cocaine exposure
scoliosis
secondary condition
sensory integration (SI)
spina bifida
spina bifida occulta
spinal muscular atrophy (SMA)
standardized testing

LEARNING OBJECTIVES

After reading this chapter, the reader will be able to:

- Describe the relationship among body structure, functional abilities, and activity limitations as presented by the World Health Organization.
- Describe the impact of federal legislation on the delivery of physical therapy services to children.
- Describe the general features of common pediatric conditions seen by a physical therapist or physical therapist assistant.
- Describe aspects of the patient/client examination that are unique to pediatric clients.
- Describe the general features of four physical therapy treatment approaches for pediatric clients.

Physical therapists who provide rehabilitation and rehabilitation services for children recognize that they are treating children, first and foremost. They are not merely scaled-down versions of adults; rather, they progress through unique age-related movement stages, or developmental milestones. Pediatric physical therapists (PTs) observe these milestones to determine whether discrepancies exist between the child's chronologic or developmental age or whether inefficient motor patterns are limiting the child's function. If so, evaluation and subsequent intervention may be appropriate. More important, pediatric PTs must evaluate each child's ability to meet the task-related challenges of that child's daily environment. This type of evaluation and intervention planning requires thoughtful, structured strategies that often involve many participants, including the child's family, caregivers, teachers, and community professionals. This chapter describes the examination and intervention techniques used by pediatric PTs. It includes common conditions and two case studies to illustrate a variety of approaches for the management of pediatric clients.

The priorities for pediatric therapists are to observe children as they utilize their individual strengths and abilities and to promote a functional, optimal developmental process. By acquiring knowledge of normal development through observation of movement patterns and transitions, the therapist can more accurately detect abnormal or inefficient movements. The challenge is differentiating normal delays from those that signal potential developmental problems.[1] For example, observations of generations of children tell us that walking is initiated at approximately 10 to 13 months, yet some infants take their first steps as early as 8 months or as late as 18 months. This type of variation occurs at all stages of child development and requires pediatric therapists to examine and provide interventions to children on a constantly changing developmental base.[2] Pediatric therapists play a crucial role in determining the absence of movement components that may impede the accomplishment of **developmental milestones** or functional motor skills for a child. In addition to child development, pediatric practice requires the therapist to acquire specific knowledge in basic areas ranging from child psychology to motor learning. The cognitive strategies and learning methods of adults are generally functionally oriented toward work, leisure, or daily living activities; whereas, children learn from a different point of view—play. The pediatric PT often uses numerous playful approaches during treatment sessions—hopping, rolling, tumbling—to engage and invite the child to participate in therapeutic activities.

Play is the medium most commonly used to promote therapeutic activities for young children, whereas for adolescents, therapy goals may be structured around social situations.[3,4] The primary goal is to identify meaningful activities that correspond to the learning style of each pediatric client, given the age, culture, and most natural social and physical environments (Figure 12-1).

Children who have health problems that require specialty or subspecialty care are often referred to as "children with special health care needs."[5,6] Pediatric therapists may provide direct or consultative therapy to these children over long periods, depending on the child's changing needs. When caring for children with special needs, PTs collaborate closely with the family and other health professionals in designing a long-term, family-centered plan of care (Figure 12-2). This plan includes a full range of services—prevention, early identification,

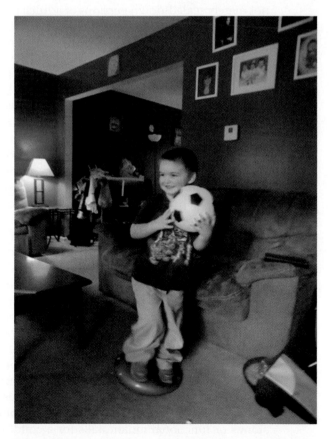

Figure 12-1 ■ Therapy services in a child's home—a natural environment.

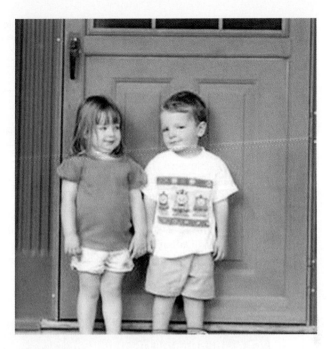

Figure 12-2 ■ Siblings incorporated into therapy sessions encourage participation and meet the family's goals. (Courtesy Karen Nolan.)

evaluation, diagnostics, treatment, habilitation, and rehabilitation.[7] Physical therapists should also recognize their responsibilities through practice under direct access as a first contact provider. The advancement of the profession to the doctor of physical therapy (DPT) degree requires that medical screening (i.e., checking for "red flags") must be included as part of any initial examination. This informs the PT to make appropriate clinical decisions for the overall plan of care for the child, including whether to provide treatment or refer to another provider for further medical evaluation.[8] Throughout service provision, emphasis is placed on recognizing each child as part of a family system, with unique cultural characteristics that must be considered when treatment goals are designed.

GENERAL DESCRIPTION

If the PT focuses solely on the child's motor strengths and needs while neglecting the cultural impact of family and community factors on that child, a successful treatment outcome is less likely. The World Health Organization (WHO) has issued an International Classification of Functioning, Disability and Health (ICF) that describes the impact of a person's health condition on body functions and structures, daily activities, and social participation.[9] This model describes the process of enablement and disablement on several levels: body structures and functions, activities, and participation (Figure 12-3 and Table 12-1).[9]

Enablement processes and **disablement processes** represent the dynamic, interactive relationships a child has within different environmental contexts. This model shows that in the disease process, impaired body functions and structures (e.g., central nervous system abnormality) directly affect the child not only

12

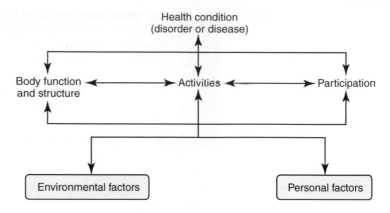

Figure 12-3 ■ Interaction among the components of the International Classification of Functioning, Disability, and Health. (Modified from *International Classification of Functioning, Disability and Health [ICF]*, Geneva, 2001, World Health Organization.)

Table 12-1
Classification of Disablement

Disablement Classification	Characteristics	Interaction Level
Impairment of body structures and body functions	Reflex development Joint motion Muscle length and strength Respiratory status Postural stability	Child
Activity limitations	Locomotion Communication Oral motor function Social and emotional	Child–daily environment
Participation restriction	Community recreation School participation Employment Access to facilities	Child–community and society

Modified from International Classification of Functioning, Disability, and Health (ICF), Geneva, 2001, World Health Organization.

physically but also in several areas of his or her life, all of which must be considered when a plan of care is being designed. The child's activity limitations (e.g., inability to speak or walk) are influenced by the body's structure and function, as well as other factors, including the child's motivational level, environment, and course of rehabilitation. In turn, the child's activity limitations may have an impact on the family system (e.g., interaction style) and peer relationships. Participation restrictions, or the influence of social or environmental restrictions on child participation (e.g., access to schools, sports), are a result of the culture, society, and environment in which the child lives.

When the WHO model is used as a guide for care of a child, all these factors are considered important elements in the design of a plan of care. It is important to note that the WHO framework is consistent with the American Physical Therapy Association's *Guide to Physical Therapist Practice 3.0*[10] and the practice model adopted by the National Center for Medical Rehabilitation Research.[11] Throughout each of these frameworks, the PT addresses body structure and function, activity limitations, and participation limitations as a result of disease or injury. Another important point is that the PT can advance a child through an enabling process by addressing the body's structural integrity so that age-appropriate movement and interactive activities can occur. In a climate of evolving health care reform and shifting venues for pediatric practice, a practitioner's understanding of the interdependence of all levels of the WHO model is relevant and applicable to the evaluation process and success in achieving outcomes.

IMPACT OF FEDERAL LEGISLATION

The scope of pediatric specialization within the profession of physical therapy is continuously evolving as a result of numerous factors that directly affect the care of children: public policy, family-centered care, and practice environments. These seemingly unrelated elements have become entwined through passage of federal legislation unique to the practice of pediatrics.

In 1975, Congress passed the Education of All Handicapped Children Act (EHCA), Public Law 94-142. This landmark legislation has continued to shape the evolution of pediatric practice for all professional disciplines.[12] The main premise of the EHCA was that all children from ages 6 to 21 years, regardless of disability, were entitled to free and appropriate public education. This premise sets the basic framework for policy and standards, which were amended in 1986 with passage of Public Law 99-457 (Amendments to the EHCA) and again in 1991 and 2004 with reauthorizations as the Individuals with Disabilities Education Act (IDEA).[13,14] These amendments provide distinct policy for children from birth until 3 years and from 3 through 5 years of age.[15] Although the states must abide by a set of regulations for implementing services, each state can establish some of its own regulations, such as the inclusion of children who are "at risk" or transitioning from early intervention to school-based services.[14] Specific language in the amendments stipulates the concept of collaboration between parent and professional, as well as a family-centered focus throughout the process of pediatric examination, intervention, and care coordination. In addition, this legislation sets forth policy guidelines requiring that children be cared for in their "least restrictive" environment or in "natural" environments, ranging from home to daycare centers, as optimal sites for physical therapy intervention (Figure 12-4).[12–14,16,17] The regulations also require schools to use evidence-based practice in the process of assisting students with learning difficulties, or determining eligibility for special education.[14]

12

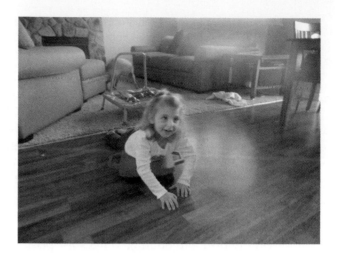

Figure 12-4 ■ Therapy in the home—a natural environment.

The focus on the family system, family-centered care, individualized child and family plans, and natural environments is now commonplace in pediatric practice. This emphasis on family and community speaks to the evolving societal and cultural contexts in which pediatric PTs collaborate in the care of children with special needs.

COMMON CONDITIONS

The full range of pediatric diagnostic conditions is beyond the scope of this chapter. Children, like adults, have conditions that require expertise in all specialty areas. Many children are seen because of acute, short-term orthopaedic needs such as an adolescent who sprains an ankle while playing soccer. The majority of these pediatric clients are seen in physical therapy outpatient orthopaedic clinics or by sports physical therapy specialists.

Another subset of pediatric clients and the group most associated with pediatric practice are children with developmental delays and disabilities. A child with a **developmental delay** has not attained predictable movement patterns or behavior associated with children of a similar chronologic age. During fetal development, a multitude of factors have the potential to cause a developmental problem. Such factors as genetic and chromosomal anomalies, environmental toxins, or premature birth may cause impairment in the central or peripheral nervous system that results in immediate or eventual developmental delays. Affected children generally require some combination of short- and long-term therapies that are adjusted in response to changes in the child's physical, cognitive, and emotional abilities.

The remainder of this section briefly describes selected developmental, orthopaedic, and neuromuscular conditions of children. The cause of many of these conditions remains unclear and may result from a combination of genetic and environmental factors. Later in the chapter, two of the conditions are described through case studies of children to provide the reader with snapshots of the many "faces" of pediatric practice.

DEVELOPMENTAL DISORDERS

Autism is a severe disorder in the group of conditions called *pervasive developmental disorders* (PDDs).[18] PDDs are characterized by impairments in social interactions with others and communication skills, commonly accompanied by the presence of unusual activities and interests such as repetitive behaviors, stereotypies, and poor play skills. A diagnosis of autism is most typically made when the child has onset of symptoms before the age of 3 years and meets six of the 12 criteria identified in the *Diagnostic and Statistical Manual of Mental Disorders, Fourth Edition* (DSM-IV).[19] Some providers expect the new codes in the DSM 5 to cause change in diagnostic practice for children with autism.[20] PDDs are currently understood to be brain-based neurologic disorders of multiple origins and can coexist with other developmental disabilities including intellectual disabilities and attention-deficit/hyperactivity disorder (ADHD).[21] Although the primary impairments for these children are in the communication, social, and behavioral domains, there can be associated motor and sensory impairments for which physical and occupational therapy can provide intervention and support. Examples include sensory integrative disorders, balance and coordination deficits, and motor development delay. These limitations in activities are influenced in some children with autism by attention deficits and tendency to perseverate on favorite objects and activities. The primary role of the physical or occupational therapist (OT) is to provide encouragement and maximize opportunities for age-appropriate movement experiences, and to address the sensory issues exhibited by many that can interfere with purposeful interactions with people and the environment. PTs and OTs work in cooperation with the other members of the medical and educational team to provide a consistent behavioral program designed for the individual child's needs.

ORTHOPAEDIC DISORDERS

Children may be born with or may acquire problems with bones, muscles, fascia, and joints. Some of the more common disorders are discussed in the following sections.

CONGENITAL MUSCULAR TORTICOLLIS

Newborn infants may be born with positional deformities that are related to their position within the intrauterine environment. **Congenital muscular torticollis (CMT)** is one condition that may be associated with these in utero constraints. CMT refers to the posture of the infant's head and neck that results from shortening of one sternocleidomastoid muscle, which causes the head to tilt toward and rotate away from the shortened muscle. If the CMT is a result of in utero positioning constraints, accompanying deformation of the craniofacial skeleton can also occur. This is described as **plagiocephaly**. The main objective for treatment of CMT is to establish full neck movement as soon as possible to stop progression or help reverse the skull deformity. Plagiocephaly can also be a result of prolonged positioning of the baby in supine, causing a flattened occipital region of the skull. This is called *positional plagiocephaly*. In the presence of plagiocephaly that persists to age 4 to 6 months, referrals to other professionals should be

12

considered if the head flattening is not responding to regular changes in the baby's position.

CLUBFOOT

The term **clubfoot** is derived from the position of the affected foot, which is turned inward and slanted upward. Because of this position, certain muscles become shortened and cause the foot to remain in a fixed position. This condition can be a positional deformity that relates to fetal position within the intrauterine environment, but can also be the result of problems that affect the nerve, muscle, and bone system (e.g., brain injury). Treatment includes progressive and prolonged casting or taping (or both), joint range-of-motion exercises, and in some cases, surgical correction.

JUVENILE RHEUMATOID ARTHRITIS

One of the many rheumatic diseases, **juvenile rheumatoid arthritis (JRA)** is characterized by inflammation of connective tissue manifested as a painful inflamed joint (arthritis). The cause of JRA is unknown, although genes associated with a variety of forms of JRA have been identified.[22] Similar to other autoimmune disorders, JRA appears to be the result of complex genetic and possibly environmental exposures.[23,24] JRA may be manifested in several distinct forms or subtypes, each with different characteristics. These subtypes vary in the number of joints affected, age at onset, male-to-female ratio, clinical findings, and prognosis. Signs and symptoms usually include joint pain, swelling, decreased motion, stiffness, and muscle atrophy. The majority of children in whom JRA is diagnosed lead active lives with the assistance of medications, therapeutic exercise, and specialized care programs. It is generally believed that an interdisciplinary team including parents, a pediatric rheumatologist, a nurse, a psychologist, a PT, and an OT is best for total care coordination.

The primary role of the PT is to assist in preventing deformity and improving the overall quality of life for the child. The focus is generally the child's musculoskeletal status, with special emphasis on needs that affect function. PTs also play a role in exercise prescription, because physical conditioning has been shown to increase functional abilities without exacerbating JRA.[25] Individualized goals are collaboratively planned to address posture, strength, mobility, and joint motion within the child's daily functional routine. Including the parent and child in decisions regarding education and instruction is vital because the home is where the majority of the child's goals will be reinforced.[26]

SCOLIOSIS

Scoliosis is characterized by a lateral curvature of the spine. The curve may vary in severity from mild to severe. Scoliosis may be idiopathic (of unknown origin), neuromuscular, or congenital (present at birth). Scoliosis is now detected more frequently because of school-based screening programs and is noted by asymmetry of the shoulders, breasts, and pelvis, among other factors. Treatment involves a wide range of external or internal fixations, and controversy has persisted over optimal management. Conclusions of a recent systematic review were in support of orthotics (bracing) over observation for adolescents with idiopathic scoliosis;

however, the authors cautioned that a curve that does not correct by 20% should not be braced.[27] Studies have shown that electrical stimulation had no effect on prevention of idiopathic curve progression; therefore, its use in clinical practice is not supported.[28] Exercise assists in reducing back pain and improving range of motion. For children with mobility limitations, positioning in appropriate seating systems is crucial to reduce the risk of scoliosis.

DEVELOPMENTAL DYSPLASIA OF THE HIP

Developmental dysplasia of the hip (DDH) results from abnormal development of the structures surrounding the hip joint such that the head of the femur can move into and out of the hip socket. The cause of DDH is unknown, but the disorder is thought to be related to a number of factors such as maternal hormonal changes during pregnancy, in utero positioning, increased birth weight, multiple gestation pregnancy, birth trauma, and family history of DDH.[29] The incidence of DDH is unclear because debate exists over methods of screening and classification.[30–32] Treatment involves manual or surgical return of the femoral head to the hip socket and stabilization with splints or casts, depending on the degree of impairment and age of the child. Intensive postsurgical exercise protocols are required for full range of joint motion, muscle strength, and function to be achieved. Children with spina bifida and certain forms of cerebral palsy (CP) are more prone to DDH and are monitored through regular physical examinations.

OSTEOGENESIS IMPERFECTA

A common and severe bone disorder of genetic origin, **osteogenesis imperfecta (OI)** affects the formation of collagen during bone development, leading to frequent fractures during the fetal or newborn period.[33] The fetal form of OI is associated with high mortality, whereas the infantile form is less severe, with increased vulnerability to frequent fractures of the long bones in early childhood. Children with OI are identified through characteristic limb deformities, dental abnormalities, stunted growth, scoliosis, loose ligaments, and an unusually shaped skull. Treatment of fractures and prevention of deformity through positioning and joint range-of-motion exercises are the major foci of intervention, as well as gentle exercise after postsurgical healing.[33,34]

NEUROMUSCULAR AND GENETIC DISORDERS

Neuromuscular disorders include all disorders that cause difficulty moving the body as a result of decreased control between the brain or central nervous system and the muscles of the body. The causes of these types of disorders are extremely variable and include trauma, genetic factors, premature birth, environmental factors, or a combination of several factors. Genetic factors include the inheritance of a trait, recessive or dominant, or a mutation that occurs during fetal development. A variety of risk factors affecting the health of either the mother or the fetus may present a risk to the newborn infant's health. Some of these factors include maternal health and nutrition (e.g., vitamin deficiency), radiation, drugs, infections, environmental toxins (e.g., lead), fetal hypoxia (lack of oxygen before or during labor), and birth trauma. Depending on the nature and the timing of the appearance of the

12

risk factor during the pregnancy, the newborn may have a variety of developmental disabilities ranging from mild to severe. A complex interplay between genetics and the environment contributes to many neuromuscular disorders.

DUCHENNE MUSCULAR DYSTROPHY

In **Duchenne muscular dystrophy (DMD),** females do not manifest symptoms, but are carriers of the disease, whereas males do manifest symptoms. Boys with DMD usually develop normally until 3 to 5 years of age, when progressive lower extremity muscle weakness and wasting become apparent and are combined with enlarged yet weak calf muscles and tight heel cords. Associated complications include muscle contractures, spinal curvature (scoliosis), and wheelchair dependence by 10 to 12 years of age. Progressive weakness, pneumonia, and cardiac myopathies reduce the life span of persons with DMD.[35] Ongoing clinical trials have reported improved outcomes, including prolonged independent and assisted walking, in individuals who have been on long-term steroid therapy.[36] The use of nighttime ventilation may increase the life span for an individual with DMD to as much as 25 years.[35,37,38] Developmental effects of this type of muscular dystrophy may include mild mental retardation or learning disabilities, low muscle tone, and delays in attainment of motor milestones.[39] Activity limitations are closely associated with muscle strength and cognitive level.[40,41] Given the increased life span for those individuals who benefited from steroid therapy and/or nighttime ventilation, emphasis on transition services and preparation for college, work, driving, and independent living are all important considerations in overall patient management.

SPINAL MUSCULAR ATROPHY

There are several different types of **spinal muscular atrophy (SMA)**, depending on the onset and severity of symptoms. Symptoms of **SMA** include severe muscle weakness in infancy and progressive respiratory failure. Children with the infantile form of SMA have a decreased life span, whereas children with the juvenile form have longer (but less than normal) life span and require aggressive physical therapy and orthopaedic management.[42,43]

NEURAL TUBE DEFECTS

A **neural tube defect** results from failure of the neural tube to close completely during the first month of gestational development. Although the cause of the neural tube defect is unclear, some hypotheses suggest that this impairment may be a result of genetic expression in combination with factors in the fetal (maternal) environment.[44] Environmental factors such as hyperthermia, maternal nutritional deprivation, and valproic acid have been suggested, and maternal folate deficiency has been determined to exert a strong influence.[45–47] Studies have shown that daily folic acid supplementation (400 mg/day) can reduce the incidence of new cases of neural tube defects by at least 50%.[42] Recent advances in surgical techniques have led to attempts to close the neural tube in utero rather than delaying intervention until the infant has been born. Outcome studies regarding the benefit of this experimental procedure are under way.[48]

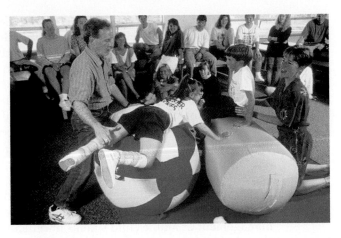

Figure 12-5 ■ Physical therapists promote interactive play to assist the movement patterns of two children with spina bifida. (Courtesy Bruce Wang.)

The following are several types of neural tube defects that differ in the level of severity depending on the degree and location of vertebral closure and spinal cord exposure.

■ Spina bifida
  ○ **Spina bifida** is the most common neural tube defect and involves mild orthopaedic malformations in its mildest form and neurologic malformations in its most severe form (Figure 12-5). In this condition, a split occurs on a section of the vertebral arches.
■ Spina bifida occulta
  ○ A common impairment of a vertebra (separation of the spinous process without entrapment of the spinal cord itself) that is not associated with disability, **spina bifida occulta** may be discovered only through diagnostic tests such as radiographic studies.
■ Meningocele
  ○ In a **meningocele**, there is a benign herniation of the meninges through the gap in the vertebra manifesting as a soft tissue cyst or lump that surrounds a normal spinal cord. This condition does not cause any neurologic deficits.
■ Meningomyelocele
  ○ **Meningomyelocele** is an open lesion with minimal to no skin protection covering the deeper nerve roots. This condition is the most severe of the spinal closure defects, with the potential for leakage of spinal fluid and infection before surgical intervention and healing. Because this impairment is usually at the lower end of the spine, loss of motor function and sensation of the lower part of the body often results, including problems with bowel and bladder function.
■ Anencephaly
  ○ **Anencephaly** is a form of neural tube defect that results from a lack of the neural tube closure at the base of the brain. This condition is not compatible with life and typically results in fetal death or death shortly after delivery.

12

DEVELOPMENTAL COORDINATION DISORDER

Children in whom **developmental coordination disorder (DCD)** is diagnosed may have a wide range of dysfunctions, including gross or fine motor coordination problems such as awkward running, frequent falling, slow reaction times, immature balance reactions, poor handwriting, and difficulty with activities of daily living such as dressing.[49-51] Although these impairments may seem mild and not easily noticed, they can cause significant functional limitations in a child's daily life. Children with DCD frequently have psychosocial problems in addition to their motor dysfunctions. The cause of DCD is unknown, but may be related to prenatal or perinatal insults to the central nervous system or damage to the neurotransmitter and receptor system.[49] DCD is more commonly diagnosed in children with ADHD and learning disabilities than in children without these conditions. Treatment for DCD includes comprehensive management of all the child's areas of difficulty.[51] Recent research on interventions for children with DCD offers encouraging results related to improved quality of life and reduced health risks that can be associated with a sedentary lifestyle of children with DCD.[52]

DOWN SYNDROME

Down syndrome is a congenital developmental disability caused by the presence of an extra copy of chromosome 21; it is also called *trisomy 21*. Routine prenatal care commonly includes screening for Down syndrome. New ultrasound techniques have increased the ability to prenatally diagnose Down syndrome in the first and second trimesters.[53] A child with Down syndrome has physical characteristics including low muscle tone, a flat facial profile, upwardly slanted eyes, short stature, varying levels of intellectual disability, slowed growth and development, a small nose with a low nasal bridge, and increased occurrence of congenital heart disease (e.g., ventricular or atrial septal defects).[54-56] Associated complications may include instability of the first and second vertebrae, lax ligaments, seizures, and leukemia; premature aging is reported in many, but not all individuals with Down syndrome.[57-62] The combination of these features is often manifested as deficiencies in balance, stability, and agility across many tasks and environmental contexts. Developmentally, a child with Down syndrome has decreased muscle tone, which improves with age. This abnormality is accompanied by loose ligaments that result in increased range of joint motion. The rate of developmental progress decreases with age in individuals with Down syndrome.[62-64]

CEREBRAL PALSY

Cerebral palsy (CP) is a group of conditions, rather than a disease, and is caused by a nonprogressive lesion of the brain. Most often, CP occurs during gestation (before birth), at birth, or immediately after birth from interruption of oxygen to the brain of the fetus or newborn.[65,66] A variety of environmental toxins, maternal or infant infections, and early childhood trauma can cause this condition. The core problem with CP is an inability of the brain to control nerve and muscle activity. Manifestations of CP depend on the cause, timing (age of the fetus or child), and location and extent of the original impairment to the brain. Often, early signs of CP include poor sucking, irritability, stiff muscles (hypertonia),

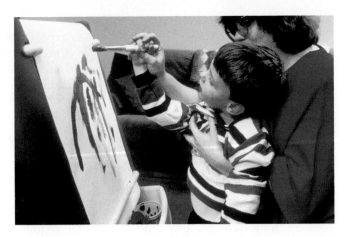

Figure 12-6 ■ Painting is a part of therapy for a child with cerebral palsy. (Courtesy Bruce Wang.)

floppy muscles (**hypotonia**), or reduced movement quality.[67] Later manifestations may include delayed motor milestones, poor coordination, involuntary movements (dyskinesia), writhing movements (athetosis), poor visual tracking (ability of the eyes to follow a moving object), and language delay.[68] Approximately one half to two thirds of children with CP have intellectual disabilities.[69] Management emphasis is on attaining optimal growth and development, while promoting functional mobility and age-appropriate participation that is safe and energy efficient for the child. A variety of specialists may be involved in caring for a child with CP, including PTs, OTs, speech-language pathologists, and developmental pediatricians. In many cases, neurosurgical intervention, orthotic devices, adaptive equipment, strengthening programs, or pharmacologic intervention is required to ameliorate or correct deformities (Figure 12-6).[70,71]

FETAL ALCOHOL SYNDROME

The most severe condition in a continuum of alcohol-induced disabilities,[72,73] **fetal alcohol syndrome (FAS)** is related to a presumed history of significant maternal alcohol consumption during pregnancy.[72,74] Recent research suggests a genetic predisposition to fetal alcohol-related syndromes.[75] FAS is one of the leading known causes of intellectual disability; of these, it is the only entirely preventable cause. Children are generally born at term (close to their due date), but are smaller than normal in weight and height. Children with FAS have distinct physical features that assist in identifying their condition. These physical features include microcephaly, widely spaced eyes, short, upturned nose, thin upper lip, flattened groove in the midline of the lips (philtrum), and large, low-set ears.[76] Complications are widespread and include an increased incidence of congenital heart defects, joint contractures, visual and auditory impairments, and hip dislocation.[77,78] A child with FAS may experience a range of developmental delays in the areas of language, fine motor control, eye-hand coordination, speech, intelligence quotient (IQ), and psychosocial behavior.[79–81]

12

PRENATAL COCAINE EXPOSURE

Prenatal cocaine exposure refers to exposure to cocaine in utero from maternal cocaine use during pregnancy.[82,83] A number of studies conducted in the 1980s documented motor problems in children who were exposed to cocaine in utero,[84] but further studies[85,86] have been unable to support these findings when controlled for the environment where the child is raised, prematurity, and other risk factors.[87]

CYSTIC FIBROSIS

The pulmonary disorder **cystic fibrosis (CF)** is the most common inherited chronic disease in white children. CF is a disorder of exocrine (secreting) gland function and involves the respiratory system, pancreas, reproductive organs, and sweat glands. CF is characterized by the production of thick mucus with progressive lung damage, and children with CF require frequent hospitalization for acute respiratory attacks. A variety of medications and therapies can help to decrease the side effects of this disease, but no cure has been found. Genetic research has resulted in isolation of the defective gene for CF.[88] The life span and quality of life of persons with CF has increased significantly in the past two decades, although they are still coping with their increasingly debilitating lung disease and accompanying respiratory infections. Some patients have received lung transplants.[89] The median life expectancy is estimated to be 40 years of age.[90–92]

PRINCIPLES OF EXAMINATION

The process of examination and evaluation of children involves measures to determine whether a child needs physical therapy intervention, in addition to monitoring the child's progress after physical therapy has been initiated. If a child is suspected of having or is at risk for a developmental disability, an examination is conducted that involves the history, a systems review, screening, and tests and measures. After the examination, the PT makes an evaluation using clinical judgment to synthesize the clinical and social information gathered during the examination. During the evaluation, a prognosis is determined, as well as a plan of care, including the child and family's goals and objectives and any intervention strategies, if indicated.

Initial information about a child, the history, is generally obtained through a review of medical records and discussions with family members. For a child up to 5 years of age, the discussion may take the form of a **family assessment.**[93] Family assessment is an essential part of the examination because the child will be treated in the context of that family system.[94] Family assessment may take the form of an interview, discussion, or standardized survey and is often initiated by the team member who will be the primary coordinator of care for the family. Regardless of the format, the purpose of family assessment is to obtain the family's insights regarding the child, including the family history, relationships, satisfactions, concerns, needs, and resources. The history has a direct impact on planning services for each child. As children get older, they may become more directly involved and state their own opinions and thoughts, thus providing vital information about their condition and areas of satisfaction or concern with their care coordination.

The administration of tests and measures, an initial and continuing part of any pediatric examination, primarily consists of two components: screening and

---

Table 12-2
Components of Tests and Measures in Pediatric Physical Therapy

Component	Description	Example
Screening	Short, inexpensive tests used to distinguish children with behavior different from that of other children of the same age; may indicate a need for further evaluation	Baylay Infant Neuromotor Screener[94] Denver II Developmental Screening Test[95]
Assessment	Instruments used to gain a comprehensive profile of a child's physical, cognitive, social, emotional, communication, and adaptive abilities to assist in determining therapeutic service needs, as well as to act as a guide for initial frequency and duration of service; assessment also involves the use of measures to determine the need for disability-related adapted equipment, as well as activity preferences addressed by the child and family	Bayley Scales of Infant and Toddler Development III[96] Gross Motor Function Measure[97] Peabody Developmental Motor Scales, ed 2[98] School Function Assessment[99] Test of Infant Motor Performance[100,101] Bruininks-Oseretsky Test of Motor Proficiency[102] Pediatric Evaluation of Disability Inventory[103] Canadian Occupational Performance Measure[104]

---

assessment. Each component has a distinct purpose in determining a child's prognosis and ultimate plan of care (Table 12-2).[95–105]

PTs may receive referrals for evaluation of children who do not have a formal diagnosis. In this clinical scenario, screening may be required as an initial measurement. Screening is usually indicated when a child is at risk for developmental delay or disability and is a quick way to determine whether the child is in need of further diagnostic services.

If a child has a definite diagnosis, screening is generally bypassed and a comprehensive assessment is recommended. Assessment measures are used to gain more in-depth information about the child's strengths and needs in all developmental domains. In the case of an orthopaedic condition, assessment may entail an examination of posture or movement, as well as special diagnostic tests such as radiographs. Assessment measures for a child with a developmental disability are generally obtained through **standardized testing**, a type of formal test in which the procedures remain the same when administered by different therapists and at variable test locations. A large variety and number of standardized measures are available for pediatric testing, and these measures are targeted according to the specific purpose of the assessment (Figures 12-7, *A* and *B*). Many standardized tests are also **norm referenced**, meaning that a large number of children have been assessed to create a comparison group for the assessment.

12

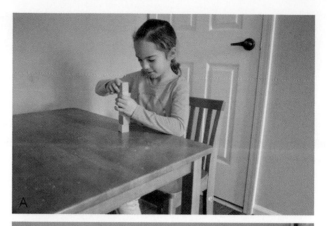

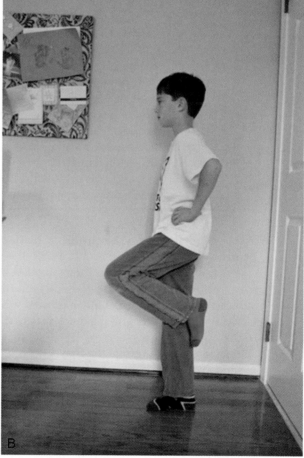

Figure 12-7 ■ Standardized testing. **A**, Assessment of eye-hand coordination and fine motor skills. **B**, Assessment of static balance.

Assessments that are norm referenced can be used to compare a child's functional abilities or activities with those of other children of the same age.

In addition to choosing an assessment tool that meets the needs of the child being tested, the physical therapist evaluator must review and judge each measure for (1) validity, or the ability of the test to measure the content area or areas that it claims to measure (e.g., evaluation of mobility); (2) reliability, or the consistency of the test among separate administrations or examiners; and (3) appropriateness of the instrument for the specific disability or culture of the child being assessed. An equally important element of objective measurement is the information provided through observation of the child and reports by the child's caregivers in a variety of natural environments (home, daycare, school).

PRINCIPLES OF EVALUATION, DIAGNOSIS, AND PROGNOSIS

The results of tests and measures performed during the examination are used in the evaluation process to confirm, revise, or establish a physical therapy (movement system) diagnosis, prognosis, and plan of care. The evaluation can be vital for the child, family, and medical professionals. In many cases, the diagnosis and corresponding prognosis provide a mechanism by which PTs can determine treatment priorities and design the plan of care. With certain conditions that have defined physical manifestations, initial therapy can be planned to counteract negative physical outcomes, or **secondary conditions** of disability (e.g., muscle contractures). Diagnosis is also important for determining clinical conditions that contraindicate specific treatment regimens. Several positive outcomes are associated with establishing a clinical diagnosis, as are negative outcomes, many of which can have psychological and social ramifications (Box 12-1). For children

BOX 12-1

Outcomes of Establishing a Diagnosis for a Pediatric Patient

Positive Outcomes
- Gives the ability to establish a prognosis
- Validates the need for services and supports
- May indicate a need for genetic counseling
- Assists in possible prevention of secondary disabilities
- May assist the family with coping mechanisms
- Aids research efforts targeted to specific conditions
- May assist in obtaining funding from government agencies for services

Negative Outcomes
- May lead to a negative stereotype (label)
- May disenfranchise the child from obtaining certain services
- May cause a state of depression or denial
- If false positive, has negative immediate consequences for both the child and the family
- If false negative, will have long-term consequences for both the child and the family
- May result in difficulty obtaining private insurance coverage

12

and their families and friends, the impact of childhood disablement is multifaceted, and all those who are touched by it repeatedly experience the phases of grief and acceptance.

During the evaluation, individualized goals and objectives are developed from the information derived from the examination (family assessment, child observations, and standardized assessment measures). The SOAP note is used as a documentation method for pediatric patients in some practice settings, such as specific hospital or rehabilitation settings (see Chapters 2 and 8 regarding the SOAP-note). However, in early intervention and school-based practice settings, federal law requires that the necessary information is contained in an **Individualized Family Service Plan (IFSP)** or an **Individualized Education Program (IEP)** developed for each child. These plans are reviewed on a regular basis as the framework for treatment and serve as a baseline by which progress is monitored.

As the name implies, the IFSP describes in detail the total plan of care for the child in the context of the family unit.[106–108] This type of plan, designed for children from birth to 3 years of age, is always determined in collaboration with the family, and therapeutic needs are integrated with family needs and priorities. This strategy recognizes that the family unit must remain healthy to provide optimum care for the child. The IFSP might include such services as special baby-sitting assistance, transportation provisions, or specialized medical care at home. The IFSP also includes the different therapeutic services that the child will receive, the specific duration and frequency of these services, and location of the intervention.

On entry into the school system, physical therapy objectives shift to interface with an educational service delivery system and become part of the IEP. Through this model, therapists often interact with the family, educators, and other health team members to provide direct intervention in the classroom setting.[109–111] The PT may work individually with the child, may work in a group setting, or may serve as a consultant to direct care providers. In the last case, the PT instructs persons who directly care for the child. Instruction may include certain positioning or movement techniques to provide therapeutic benefit throughout the day. The school-based physical therapy plan of care must address skills and activities that support the child's successful participation in the educational program, in the least restrictive environment.

Young children may be seen by a PT at a variety of locations with different therapist-child ratios, depending on the particular objectives of therapy. Generally, the site of choice is the child's most natural environment, which may be the home, school, or a daycare setting. Therapists may choose to work with a child in a 1:1 ratio, in a group with other children, or with the parents. Often, some mixture of formats and environments provides treatment variety and the greatest benefit for the child.

It is important to remember that the initiation of therapy does not signal the end of examination. Examination is an ongoing process that begins with the history and continues throughout each therapy session. It includes assessment of each child's strengths and needs and evolves as the child, family, and therapist continue to determine appropriate therapeutic activities. Annual, biannual, or monthly reexamination is extremely important for monitoring the child's progress and redirecting intervention if necessary and is usually required by insurance companies. By applying the results of the examination and subsequent evaluation, the health care team and family work in a partnership to determine a well-coordinated plan of care for each child.

PRINCIPLES OF INTERVENTION

Intervention in pediatric physical therapy involves helping each child gain abilities to assist in meeting the daily challenges of the most natural environments. As mentioned earlier, the initial task of the therapist, in collaboration with the family, is an examination of the child's individual strengths and needs. With this information, a unique plan of care is developed that supports the child's strengths while facilitating skills in needed areas. Depending on the child's needs or diagnosis, intervention may involve a variety of approaches.

To initiate therapy with pediatric orthopaedic patients, PTs will find it useful to have specific knowledge in the area of pediatric orthopaedics (Box 12-2).[112] Orthopaedic examination and intervention vary according to the condition, but certain procedures are common to all orthopaedic clients such as measurement of range of motion, muscle and sensory testing, gait assessment, and postural evaluation (see Chapter 8 for a further description of these procedures). Children may require specialized orthopaedic management for acute and long-term orthopaedic conditions, as well as for neuromuscular diseases. Intervention in both cases requires knowledge of the specific diagnoses, as well as of protocol for condition management if any exists. For example, specialized surgical procedures often require the therapist to know specific postoperative management protocols (e.g., positioning or weight bearing) in order to maintain the surgical correction. Often, PTs are requested to fabricate splints or casts for a pediatric patient to assist in muscle lengthening, joint stabilization, or improved alignment (Figure 12-8).

In addition to orthopaedic techniques, PTs use a range of therapeutic techniques to enhance the rehabilitation process. A variety of neuromotor approaches may be used to treat a child with neurologic and orthopaedic disabilities. Some of these approaches were primarily developed between 1950 and 1980 and were based on the theory, literature, and patient observations current at that time. These approaches have been and continue to be reviewed and

BOX 12-2

Knowledge Base for Pediatric Orthopaedic Assessment and Treatment

- Normal pediatric biomechanical alignment
- Specific orthopaedic assessment procedures
- Presurgical evaluation of posture and movement
- Postoperative management of specialized surgical interventions
- Rationale, indications, and contraindications for using manual therapy
- Use of casts and orthotics for correction or management of musculoskeletal misalignment
- Appropriate use of modalities and exercise protocols for children

From *Journal of Pediatric Orthopaedics*, 1992, Lippincott-Raven Publishers.

12

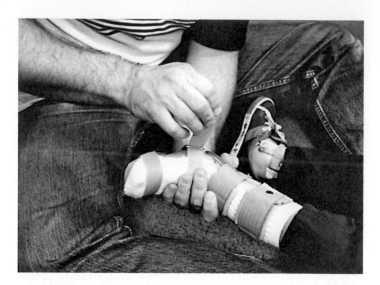

Figure 12-8 ■ Ankle-foot orthosis is used to assist the orthopaedic needs of a child. (Courtesy Bruce Wang.)

adapted in light of current nervous system theories.[113–115] A primary task for both new and veteran pediatric PTs is to continue to research the effectiveness of each approach and assess the use of these approaches in a variety of settings and their ability to facilitate the neuromotor changes they are claimed to achieve. It is also essential that PTs evaluate the effectiveness of each approach in facilitating the child's achievement of targeted goals.

Most pediatric PTs continue to rely on an "eclectic," or multiple-method, approach when providing therapy. An **eclectic approach** includes some combination of therapeutic strategies used by the PT that are thought to be helpful in the treatment of a given client.[116–119] Although the common use of eclectic practice has made it difficult to isolate and study the effectiveness of each specific approach, numerous published articles have discussed both the controversial nature and the effectiveness of a variety of neuromotor approaches.[120–134] Additional clinical research is necessary to achieve a sound basis of support for the continued use of many therapeutic approaches. Regardless of the type of intervention, pediatric therapy should pave the way for a healthy, high-quality life for each child. Campbell outlined a checklist, or "defining strategy," for the evaluation of pediatric interventions.[135] The questions she poses can be used to evaluate intervention collaborations in the home, school, or other community venues. The answers to these questions provide a litmus test for successful pediatric intervention.

1. Does the intervention encourage the child to initiate a program of lifelong fitness activities, including proper nutrition, exercise, weight control, and stress management?
2. Does the intervention encourage the child to assume responsibility for personal health, including knowledge of the condition? Is the child encouraged to become personally involved in decisions regarding rehabilitation?

3. Does the intervention motivate the child and foster self-esteem?
4. Does the intervention promote meaningful pursuits that will foster the prevention of secondary conditions and thereby lead to lifelong musculoskeletal health and improved cardiovascular fitness?

A variety of approaches continue to be used to habilitate and rehabilitate pediatric clients. The following brief descriptions provide an objective overview of the more common neuromotor approaches in use.

DYNAMICAL SYSTEMS THEORY

In the **dynamical systems theory**, both the internal components of the patient and the external context of the task are equally important and contribute to functional movement.[136,137] This theory emphasizes the process of moving rather than the product of a movement. Cooperating systems include, but are not limited to the musculoskeletal system, sensory system, cardiovascular/pulmonary system, and limbic system. The interactions of all the body's systems with the environment facilitate or inhibit movements. Therapists must work with the interplay of all systems rather than each system in isolation. To improve a child's ability to move independently, a therapist may modify the task or the environment (e.g., using an assistive device, adjusting surface texture) in addition to helping a child improve strength, endurance, and motor control (Figure 12-9).

NEURODEVELOPMENTAL TREATMENT APPROACH

The **neurodevelopmental treatment (NDT)** approach was originated by Berta and Karel Bobath in England more than 60 years ago to both analyze and treat neurologic disorders of posture and movement.[138–140] Through the use of a motivating environment and the child's active participation, the therapist uses manual facilitation and inhibition techniques to present the child with a "normal" sensory experience and thereby encourage facilitation of a more functional motor response.[140–142] Continued active repetition of normal developmental skills is theorized to assist the child in establishing more coordinated, efficient movement

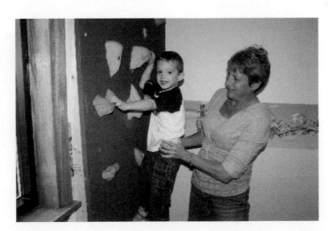

Figure 12-9 ■ Use of environment can improve strength, endurance, and motor control.

patterns.[139,141–144] The primary emphasis of the NDT approach is on movement quality, and training of the parent or provider is stressed for the purpose of incorporating movement concepts into the child's functional daily routines. Pediatric therapists using this approach should realize that although some studies have demonstrated the efficacy of NDT,[144,145] other studies do not support its usefulness as a treatment approach.[146,147] Despite the controversy, NDT continues to be a frequently used and documented therapeutic approach in the United States for the treatment of upper motor neuron lesions such as CP.[146,148,149]

SENSORY INTEGRATION THEORY

The **sensory integration (SI)** technique is based on the theory that poor integration of sensory information (e.g., tactile, vestibular, or visual feedback) prevents the organization of resultant motor behavior (e.g., walking or jumping). This approach assesses the child's sensory systems through reports by the parent and child, clinical observations of limited tolerance for sensory experiences, and tests before initiation of therapy. The provision of controlled vestibular and somatosensory experiences within meaningful environments is believed to enable the child to integrate the sensory information and evoke a spontaneous motor or sensory adaptive response that is functional and appropriate to the situation (Figures 12-10 through 12-12).[131,150–153]

NORMAL DEVELOPMENTAL THEORY

Therapy goals and objectives are designed to follow the progression of normal motor development (developmental milestones), as well as developmental theory (e.g., development proceeds in a proximal-to-distal direction). This **normal developmental theory** approach is based on a model of higher level cortical control that dictates the maturation process. The theory assumes that children with central nervous system damage will acquire motor skills in a fashion similar to that of children with normally developing nervous systems.[116] Many of the neuromotor therapies used today were originally based on this theoretical foundation.[154]

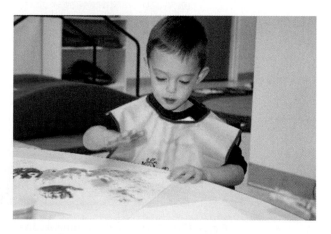

Figure 12-10 ■ Sensory integration can improve body awareness.

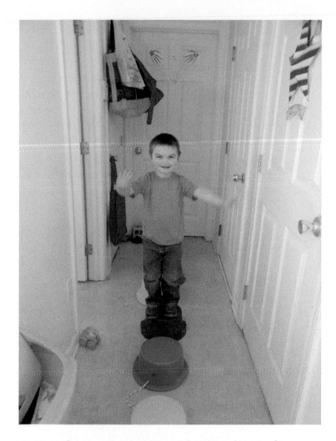

Figure 12-11 ■ Sensory integration and postural control.

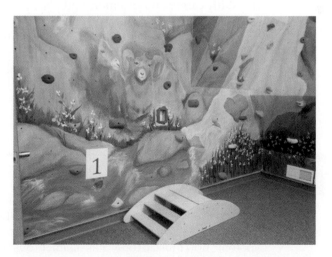

Figure 12-12 ■ By using a climbing wall/mural, sensory integration can be fun.

12

TASK-ORIENTED MOVEMENT MODEL

Based on the work of Gentile,[155] a **goal-directed movement approach** to intervention has been established by Shepherd[156] and by others[157] who were seeking to use environmental task conditions as a stimulus for improved motor control and motor learning. In Gentile's paradigm, goal-directed movements include both the investigative and the adaptive behaviors resulting from a child's interactions with the environment. In observing such behavior, the pediatric PT can orient therapy so that it focuses on the child's impairments, on task reorganization, and on environmental modifications that may improve child outcomes. Therapy is specific to the environment and task and is designed to promote a child's development of solutions to movement problems.

SUMMARY

PTs who work with pediatric patients focus on child development, psychology, and learning. They may provide services to the patient for a long period, for a short time, or on a consultant basis. Intervention is family centered and usually incorporates activities adapted to play. Physical therapy is frequently provided in the home or school setting as directed by federal entitlement programs.

Common conditions seen by pediatric PTs are generally classified as orthopaedic or neuromuscular disorders. Screening, examination, and assessment techniques are used to complete an evaluation and establish functional goals and objectives, which are incorporated into an IFSP or IEP. Intervention is often eclectic—that is, it combines components from a variety of approaches, including dynamic systems theory, NDT, SI, normal developmental theory, and a task-oriented model. Early and continuing intervention programs for children are designed to incorporate a child's motivation and desire to play or participate in community-based recreation and leisure activities. Parents are active partners in assessing their child's individual interests and helping to design the optimal environment(s) that will support therapy goals while matching the child's interests. With careful observation and the use of environmental adaptations and assistive devices, community activities (e.g., soccer, art class) can be modified to be accessible and inclusive for a child with special needs. Pediatric physical therapy is challenging and rewarding. Research, legislation, and new techniques create a changing practice environment to enhance the quality of care. The result is an exciting specialty in physical therapy.

CASE STUDIES

CASE STUDY ONE

Matthew is 3 years old and is one of many preschoolers at Rosedale Preschool. He has Down syndrome.

Matthew attends preschool with other infants and toddlers. He plays with balls and puzzles and loves to swim. A formal evaluation revealed that Matthew has many strengths as well as needs in the gross and fine motor domains. Matthew is severely hypotonic (low muscle tone), has ligamentous laxity, and has difficulty running without falling. This problem was noted on the formal examination as well as in observations by Matthew's parents and preschool teacher. It was also noted that his automatic reactions to disturbances in balance (righting reactions and protective responses) were delayed, especially when moving into and out of various positions (transitions). Matthew was able to grasp objects in a manner appropriate for other 3-year-olds and enjoys drawing and playing with building blocks. He continues to exhibit needs in feeding skills because of the low muscle tone in muscles used for chewing and mouth closure. His medical history reveals that Matthew has a congenital heart problem, as well as several other features associated with Down syndrome.

Researchers have attempted to determine appropriate physical therapy interventions for children with Down syndrome.[158] Conclusions drawn from this research indicate that it appears most important to provide a child with Down syndrome opportunities to explore a variety of environments requiring different postural adjustments or movement patterns in response to changing task conditions. In accordance with this research, the therapist must observe the individual motor learning style of each child and respond by creating motivating and challenging learning situations. Research has also shown support for the effects of lower extremity orthotics on balance performance in young children with Down syndrome. Supra-malleolar orthotics may be considered if his parents/caregivers and primary care physician support this addition to his plan.[159]

In Matthew's case, the PT will provide therapy in the school as designed in his IEP and collaborate with his preschool staff by instructing them to carry out physical therapy goals throughout his daily school routine. An inclusion program, such as the one at Rosedale Preschool, maintains a philosophy that children with a variety of developmental abilities should play and learn together in an atmosphere that fosters a sense of belonging and personal growth for all its members. This type of environment is naturally where a child as special as Matthew belongs.

MATTHEW'S INDIVIDUALIZED EDUCATION PLAN
Because of Matthew's diagnosis of a congenital heart defect, it is important that he avoid excessive exertion and fatigue. Activities that involve impact to the cervical vertebrae should also be avoided because of his ligamentous laxity, which can be associated with vertebral instability. In designing a plan for Matthew, the therapist focuses on family goals and Matthew's current interests. Several pediatric assessment tools can assist in identifying and prioritizing Matthew's therapy goals. The Canadian Occupational Performance Measure is one measure designed specifically to identify and determine the importance of the child's and family's goals for therapy.[160] It is from this frame of reference that therapeutic goals and objectives will be designed. Specific objectives might involve achieving a task that is appropriate for Matthew's developmental abilities as well as his functional level. Most objectives target a particular skill, the manner of performance or assistance, and the criterion to be met (Box 12-3).

BOX 12-3 | *Example of a Goal and Criterion for Matthew* | **12**

Goal: Matthew will run across a level (hard) mat surface without falling when prompted with his favorite toy.
Criterion: Three to four times during four play sessions.

BOX 12-4

Goal Attainment Scaling

■ −2 Matthew will walk across a level mat surface without falling when prompted with his favorite toy.

■ −1 Matthew will run across a level mat surface with one stop to regain his balance (hands down on mat) when prompted with his favorite toy.

■ 0 Matthew will run across a level mat surface without falling when prompted with his favorite toy.

■ +1 Matthew will run across a level mat raised by a 10-degree angle with one stop to regain his balance (hands down on mat) when prompted with his favorite toy.

■ +2 Matthew will run across a level mat raised by a 10-degree angle without a stop or fall when prompted with his favorite toy.

The same skill can also be scaled[131] so that Matthew will always achieve different measures of success and his individual progress can be monitored over time (Box 12-4). Initial therapeutic goals are vital for assessing his response to intervention, as well as for maintaining treatment consistency. Through the ongoing assessment process, Matthew's progress will be monitored, with alterations made to his care plan if warranted.

INTERVENTION

Physical therapy intervention may first involve assisting Matthew in developing a relationship with his environment. Matthew may initially move too quickly or slowly, take steps that are too large or uneven, or resist the challenge to ambulate altogether. During an activity, the therapist may use NDT techniques such as guided handling to assist with movement. Another strategy may involve Matthew's active participation through the use of cognitive and verbal reinforcement during a motivating recreational activity to reinforce learning. As mentioned previously, some combination of techniques may best accomplish the task (see the section on principles of direct intervention). If each of Matthew's goals can be designed according to his motivations (e.g., eating, playing, recreation), the inclusion of therapeutic approaches and techniques becomes more functional and more likely to meet with success.

CASE STUDY TWO

Emmie began her life in the neonatal intensive care unit of Eastern Shore Memorial Hospital. Her first experiences were the sounds of the slow beeps and hums of the infant monitors. Her first visions were obstructed by glass, and her human touch was limited to persons performing routine checks of her medical status. Unlike other newborn infants who experience the sounds of home and the arms of friends or siblings, Emmie will have to wait until she has surgery, because she was born with spina bifida (meningomyelocele). Children with spina bifida have no choice but to begin their lives in the hospital environment. Although diligent efforts have improved the comfort and familiarity of hospital neonatal intensive care and pediatric units, they continue to be a threatening, imposing environment for families.

MANAGEMENT

The general goals of physical therapy management for Emmie and other children with spina bifida are (1) to prevent her body structure from causing participation limitations that are a potential consequence of activity limitations (e.g., "can't crawl") and (2) to improve the quality of life for her and her family by preventing activity limitations from limiting her participation in daily activities and social events (e.g., "can't go to the school dance").[161] Accomplishing these goals requires a collaborative approach involving the child, the family, and the health care team. Physical therapy examination should be comprehensive and take into account the observations and examinations of other health care team and family members. Evaluation and continued follow-up (monitoring) should include the following specific objectives:

- General multidomain screening and evaluation of developmental level
- Neurologic examination, including monitoring for signs of increased intracranial pressure or tethered spinal cord
- Orthopaedic examination for joint range and mobility, kyphosis, scoliosis, or hip dislocations
- Examination of bowel and bladder function
- Examination of skin integrity
- Assessment of activities of daily living
- Examination of mobility
- Promotion of recreational activities

EMMIE'S INDIVIDUALIZED FAMILY SERVICE PLAN

Activities are generally centered on the goals and objectives indicated in the child's individualized plan. For a child of Emmie's age, the format would be an IFSP. A child with spina bifida often has a range of cognitive delays and delayed skills in the psychosocial area. Consideration of these abilities, as well as physical and environmental factors, is essential when a plan of care is designed. During the first few years of life, Emmie will develop a sense of her autonomy and self-esteem, so physical therapy will focus on her ability to explore her environment.

Depending on each child's abilities, the PT will explore options to accomplish mobility goals. Many children with spina bifida use orthoses or braces to assist in locomotion. Therapy goals may also focus on other functional activities such as position transitions, muscle strengthening, and self-care activities. Assistive technology devices, such as an adapted computer keyboard, will be especially useful in creating a more accessible environment for Emmie as she enters school.[162] As Emmie reaches adolescence, she will probably choose to use a wheelchair that allows greater speed and efficiency for daily living. The team should encourage Emmie to explore a variety of recreational activities that are motivating and will improve general fitness and quality of life. She may continue to be seen on a periodic basis through the hospital's outpatient clinic or may opt for private outpatient care. Therapy will continue only on an "as-needed" basis to assist with problems that arise during transitional developmental phases.

12

Acknowledgment   The author wishes to acknowledge Cassidy Goepel, PT, DPT for her contributions to the chapter, and the staff, children, and families of Bright Start Pediatric Services of Fairport, New York for their assistance.

REFERENCES

1. Cherry DB: Pediatric physical therapy: philosophy, science and techniques, *Pediatr Phys Ther* 3(2):70–76, 1991.
2. Bottos M, Dalla Barba B, Stefani D, et al.: Locomotor strategies preceding independent walking: prospective study of neurological and language development in 424 cases, *Dev Med Child Neurol* 31:25–34, 1989.
3. Eagleton M, Iams A, McDowell J, et al.: The effects of strength training on gait in adolescents with cerebral palsy, *Pediatr Phys Ther* 16(1):22–30, 2004.
4. Linder TW: *Transdisciplinary play-based assessment: a functional approach to working with young children,* Baltimore, 1990, Brookes.
5. McPherson M, Arango P, Fox H, et al.: A new definition of children with special health care needs, *Pediatrics* 102:137–140, 1998.
6. Surgeon General's Report: *Children with special health care needs,* Rockville, MD, 1987, U.S. Department of Health and Human Services, Public Health Service.
7. National Maternal and Child Health Resource Center: *Community-based service systems for children with special health care needs and their families,* Washington, DC, 1988, U.S. Department of Health and Human Services.
8. Rodeghero JR, Denniger TR, Ross MD: Abdominal pain in physical therapy practice: 3 patient cases, *J Orthop Sports Phys Ther* 43(2):44–53, 2013.
9. World Health Organization (WHO): *International classification of functioning, disability and health,* Geneva, 2001, WHO.
10. *Guide to Physical Therapist Practice 3.0* American Physical Therapy Association. http://guidetoptpractice.apta.org/. Accessed November 27, 2014.
11. National Advisory Board of Medical Rehabilitation Research: *Research plan for the national center for medical rehabilitation,* Bethesda, Md, 1993, National Institute of Child Health and Human Development, National Institutes of Health.
12. Education of All Handicapped Children Act of 1975, Public Law:94-142, 1975:20 USC 1401.
13. Individuals with Disabilities Education Act Amendments of 1991, Public Law:102-119, 1991:105 STAT.587.
14. Individuals with Disabilities Education Improvement Act of 2004, Public Law:108-443, 2004: STAT. 2647.
15. Fischer J: Physical therapy in education environments: moving through time with reflections and visions, *Pediatr Phys Ther* 6(3):144–147, 1994.
16. Individuals with Disability Education Act Amendments of 1997 [IDEA]. (1997) http://thomas.loc.gov/home/thomas.php. Accessed September 14, 2014.
17. Strain P: Least restrictive environments for preschool children with handicaps: what we know, what we should be doing, *J Early Interv* 14:291–296, 1990.
18. Bauer S: Autism and the pervasive developmental disorders, *Pediatr Rev* 16(130–136):168–176, 1995.
19. American Psychiatric Association (APA): *Diagnostic and statistical manual of mental disorders,* ed 4, Washington, DC, 1994, APA.
20. American Psychiatric Association (APA): *Diagnostic and statistical manual of mental disorders,* ed 5, Washington, DC, 2013, APA.
21. Mauk JE, Reber M, Batshaw ML: Autism and other pervasive developmental disorders. In Batshaw ML, editor: *Children with disabilities,* Baltimore, 1997, Brookes.
22. Miterski B, Drynda S, Boschow G, et al.: Complex genetic predisposition in adult and juvenile rheumatoid arthritis, *BMC Genet* 5:2, 2004.
23. Prahalad S: Genetics of juvenile idiopathic arthritis: an update, *Curr Opin Rheumatol* 16:588–594, 2004.
24. Thompson SD, Moroldo MB, Guyer L, et al.: A genome-wide scan for juvenile rheumatoid arthritis in affected sibpair families provides evidence of linkage, *Arthritis Rheum* 50 (9):2920–2930, 2004.

25. Klepper SE: Effects of an eight-week physical conditioning program on disease signs and symptoms in children with chronic arthritis, *Arthritis Care Res* 12:52–60, 1999.
26. Klepper SE: Juvenile idiopathic arthritis. In Tecklin JS, editor: *Pediatric physical therapy*, Philadelphia, 2008, Wolters Kluwer, Lippincott, Williams and Wilkins.
27. Stokes OM, Lukes KDK: The current status of bracing for patients with adolescent idiopathic scoliosis, *J Bone Joint Surg* 95B:1308–1316, 2013.
28. Bertrand SL, Drvaric DM, Lange N, et al.: Electrical stimulation for idiopathic scoliosis, *Clin Orthop Relat Res* 276:176–181, 1992.
29. Omeroglu H, Koparal S: The role of clinical examination and risk factors in the diagnosis of developmental dysplasia of the hip: a prospective study in 188 referred young infants, *Arch Orthop Trauma Surg* 121:7–11, 2001.
30. Bialik V, Bialik GM, Blazer S, et al.: Developmental dysplasia of the hip: a new approach to incidence, *Pediatrics* 103:93–99, 1999.
31. Goldberg MJ: Early detection of developmental hip dysplasia: synopsis of the AAP clinical practice guideline, *Pediatr Rev* 22:131–134, 2001.
32. Patel H: Preventive health care, 2001 update: screening and management of developmental dysplasia of the hip in newborns, *CMAJ* 164:1669–1677, 2001.
33. Zeitlin L, Fassier F, Glorieux FH: Modern approach to children with osteogenesis imperfecta, *J Pediatr Orthop B* 12:77–87, 2003.
34. Binder H: Rehabilitation of infants with osteogenesis imperfecta, *Connect Tissue Res* 31:S37–S39, 1995.
35. Eagle M, Baudouin SV, Chandler C, et al.: Survival in Duchenne muscular dystrophy: Improvements in life expectancy since 1967 and the impact of home nocturnal ventilation, *Neuromuscul Disord* 12:926–929, 2002.
36. Biggar WD, Gingras M, Fehlings DL, et al.: Deflazacort treatment of Duchenne muscular dystrophy, *J Pediatr* 138:45–50, 2001.
37. Labbe A: *New DMD care recommendations*, http://quest.mda.org/news/new-dmd-care-recommendations/, Accessed on July 22, 2010.
38. Manzur AY, Kinali M, Muntoni F: Update on the management of Duchenne muscular dystrophy, *Arch Dis Child* 93(11):986–990, 2008.
39. Hyser CL, Mendell JR: Recent advances in Duchenne and Becker muscular dystrophy, *Neurol Clin* 6:429–453, 1988.
40. Nair KP, Vasanth A, Gourie-Devi M, et al.: Disabilities in children with Duchenne muscular dystrophy: a profile, *J Rehabil Med* 33:147–149, 2001.
41. Uchikawa K, Liu M, Hanayama K, et al.: Functional status and muscle strength in people with Duchenne muscular dystrophy living in the community, *J Rehabil Med* 36:124–129, 2004.
42. Chung BH, Wong VC, Ip P: Spinal muscular atrophy: survival pattern and functional status, *Pediatrics* 114:e548–e553, 2004.
43. Wang CH, Finkel RS, Bertini ES, et al.: Consensus statement for standard of care in spinal muscular atrophy, *J Child Neurol* 22:1027–1049, 2007.https://smaregistry.iu.edu/Links/Downloads/ICC_SMA_SoC_Consensus_Statement_EN.pdf. Accessed on July 22, 2010.
44. Mitchell LE, Adzick NS, Melchionne J, et al.: Spina bifida, *Lancet* 364:1885–1895, 2004.
45. Blatter BM, Roeleveld N, Bermejo E, et al.: Spina bifida and parental occupation: results from three malformation monitoring programs in Europe, *Eur J Epidemiol* 16:343–351, 2000.
46. Cragan JD, Roberts HE, Edmonds LD, et al.: Surveillance for anencephaly and spina bifida and the impact of prenatal diagnosis—United States, 1985-1994, *MMWR CDC Surveill Summ* 44:1–13, 1995.
47. Shaw GM, Lammer EJ, Zhu H, et al.: Maternal periconceptional vitamin use, genetic variation of infant reduced folate carrier (A80G), and risk of spina bifida, *Am J Med Genet* 108:1–6, 2002.
48. Bruner JP, Tulipan N, Reed G, et al.: Intrauterine repair of spina bifida: Preoperative predictors of shunt-dependent hydrocephalus, *Am J Obstet Gynecol* 190:1305–1312, 2004.
49. Barnhart RC, Davenport MJ, Epps SB, Nordquist VM: Developmental coordination disorder, *Phys Ther* 83:722–731, 2003.
50. Dewey D, Wilson BN: Developmental coordination disorder: What is it? *Phys Occup Ther Pediatr* 20:5–27, 2001.
51. Dewey D, Kaplan BJ, Crawford SG, Wilson BN: Developmental coordination disorder: associated problems in attention, learning, and psychosocial adjustment, *Hum Mov Sci* 21:905–918, 2002.

12

52. Kane K, Bell A: A core stability group program for children with developmental coordination disorder: 3 clinical case reports, *Pediatr Phys Ther* 21(4):375–382, 2009.
53. Filkins K, Koos BJ: Ultrasound and fetal diagnosis, *Curr Opin Obstet Gynecol* 17:185–195, 2005.
54. Batshaw M, Perret Y, Shapiro B: Normal and abnormal development. In Batshaw M, Perret Y, editors: *Children with disabilities: a medical primer*, 4 ed., Baltimore, 1997, Brookes.
55. Roche AF: The cranium in mongolism, *Acta Neurol* 42:62–78, 1966.
56. Spicer RL: Cardiovascular disease in Down syndrome, *Pediatr Clin North Am* 31:1331–1343, 1984.
57. Agha MM, Williams JI, Marrett L, et al.: Congenital abnormalities and childhood cancer, *Cancer* 103:1939–1948, 2005.
58. American Academy of Pediatrics: Committee on sports medicine: atlantoaxial instability in down syndrome, *Pediatrics* 74:152–154, 1984.
59. Barden HS: Growth and development of selected hard tissues in Down syndrome: a review, *Hum Biol* 55:539–576, 1983.
60. Menendez M: Down syndrome, Alzheimer's disease and seizures, *Brain Dev* 27:246–252, 2005.
61. Pueschel SM: Clinical aspects of Down syndrome from infancy to adulthood, *Am J Med Genet Suppl* 7:52–56, 1990.
62. Zigman WB: Atypical aging in Down syndrome, *Dev Disabil Res Rev* 18(1):51–67, 2013.
63. Cooley WC, Graham JM Jr, : Common syndromes and management issues for primary care physicians: Down's syndrome: an update and review for the primary pediatrician, *Clin Pediatr* 30:233–253, 1991.
64. Galley R: Medical management of the adult patient with Down syndrome, *JAAPA* 18:45–46, 2005, 48, 51–52.
65. Murase M, Ishida A: Early hypocarbia of preterm infants: Its relationship to periventricular leukomalacia and cerebral palsy, and its perinatal risk factors, *Acta Paediatr* 94:85–91, 2005.
66. Scher MS, Belfar H, Martin J, Painter MJ: Destructive brain lesions of presumed fetal onset: antepartum causes of cerebral palsy, *Pediatrics* 88:898–906, 1991.
67. Einspieler C, Prechtl HF: Prechtl's assessment of general movements: a diagnostic tool for the functional assessment of the young nervous system, *Ment Retard Dev Disabil Res Rev* 11:61–67, 2005.
68. Allen MC, Capute AJ: Neonatal neurodevelopmental examination as a predictor of neuromotor outcome in premature infants, *Pediatrics* 83:498–506, 1989.
69. Pelligrino L: Cerebral palsy. In Batshaw ML, editor: *Children with disabilities*, Baltimore, 1997, Brookes.
70. Morton JF, Brownlee M, McFadyen AK: The effects of progressive resistance training for children with cerebral palsy, *Clin Rehabil* 19:283–289, 2005.
71. Styer-Acevedo J: The infant and child with cerebral palsy. In Tecklin JS, editor: *Pediatric physical therapy*, Baltimore, 2008, Lippincott Williams and Wilkins.
72. Kvigne VL, Leonardson GR, Neff-Smith M, et al.: Characteristics of children who have full or incomplete fetal alcohol syndrome, *J Pediatr* 145:635–640, 2004.
73. National Institute on Alcohol Abuse and Alcoholism (NIAA): *Sixth special report to the U.S. congress on alcohol and health*, Washington, DC, 1987, U.S. Department of Health and Human Services.
74. Stratton K, Howe C, Battaglia F: *Fetal alcohol syndrome: diagnosis, epidemiology, prevention, and treatment*, Washington, DC, 1996, National Academies Press.
75. Warren KR, Li TK: Genetic polymorphisms: impact on the risk of fetal alcohol spectrum disorders, *Birth Defects Res A Clin Mol Teratol* 73(4):195–203, 2005.
76. Batshaw ML, Conlon CJ: Substance abuse. A preventable threat to development. In Batshaw ML, editor: *Children with disabilities*, Baltimore, 1997, Brookes.
77. Graham JM Jr, Hanson JW, Darby BL, et al.: Independent dysmorphology evaluations at birth and 4 years of age for children exposed to varying amounts of alcohol in utero, *Pediatrics* 81:772–778, 1988.
78. Streissguth A: *Fetal alcohol syndrome: a guide for families and communities*, Baltimore, 1997, Brookes.
79. Faden VB, Graubard BI: Maternal substance use during pregnancy and developmental outcome at age three, *J Subst Abuse* 12:329–340, 2000.
80. Larkby C, Day N: The effects of prenatal alcohol exposure, *Alcohol Health Res World* 21:192–198, 1997.
81. Streissguth AP, Barr HM, Sampson PD, et al.: Attention, distraction and reaction time at age 7 years and prenatal alcohol exposure, *Neurobehav Toxicol Teratol* 8:717–725, 1986.

82. Chasnoff IJ, Burns KA, Burns WJ: Cocaine use in pregnancy: perinatal morbidity and mortality, *Neurotoxicol Teratol* 9:291–293, 1987.
83. Schneider JW, Griffith DR, Chasnoff IJ: Infants exposed to cocaine in utero: implications for developmental assessment and intervention, *Infants Young Child* 2(1):25–36, 1989.
84. Newald J: Cocaine infants: a new arrival at hospitals' step? *Hospitals* 60:96, 1986.
85. Doberczak TM, Shanzer S, Senie RT, Kandall SR: Neonatal neurologic and electroencephalographic effects of intrauterine cocaine exposure, *J Pediatr* 113:354–358, 1988.
86. Schneider JW, Chasnoff IJ: Cocaine abuse during pregnancy: its effects on infant motor development: a clinical perspective, *Top Acute Care Trauma Rehabil* 2:59–69, 1987.
87. Blanchard Y: Neurobehavioral and neuromotor long-term sequelae of prenatal exposure to cocaine and other drugs: an unresolved issue, *Pediatr Phys Ther* 11:140–146, 1999.
88. Rommens JM, Iannuzzi MC, Kerem B, et al.: Identification of the cystic fibrosis gene: chromosome walking and jumping, *Science* 245:1059–1065, 1989.
89. Kirkby S, Hayes D Jr, : Pediatric lung transplantation: indications and outcomes, *J Thorac Dis* 6 (8):1024–1031, 2014.
90. Frank DA, Augustyn M, Knight WG, et al.: Growth, development, and behavior in early childhood following prenatal cocaine exposure: a systematic review, *JAMA* 285:1613–1625, 2001.
91. Jaffe A, Bush A: Cystic fibrosis: review of the decade, *Monaldi Arch Chest Dis* 56:240–247, 2001.
92. Messinger DS, Bauer CR, Das A, et al.: The maternal lifestyle study: cognitive, motor, and behavioral outcomes of cocaine-exposed and opiate-exposed infants through three years of age, *Pediatrics* 113:1677–1685, 2004.
93. Bailey D, Simeonsson R: *Family assessment in early intervention: rationale and model for family assessment in early intervention,* Columbus, Ohio, 1988, Merrill.
94. Foster M, Phillips W: Family systems theory as a framework for problem solving in pediatric physical therapy, *Pediatr Phys Ther* 4(2):70–73, 1992.
95. Aylward G: *Bayley infant neurodevelopmental screener (BINS),* San Antonio, TX, 1995, Psychological Corporation.
96. Frankenburg WK: *Denver Developmental Screening Test Manual II,* Denver, 1992, LADOCA Project & Publishing Foundation.
97. Bayley N: *Bayley Scales of Infant Development III,* San Antonio, TX, 2006, PsychCorp.
98. Russell D, Rosenbaum P, Cadman D, et al.: The gross motor function measure: a means to evaluate the effects of physical therapy, *Dev Med Child Neurol* 31:341–352, 1989.
99. Folio RM, Fewell RR: *Peabody developmental motor scales. examiner's manual,* ed 2, Austin, Tx, 2000, Pro-Ed.
100. Campbell SK, Hedeker D: Validity of the test of infant motor performance for discriminating among infants with varying risk for poor motor outcome, *J Pediatr* 139:546–551, 2001.
101. Coster W, Deency T, Haltiwanger J, Haley S: *School function assessment,* Austin, Tx, 1998, Pro-Ed.
102. Campbell SK, Kolobe TH, Wright BD, Linacre JM: Validity of the test of infant motor performance for prediction of 6-, 9- and 12-month scores on the Alberta infant motor scale, *Dev Med Child Neurol* 44:263–272, 2002.
103. Bruininks-Oseretsky Test of Motor Proficiency 2, Circle Pines, Minn, AGS, 2005.
104. Haley SM, Coster WJ, Ludlow LH, et al.: *Pediatric evaluation of disability inventory (PEDI): development, standardization and administration manual,* Boston, 1992, New England Medical Center Hospitals and PEDI Research Group.
105. Law M, Baptiste S, McColl M, et al.: The Canadian occupational performance measure: an outcome measure for occupational therapy, *Can J Occup Ther* 57(2):82–87, 1990.
106. American Academy of Pediatrics, Committee on Children with Disabilities: The pediatrician's role in development and implementation of an individual education plan (IEP) and/or an individual family service plan (IFSP), *Pediatrics* 104:124–127, 1999.
107. Bailey DB Jr, Hebbeler K, Scarborough A, et al.: First experiences with early intervention: a national perspective, *Pediatrics* 113:887–896, 2004.
108. McGonigel MJ, Garland CW: The individualized family service plan and the early intervention team: team and family issues and recommended practices, *Infants Young Child* 1 (1):10–21, 1988.
109. Giangreco M: Delivery of therapeutic services in special education programs for learners with severe handicaps, *Phys Occup Ther Pediatr* 6(2):5–15, 1986.

110. Henry B: The role of physical therapists in development of individualized educational plans, *Totline* 12:13–15, 1986.

111. Krehbiel R, Munsick-Bruno G, Lowe JR: NICU infants born at developmental risk and the individualized family service plan/process (IFSP), *Child Health Care* 20:26–33, 1991.

112. American Physical Therapy Association: *Pediatric orthopedics,* Alexandria, VA, 1992, American Physical Therapy Association.

113. Kleim JA: Principles of experience-dependent neural plasticity: implications for rehabilitation after brain damage, *J Speech Lang Hear Res* 51(1):S225–S239, 2008.

114. Montgomery P: Neurodevelopmental treatment and sensory integrative theory. In Lister MJ, editor: *Contemporary management and motor control problems: proceedings from the II step conference,* Alexandria, Va, 1991, Foundation for Physical Therapy.

115. Umphred D: Merging neurophysiologic approaches with contemporary theories. In Lister MJ, editor: *Contemporary Management of motor control problems: proceedings from the II step conference,* Alexandria, Va, 1991, Foundation for Physical Therapy.

116. Campbell PH: Posture and movement. In Tingey C, editor: *Implementing early intervention,* Baltimore, 1989, Brookes.

117. Fetters L, Kluzik J: The effects of neurodevelopmental treatment versus practice on the reaching of children with spastic cerebral palsy, *Phys Ther* 76:346–358, 1996.

118. O'Flaherty S: International perspectives on paediatric rehabilitation—Australia, *Pediatr Rehabil* 7:267–270, 2004.

119. Stuberg W, Harbourne R: Theoretical practice in pediatric physical therapy: past, present, and future considerations, *Pediatr Phys Ther* 9(3):119–123, 1994.

120. Arndt SW, Chandler LS, Sweeney JK, et al.: Effects of a neurodevelopmental treatment-based trunk protocol for infants with posture and movement dysfunction, *Pediatr Phys Ther* 20 (1):11–22, 2008.

121. Bartlett DJ, Palisano RJ: Physical therapists' perceptions of factors influencing the acquisition of motor abilities of children with cerebral palsy: Implications for clinical reasoning, *Phys Ther* 82:237–248, 2002.

122. Cotton E: Improvement in motor function with the use of conductive education, *Dev Med Child Neurol* 16:637–643, 1974.

123. DeGangi GA, Royeen CB: Current practice among NeuroDevelopmental treatment association members, *Am J Occup Ther* 48:803–809, 1994.

124. Golden GS: Nonstandard therapies in the developmental disabilities, *Am J Dis Child* 134:487–491, 1980.

125. Golden GS: Controversial therapies in developmental disabilities. In Gottlieb MI, Williams JE, editors: New York, 1990, PlenumDevelopmental behavioral disorders: selected topics, vol 3.

126. Goodgold-Edwards SA: Principles for guiding action during motor learning: a critical evaluation of neurodevelopmental treatment, *Physiother Ther Pract* 2(4):30–39, 1993.

127. Harris S: Early intervention: does developmental therapy make a difference? *Topics Early Child Spec Educ* 7:20–32, 1988.

128. Harris SR, Atwater SW, Crowe TK: Accepted and controversial neuromotor therapies for infants at high risk for cerebral palsy, *J Perinatol* 8:3–13, 1988.

129. Kaminker MK, Chiarello LA, O'Neil ME, Dichter CG: Decision making for physical therapy service delivery in schools: a nationwide survey of pediatric physical therapists, *Phys Ther* 84:919–933, 2004.

130. Ketelaar M, Hart Bermeer A, Beck E, et al.: Effects of a functional therapy program on motor abilities of children with cerebral palsy, *Phys Ther* 81:1534–1545, 2001.

131. Ottenbacher K: Sensory integration therapy: affect or effect, *Am J Occup Ther* 36:571–578, 1982.

132. Ottenbacher KJ, Biocca Z, DeCremer G, et al.: Quantitative analysis of the effectiveness of pediatric therapy: emphasis on the neurodevelopmental treatment approach, *Phys Ther* 66:1095–1101, 1986.

133. Palisano RJ, Haley SM, Brown DA: Goal attainment scaling as a measure of change in infants with motor delays, *Phys Ther* 72:432–437, 1992.

134. Thorpe DE, Valvano J: The effects of knowledge of performance and cognitive strategies on motor skill learning in children with cerebral palsy, *Pediatr Phys Ther* 14(1):2–15, 2002.

135. Campbell S: Physical therapy programs that last a lifetime, *Phys Occup Ther Pediatr* 17(1):115, 1997.
136. Kamm K, Thelen E, Jensen JL: A dynamical systems approach to motor development, *Phys Ther* 70:763–775, 1990.
137. Ulrich BD: Dynamic systems theory and skill development in infants and children, *Clin Dev Med* 143/144:318–345, 1997.
138. Bobath B: A neuro-developmental treatment of cerebral palsy, *Physiotherapy* 49:242–244, 1963.
139. Bobath K: *A Neurophysiological basis for the treatment of cerebral palsy,* Philadelphia, 1980, Lippincott.
140. Bobath K, Bobath B: The neuro-developmental treatment. In Scrutton D, editor: *Management of motor disorders in children with cerebral palsy,* Philadelphia, 1984, Lippincott.
141. Bly A: Historical and current view of the basis of NDT, *Pediatr Phys Ther* 3:131–135, 1991.
142. Bobath K, Bobath B: The facilitation of normal postural reactions and movements in the treatment of cerebral palsy, *Physiotherapy* 50:246–262, 1964.
143. Cammisa K, Calabrese D, Myers M, et al.: NDT theory has been updated, *Am J Occup Ther* 49:176, 1995.
144. Tsorlakis N, Evaggelinou C, Grouios G, Tsorbatzoudis C: Effect of intensive neurodevelopmental treatment in gross motor function of children with cerebral palsy, *Dev Med Child Neurol* 46:740–745, 2004.
145. Girolami GL, Campbell SK: Efficacy of a neuro-developmental treatment program to improve motor control in infants born prematurely, *Pediatr Phys Ther* 6(4):175–184, 1994.
146. Butler C, Darrah J: Effects of neurodevelopmental treatment (NDT) for cerebral palsy: an AACPDM evidence report, *Dev Med Child Neurol* 43(11):778–790, 2001.
147. Palisano R: Research on the effectiveness of neurodevelopmental treatment, *Pediatr Phys Ther* 3(3):143–148, 1991.
148. Conner F, Williamson G, Sieff JA: *Programming for the infants and toddlers with neuromotor and other developmental disabilities,* New York, 1978, Teachers College Press.
149. Finnie N: *Handling your young cerebral palsied child at home,* Philadelphia, 1997, Elsevier.
150. Ayres AJ: *Sensory integration and learning disorders,* Los Angeles, 1972, Western Psychological Services.
151. Fisher AG, Bundy AC: Sensory integration theory, *Med Sport Sci* 36:16, 1992.
152. Miller LJ, Coll JR, Schoen SA: A randomized controlled pilot study of the effectiveness of occupational therapy for children with sensory modulation disorder, *Am J Occup Ther* 61(2):228–238, 2007.
153. Olson LJ, Moulton HJ: Use of weighted vests in pediatric occupational therapy practice, *Phys Occup Ther Pediatr* 24:45–60, 2004.
154. Campbell PH, Finn D: Programming to influence acquisition of motor abilities in infants and young children, *Pediatr Phys Ther* 3(4):200–205, 1991.
155. Gentile AM: Skill acquisition: action, movement, and neuromotor processes. In Carr JA, Shepherd R, editors: *Movement science: foundations for physical therapy in rehabilitation,* Rockville, MD, 1987, Aspen.
156. Shepherd RB: Training motor control and optimizing motor learning. In Shepherd RB, editor: *Physiotherapy in paediatrics,* 3 ed., Oxford, 1995, Butterworth-Heinemann.
157. Shumway-Cook A, Woollacott M: *Motor control: theory and practical applications,* Baltimore, 1995, Williams and Wilkins.
158. Shea AM: Motor attainments in Down's syndrome. In Lister MJ, editor: *Contemporary management of motor control problems: proceedings of the II Step conference,* Alexandria, Va, 1991, Foundation for Physical Therapy.
159. Martin K: Effects of supramalleolar orthoses on postural stability in children with Down syndrome, *Dev Med Child Neurol* 46:406–411, 2004.
160. Law M, Narrah J, Pollock N, et al.: Family-centered functional therapy for children with cerebral palsy: an emerging practice model, *Phys Occup Ther Pediatr* 18(1):83–102, 1998.
161. Hirst M: Patterns of impairment and disability related to social handicap in young people with cerebral palsy and spina bifida, *J Biosoc Sci* 21:1–12, 1989.
162. Langone J, Malone MD, Kinsley T: Technology solutions for young children with developmental concerns, *Infants Young Child* 11(4):65–78, 1999.

13

Physical Therapy for the Older Adult

Teresa A. Hoppenrath

KEY TERMS

adaptive equipment
assistive devices
bariatric
dynamic balance
extrinsic factors
Functional Reach test
hypokinesis
instrumental activities of daily living (IADLs)
intrinsic factors
osteoarthritis
osteoporosis
presbycusis
rheumatoid arthritis
sarcopenia
static balance
stereognosis

LEARNING OBJECTIVES

After reading this chapter, the reader will be able to:
- Differentiate between "older adult" and "oldest old"
- List examples of ADLs and IADLs

■ Identify three specific reasons that a physical therapist would modify an intervention for an older person
■ Differentiate between static and dynamic balance
■ Describe the primary role for the physical therapist or the physical therapist assistant in each of the common conditions discussed in this chapter
■ Explain why an interdisciplinary approach is important when developing a plan of care for an older person

*S*enior citizen, older adult, elderly person, frail elderly, aged: what kind of individual comes to mind when you see or hear these words? Is it an 83-year-old bedridden white-haired gentleman? Is it an 83-year-old silver-haired woman swimming laps at the community pool? Both of them should come to mind, as well as countless other descriptions of appearance and abilities. In health care, professionals tend to think first of the multiple medical problems affecting older people. But physical therapists (PTs) and physical therapist assistants (PTAs) may be as likely to intervene with an 85-year-old athlete as with a 70-year-old person who experienced a stroke. To avoid stereotypes and ageism "older adult" or "older person" are used for this population group, bearing in mind the wide variation of *functional abilities* that may be present. While keeping this individual variation in mind, also recognize the commonality that we are *all* part of the aging population!

GENERAL DESCRIPTION

DEMOGRAPHICS

PTs have provided services to individuals with conditions common to people over the age of 65 for many decades. However, only in the past 2 decades have PTs and PTAs worked with older persons in such large (and growing!) numbers. Current trends in health care and life expectancy have rapidly increased the numbers of older adults requiring some type of physical therapy service whether rehabilitative or preventative. For example, according to the U.S. Census Bureau, in 2013 there were 44.5 million people over the age of 65 in the United States, or 14.1% of the population.[1] The Baby Boomers (born between 1946 and 1964) will continue to join the older adults (age 65 and over) increasing the number to 72 million by 2030. It is expected the number of people 85 and older (oldest old) will increase from 5.8 million in 2010 to 19 million by 2050.[2] For an individual born in 2012, the life expectancy is 76.4 years for a male and 81.2 years for a female, the longest life expectancy ever experienced in the United States; however, for a male aged 65 years in 2012, life expectancy is 82.9 years and for a female it is 85.5 years (Figure 13-1).[3]

As people live longer, they tend to develop physical or medical conditions that require a PT's expertise to maximize movement function in their daily activities. Although each individual requiring physical therapy benefits from specific, unique interventions, the goals for most people will include skills to independently perform fundamental activities such as bathing, feeding, toileting, and dressing. These activities are described as activities of daily living (ADL),

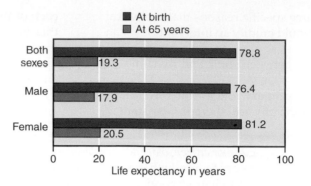

Figure 13-1 ▪ Life expectancy in the United States by sex at birth (2012) and age 65. (From Mortality in the United States, 2012. NCHS data brief, no. 168. October 2014.)

whereas more complex activities necessary for community living are called **instrumental activities of daily living (IADL)**. Examples of IADLs include using public transportation, shopping, laundry, housekeeping, and managing finances (see Box 8-2 for examples of ADLs).

ADLs and IADLs are the skills that allow an older person to be less dependent on caregivers. For instance, shopping is a difficult skill for many older adults with physical impairments. If therapists assist older adults in improving balance and provide an appropriate assistive device, more individuals may be able to complete shopping trips with less assistance.

Almost half of non-institutionalized persons, 70 years of age and older, have difficulty with at least one ADL. This percentage increases with age and is higher for women in physical activities, confirming that physical therapy plays an important role in improving functional performance and patient independence.[4] Normal aging processes include changes that are common in all persons. Professionals differentiate older persons based upon changes in body structure and function, limitations in activities, and the impact on a person's ability to participate at a societal level. The 91-year-old woman in Figure 13-2 is a good example of a person who has documented medical issues yet functions on an independent level. The primary goal related to physical therapy for someone like her is to achieve optimal physical function and prevent conditions that might limit her ability to continue at this level. This is accomplished by regular physical activity such as daily walking as demonstrated in Figure 13-3. In contrast, older persons with conditions that significantly impair daily function or require frequent medical intervention may need physical therapy to regain mobility skills or modify the environment to maximize the individual's function.

SETTINGS

As the abilities of older adults are diverse, so are the environments in which these individuals live. PTs and PTAs will encounter older individuals in a wide variety of settings. Those with acute medical conditions such as pneumonia,

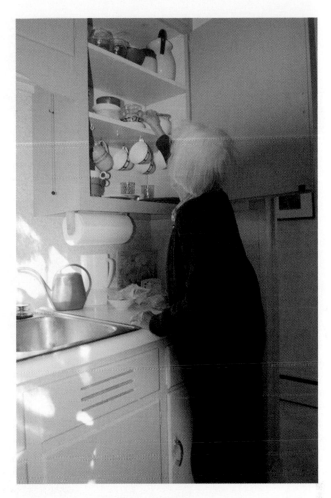

Figure 13-2 ■ An example of an older person who functions independently at home. (Courtesy Terri Hoppenrath.)

cardiovascular dysfunction, or fractures will be treated in a hospital. Older people with conditions such as cerebrovascular accident (CVA) (stroke), Parkinson's disease, or amputation may be seen for physical therapy in a rehabilitation center once they are medically stable. A variety of long-term care (LTC) centers such as skilled nursing facilities (SNF) or assisted living facilities (ALF) provide services to people who are not acutely ill but require nursing care or assistance with ADLs. PTs and PTAs in LTC settings generally provide two types of services: (1) rehabilitative services to improve skills so people may return to their prior level of function (PLOF) or allow less dependence on caregivers and (2) functional maintenance programs developed by PTs and implemented by facility staff to assist older adults in maintaining their current skills and preventing further limitations or disability.

Many older people with functional limitations are healthy enough to live at home independently or have family members who are able to care for them.

13

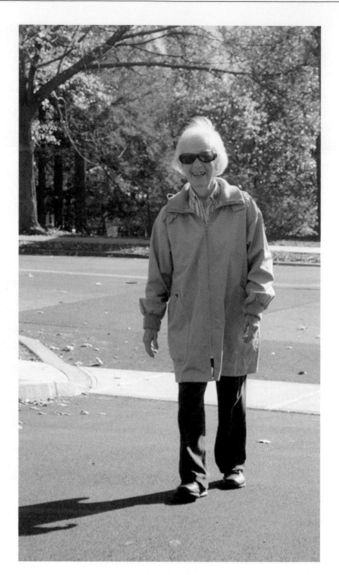

Figure 13-3 ■ Daily physical activity such as walking can maintain or improve physical function. (Courtesy Terri Hoppenrath.)

Depending on the medical condition of the individual and availability of appropriate transportation, older people living at home who require physical therapy may receive those services at an outpatient clinic, through a home health care agency, or an adult day care facility.

Healthy older people who want to maintain, regain, or improve their optimum physical status may attend exercise classes at community fitness centers or sponsored by groups such as the Arthritis Foundation. Figure 13-4 demonstrates a variety of exercises that can be performed in the home with no additional equipment. Traditional or aquatic exercise programs, tai chi, or yoga

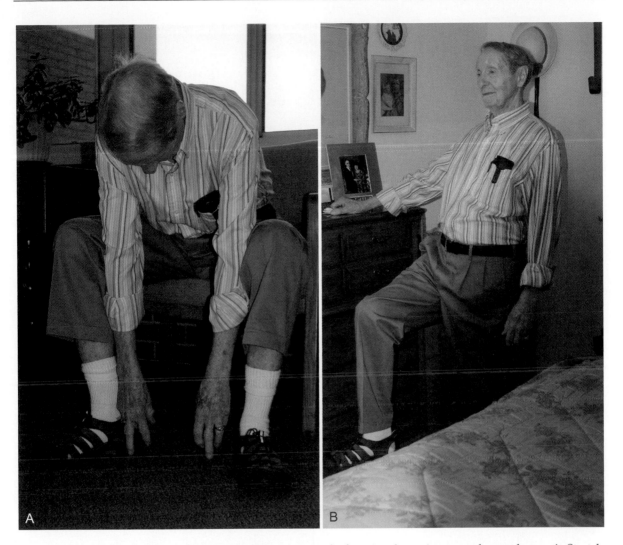

Figure 13-4 ■ A physical therapist has taught this man simple, functional exercises to perform at home. **A**, Stretching low back muscles. **B**, Standing hip flexion for strengthening and balance.

Continued

may be conducted, supervised, or developed by PTs. These exercise programs may be aimed at general fitness and health promotion or at the prevention of specific conditions responsive to exercise, such as osteoporosis or poor balance.

ROLES FOR PTS WITH OLDER ADULTS

It is easy to envision the PT as a clinician who provides hands-on services (primary intervention) to older adults. However, in each of the settings described

13

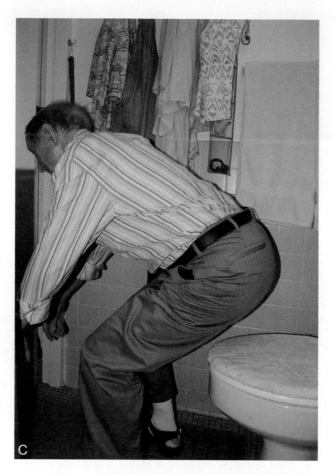

Figure 13-4—*Cont'd* **C**, Sit to stand from toilet without using hands to push up. (Courtesy Terri Hoppenrath.)

earlier, PTs are also educators. With valuable knowledge of the physiologic aging process, PTs are the ideal professionals to educate patients, family members, and other professionals to prevent and minimize impairments, activity limitations, and participation restrictions. Armed with facts, older people will be better able to exercise appropriately and maintain or regain skills. For example, the woman in Figure 13-5 is being taught how to use her arms to more easily get up from a reclined position.

Why wait until an older person has limitations? PTs promote prevention activities and provide education in health, wellness, and fitness promotion using evidence-based research creating opportunities for productive and healthy lifestyles.[5]

PTs may act as expert consultants to individuals and organizations. PTs are effective advocates for older people in identifying problems and providing solutions, performing environmental assessments, developing appropriate activity

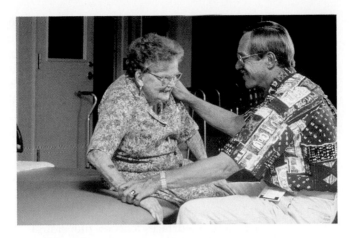

Figure 13-5 ■ Instruction is a major component of physical therapy. The woman in the photo is being taught how to use her arms to sit up from a reclined position. (Courtesy Bruce Wang.)

programs, and in ensuring accessibility to all environments.[6] For an individual, the PT provides the knowledge necessary to acquire appropriate **adaptive equipment** or **assistive devices** that provide for both safety and convenience. Adaptive equipment allows an individual to perform a functional task with increased ease and/or independence. An example is a grab bar secured to the wall in the bathroom near the shower or toilet so the individual can safety attend to ADLs without assistance from a caretaker. An assistive device is one that provides the individual with assistance during periods of mobility. For example, a cane may assist an individual in climbing stairs safely. As an organization consultant, the PT performs environmental assessments to minimize the risk of falls. The PT acts as a resource for other health care providers to determine how to incorporate goals related to mobility into other components of the rehab program.

Other roles PTs may assume relating to the older adult are those of administrator and researcher. PTs are prepared to assume such roles as managers of rehabilitation services or supervising PTAs, aides, or other support personnel. In each of these positions, the PT's educational background in managing resources and leadership allows them to combine knowledge of the aging issues and management skills to take on additional responsibilities to serve clients. Research related to topics such as the aging process, prevention of disability related to aging, and effective interventions for the older adult is a priority in the health care field. Discipline-specific studies of the cost effectiveness of particular interventions are essential in the determination of reimbursement policies for health care for older individuals. PTs are also essential team members in interdisciplinary studies that expand the knowledge of all health care professionals related to aging.

AGING-RELATED CHANGES

PTs and PTAs must be familiar with the changes that occur in "normal" aging in order to distinguish them from pathologic changes. Aging-related changes,

13

which vary with each individual, are considered when PTs conduct an examination, formulate an evaluation that includes a diagnosis, prognosis, plan of care with clinical interventions, and goals for people over 65 years of age. Although there are biologic changes associated with aging, many changes once thought to be an inevitable part of aging are now related to the reduced activity and sedentary lifestyle of many older people. The PT, with the health care team, has an important role in evaluating older adults to determine what body structures and functions and functional activities can be addressed or what participation restrictions can be minimized through physical therapy. Changes that are not amenable to improvement may be addressed through adaptation, accommodation, or compensation. For example, a PT may conclude that an elderly person who has experienced multiple falls needs an assistive device. The PT or PTA would then adjust the height of the device and teach the patient how to use it on a variety of surfaces (carpet, tile, stairs).

The physical changes observed in older adults that affect the musculoskeletal system (bones, muscles, and joints) often result in poor posture, changes in gait pattern, and decreased strength and flexibility. Decreased strength is often related to **hypokinesis** (decreased activity or movement) and **sarcopenia** (decreased muscle mass) typically seen in older people. Muscle mass is reduced because of a decrease in the number of muscle fibers.[7] The reduction in fibers is related to loss of motor neurons (nerves innervating muscles) and active motor units (a single motor neuron and all the muscle fibers it innervates).[8]

Decreased flexibility with age is related to both hypokinesis and biologic changes in connective tissue. Connective tissue tends to become less hydrated thus stiffer with aging. With less activity, muscles are not required to lengthen as often and actually become shorter over time. As muscles shorten, individuals tend to assume more flexed positions leading to postural changes.

Bone also undergoes changes with age. In studies of vertebral bodies, bone mass was shown to decrease by 35% to 40% between the ages of 20 and 80 years.[9] This finding suggests that bone is weaker in older people. Declining bone mass may eventually advance to osteoporosis.

Weight-bearing joints such as hips or knees degenerate over time. Excessive wear and tear destroys articular cartilage (which covers the ends of bones) causing impairments such as pain, inflammation, and deformities. Obesity is a risk factor that causes additional stress to these joints facilitating rapid deterioration[10] (see the discussion of arthritis in the section on common conditions).

The central nervous system shows a reduction in conduction velocity associated with age.[7] The reduction affects the ability of the nerve to transmit impulses. This change tends to make movement responses slower in older persons and may explain the reduced ability to respond rapidly to loss of balance or the slowed gait pattern often seen in later life.

Several of the sensory systems display changes that significantly affect balance, mobility, and the ability to detect environmental hazards. To move safely, the visual system provides accurate information regarding the environment. In the older person, the lens can become cloudy (cataract), and the muscles around the lens decrease in their ability to accommodate rapidly from seeing far to near distance.[11] Visual acuity is also reduced. These changes make lighting and contrasting colors important in offering the older person cues about objects or surfaces that might interfere with safe mobility. Macular degeneration is a condition that affects the retina resulting in a loss of central vision. Visual changes can cause fear of falling and an increase in falls in the older population.[12]

Age-related hearing loss is called **presbycusis**. This term refers to the decreased ability to perceive high-pitched sounds and to distinguish between similar sounds.[11] Auditory acuity is also reduced. These changes must be considered and strategies need to be adopted (such as lowering of the voice, talking more slowly, or looking directly at the patient at all times) when instructions are given in a physical therapy session.

The tactile system is another sensory system whose changes may affect mobility. The tactile system provides important information regarding the texture and changes in the walking surface. Age-related changes reduce the amount of touch, pressure, and pain the individual receives from the environment. If an older person does not receive accurate information regarding the surface underfoot, the gait pattern may become altered or a loss of balance may occur.

Age-related changes occur in the cardiovascular and pulmonary systems. For example, 64% of people over the age of 65 have hypertension (high blood pressure), women being at higher risk than men.[13,14] Non-Hispanic blacks (men and women) are more likely to be hypertensive than people of any other racial or ethnic group.[15] It appears, however, that overall cardiac performance at rest is not altered by age in healthy people, although cardiac response to stress does differ. This is demonstrated by a decrease in maximum cardiopulmonary function and work capacity.[16] Increased stiffness in the chest wall affects the respiratory system, which further reduces the effectiveness of cardiopulmonary function. These changes should be considered carefully in the design of exercise programs for individuals over 65 years of age.

Balance is a skill essential for safe and independent daily function. Limitation in balance and an increase in the risk of falling are common problems in older adults. One out of every three adults over the age of 65 will experience a fall.[17] Static balance and dynamic balance are the result of a complex interaction of multiple systems subject to age-related changes mentioned previously. If any of these systems undergoes change balance may be affected. A fall resulting from a loss of balance could expose the person to a multitude of subsequent impairments, such as fracture, traumatic brain injury, pneumonia, decubitus ulcers, and loss of strength or range of motion. The psychosocial impact on the individual can also be disabling. Fear of falling and loss of confidence may cause the individual to become isolated or more sedentary.[18] If the fall is serious enough to cause injury, the older person could lose the ability to safely live independently.

For many years, one of the most common myths of aging was that cognitive function always significantly decreases with advanced age. In fact, people seemed to assume that dementia was inevitable. It is now known that deterioration of cognitive function characterized as dementia is related to Alzheimer's disease or some other pathologic condition, not to aging itself, although age remains a risk factor.[19] In 2013 it was estimated that approximately 5 million Americans had Alzheimer's disease.[20] Health professionals serving older people are aware of how to recognize and interact with people who have dementia.

13

Significant cognitive changes that do fall in the category of normal aging are in memory and conceptualization (tasks requiring abstract thinking).[21] Specifically, the manner in which new information is stored (encoded) in the memory is altered. This leads to difficulty in retrieving newer information. Studies show that training in memory techniques such as list organization can improve recall in older persons.[22]

Psychosocial changes affect people in older population groups, varying widely based on the individual, family, environment, and presence of other changes or actual disease. What is important for the PT and PTA to remember is that understanding psychosocial issues is crucial to the success of any rehabilitation program. For example, LGBT (lesbian, gay, bisexual, transgender) older adults may face discrimination barriers that health care providers must understand and address.[23] Social considerations such as adjustment to retirement, loss of lifetime roles, social isolation, and absence of health insurance have a tremendous impact on quality of life. Loss of a spouse, sibling, child or friend, or dealing with chronic illness requires considerable adjustment. Psychiatric disorders such as depression and anxiety are more common among homebound older people than those who are able to be out in the community.[24] The PT or PTA has a responsibility to bring signs of psychological problems to the attention of other members of the health care team.

COMMON CONDITIONS

Many impairments prevalent in older people can benefit from physical therapy intervention. Individuals with the following common conditions are frequently seen by PTs and PTAs. Problems for older adults that are neurologic in nature, such as Parkinson's disease and CVA, are discussed in Chapter 9.

Therapists should be aware of the impact of medical conditions on the older person's ability to recover from functional limitations. A retrospective analysis of a group of more than 1000 people older than age 65 showed that an older person who has two or more medical conditions is less likely to recover function in such tasks as dressing or carrying 10 lb. Diabetes mellitus, stroke, depression, and hip fracture had the greatest effect on recovery.[25]

OSTEOARTHRITIS

The most common orthopaedic problem for older people is degenerative joint disease described as **osteoarthritis (OA)**. Based on a survey from 2010-2012, 22.7% (52.5 million) of Americans were diagnosed with OA.[26] OA most commonly occurs in weight-bearing joints of the knees, hips, and spine; however, it is also common in the hands and the big toe. OA occurs when the cartilage deteriorates owing to advancing age and/or obesity. Patients often complain of morning stiffness and pain with movement. This may alter the gait pattern or make simple tasks such as buttoning a blouse very difficult. Therapists should encourage patients to maintain at least a moderate activity level while protecting the joints. PTs and PTAs can teach appropriate exercise routines (such as aquatic exercises) to maintain flexibility without excessively stressing the joints. For people who are excessively overweight, programs that address weight loss as well as exercise and joint protection are beneficial to reduce the stress on the joints. There are some facilities and therapists that specialize in treating such individuals.

Their services may be referred to as *bariatric* programs.[10] With an aging population and the increase of obesity, the economic burden of arthritis is likely to continue to escalate.

Total joint replacements of the hip and knee are common surgeries for older adults to alleviate pain and to improve function. When joint replacements are performed for a person with OA, the PT is involved with the patient before surgery as well as during the rehabilitation process. Before surgery the PT teaches strengthening and flexibility exercises so the patient will go into surgery in optimal condition. The therapist also teaches the individual important guidelines to follow after surgery, orders assistive devices, and reinforces the importance of exercise and rehabilitation after surgery. After joint replacements, the PT and PTA provide interventions for maximizing muscle strength, joint motion, and ability to perform ADLs.

RHEUMATOID ARTHRITIS

In contrast to OA, **rheumatoid arthritis (RA)** is a chronic autoimmune disease that causes inflammation of the joints. It is more common in women than men, and the peak incidence occurs at 40 to 60 years of age.[27] RA is characterized by enlarged joints that are often reddened and warm to the touch. The affected joints are stiff and painful, usually more so in the morning or after extended periods of inactivity. This disease process leads to limited range of motion, joint deformities, and eventually progressive joint destruction. Older persons with RA have increased mortality from cardiovascular disease.[28] Typical physical therapy goals for the person with RA are pain relief, increased joint movement, assistive devices to facilitate independent function, cardiovascular fitness, and rehabilitation when joint surgery is required.

Pain relief may be provided by heat modalities such as a paraffin bath. The PT or PTA may teach the individual positioning principles for pain relief when in resting postures. Active range of motion exercises assist the individual in maintaining movement and flexibility necessary for function, and when done as aquatic exercises in a warm pool, these can be quite beneficial. Assistive devices such as canes or walkers may reduce pain in the affected joints during ambulation.

OSTEOPOROSIS

Osteoporosis is not a part of the normal aging process. Yet, the National Osteoporosis Foundation estimates that approximately 54 million American women and men have osteoporosis or low bone mass.[29] Osteoporosis is characterized by decreased mineralization of the bones, which results from decreased production of new bone cells (osteoblasts) and an increased resorption of bone. The condition is measured by dual-energy X-ray absorptiometry (DEXA scan), and it is defined in terms of bone mineral density (BMD) of 2.5 standard deviations or more below the mean peak bone mass of young, healthy adults.[30] Osteoporosis is more common in women than men. Risk factors that predispose people to osteoporosis are postmenopausal state, malnutrition, alcoholism, sedentary lifestyle, smoking, lack of calcium, and certain medications.[11] Once again, ethnicity and race play an important role. Caucasian Americans are more likely to have osteoporosis than African Americans.[31] Minimal trauma fracture typically affects the femoral

13

neck, vertebrae, and wrist.[32] Physical therapy's primary role in osteoporosis is *prevention*. This is discussed in the next section that addresses hip fracture.

HIP FRACTURE

The combination of osteoporosis and accidental falls has made hip fracture one of the most important health care issues for older adults. People over age 65 sustain 86% of the hip fractures in the United States. Annually more than 258,000 persons are hospitalized for these fractures with a mortality rate of nearly 30% and at a cost of $30 billion.[33,34] As larger proportions of the population enter the over 65 age group these numbers are likely to increase. Hip fracture is considered by many to be a major public health problem. A study conducted in Boston illustrates the significant impact that hip fracture has on the functional skills an elderly person may hope to regain after surgery to repair the hip. Only 33% of the people in that study had regained their prefracture status in five basic ADLs 1 year after the fracture.[35] Another study showed that 2 months after hospital discharge about 40% had regained the ability to perform ADLs, but only 18% had returned to previous levels of performance of IADLs. An older adult who sustains a hip fracture has a 1-year post-op mortality rate of 27.3%.[36]

PTs are essential in the rehabilitation of patients after hip fracture. Early mobilization is important to minimize risk of respiratory problems. Transfer skills, gait training, teaching weight-bearing precautions, and selection of an assistive device are initiated in the hospital. Working toward returning the patient to his or her PLOF occurs at a rehabilitation center, SNF, or the person's home (Figure 13-6). As these basic skills are attained, PTs teach the person to regain additional functional skills such as showering, or transfers to and from an automobile.

Physical therapy plays an important role in preventing both osteoporosis and hip fractures. The most beneficial programs address activity level,

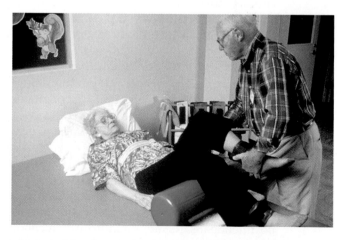

Figure 13-6 ■ After instruction by the physical therapist, a spouse provides assistance in an exercise program to regain hip and knee strength after surgery to repair a hip fracture. (Courtesy Bruce Wang.)

Table 13-1
Examples of Intrinsic and Extrinsic Factors That Contribute to Falling

Intrinsic Factors	Extrinsic Factors
Age	Poor lighting
Previous history of falls	Uneven or slippery surfaces
Cognitive changes	Medications
Sensory problems (vision or dizziness)	Improper assistive device/improper use of device
Multiple medical conditions	Improper footwear
Muscle weakness	Throw rugs
Orthostatic hypotension	Lack of handrails or grab bars

weight-bearing activities, flexibility, strengthening, and education regarding a safe physical environment. Prevention of falls requires input from the entire health care team. Falls are multifactorial and are often related to both **intrinsic factors** (within the individual) and **extrinsic factors** (within the environment) (Table 13-1). Tool kits such as STEADI (Stopping Elderly Accidents, Deaths, and Injuries) are available for healthcare providers to assess risk.[37] Routine opportunities for weight bearing and walking are important prevention strategies (Figure 13-7).

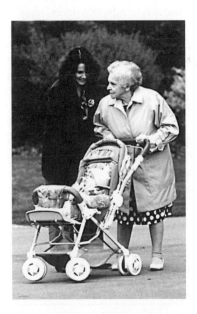

Figure 13-7 ■ The home care physical therapist uses another family member (child) as a meaningful approach to increasing the strength and endurance of an older individual. (Courtesy Bruce Wang.)

13

DIABETES

Diabetes mellitus affects 11.2 million (25.9%) of Americans over the age of 65 years.[38] Diabetes is a chronic disorder with serious effects on many body systems. It is a disease of insufficient insulin action, affecting the efficient transport of glucose into muscle, adipose, and liver cells. Instead, excessive glucose accumulates in the blood. Common complications of diabetes include renal failure, peripheral neuropathies, poor circulation leading to skin ulcerations, coronary artery disease (making heart attack and stroke prevalent in people with diabetes), and retinopathies (leading to blindness). Physical therapy can address specific problems for the person with diabetes. PTs must consider these issues when designing an exercise program. A health care team approach can address and monitor an exercise program, diet, prescribed medications, and appropriate footwear.

For people with non-insulin-dependent diabetes, studies support management of the disease through diet and exercise.[39,40] PTs play an important role in developing exercise programs that consider the problems associated with diabetes.

PRINCIPLES OF EXAMINATION

EXAMINATION

Physical therapy for an older adult begins with examination and evaluation. The PT's examination is one component of a team evaluation. It is necessary for professionals from a variety of disciplines to critically examine the older person. By sharing their findings each will be better able to serve the individual with optimum care.

Some settings, however, may not have every health care discipline available to their clients. In these situations the PT should be able to make observations about the individual that include not only musculoskeletal, neurologic, cardiovascular and pulmonary, and integumentary status, but also basic information regarding cognitive status, social situation, and communication abilities. The *Guide to Physical Therapist Practice 3.0* contains a comprehensive list of tests and measures for use in examination.[6]

Examination and evaluation should be specifically oriented to the skills and capabilities needed for maximum independence. These capabilities will differ for each older person. For example, a 70-year-old who has been inactive and sedentary since retirement at age 55 will have very different needs for rehabilitation from those of a 78-year-old who walks 2 miles every day and continues to work 4 hours a day as a volunteer in a recreation program. In each case the health care team considers how the individual functioned before the condition requiring therapy. A thorough examination includes information related to the person's typical daily function and what the person hopes to accomplish after the intervention.

HISTORY

During the initial session, the PT begins the examination process by gathering information obtained through a patient questionnaire form (including nature of current condition, medical/surgical history, medications) and interview with the patient (and possibly family members). Consider a quiet space with adequate lighting when possible. When interviewing, the PT seeks information about how the patient views the current problem and its impact on function. A person's perceptions of the seriousness of the problem and expectations of therapy are important to consider when the plan of care is being developed. Information from the person regarding any culturally based beliefs about illness, disability, and health should be considered.

The interview gives the PT a general impression of cognitive function to determine whether a more formal examination of cognition is necessary. The individual should be able to give the PT information about family support, typical activity level, occupation or former occupation, and the living environment.

A thorough social history is important for understanding the patient's previous function, amount and type of support, and need for goals. Issues such as previous or current employment, recreation and hobbies, availability of transportation, and insurance coverage are all important considerations for developing a relevant plan of care. The availability of caregivers or other support systems may be needed.

Input from family members and other caregivers may supplement or clarify the poor historian. This information can determine the amount of assistance a person may need from other sources. In Figure 13-8 both the patient and her spouse are providing essential information to the PT. A thorough chart review in an inpatient setting is critical for a complete history. Objective information is gained from the patient's chart, reports, records including information such as the medical diagnosis, dates of hospitalization, laboratory reports, and other documented facts about the present illness or complaint, as well as past problems that could influence the plan of care for the current problem.

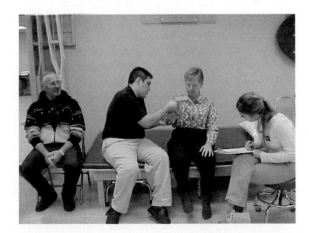

Figure 13-8 ■ The spouse (on the far left) is able to provide additional important information for the physical therapist during the history portion of the examination.

13

SYSTEMS REVIEW

The examination continues with a systems review, which entails a brief examination of the individual's systems to provide the PT with information regarding the older adult's general health. Systems include cardiovascular and pulmonary, integumentary, musculoskeletal, neuromuscular, and communication ability. The information from the brief examination helps the PT to select the most appropriate tests and measures for the individual.

TESTS AND MEASURES

The examination of an older person proceeds much like the PT's examination of any individual except that the PT is especially alert to the common problems of this age group. The PT may adapt some examination procedures to be more appropriate to the older individual. Tasks that are requested of the individual are explained as they relate to function. Tests and measures help the PT to verify or disprove factors regarding impairment or functional limitations and support their clinical judgment for a PT diagnosis, prognosis, and plan of care.

In examining the muscle performance of the older person, the PT keeps in mind the potential for age-related changes described earlier. The therapist examines strength as it relates to activities the individual wants or needs to perform. In other words, strength is examined in terms of function. Norms for range of motion in people over 65 years old have not been established, nor are any norms universally accepted. Based on the person's activity level some deficits may be expected. The therapist determines, with the patient, how much limitation of movement at the joints is acceptable. Posture of the older adult is examined in the same way as for other patients. The PT determines whether the observed posture is a result of actual structural changes or whether it is a result of habit or functional issues. If the changes are not structural, education and exercise may significantly improve abnormal postural findings.

The neurologic examination of the older person is similar to that of any individual. Some responses may be slow as described earlier, but it is a matter of determining what impact, if any, this has on the person's quality of life. The neurologic examination includes sensory integrity testing, such as cutaneous sensation, proprioception, **stereognosis** (perception of form through touch) and results of visual and auditory testing performed by other members of the health care team. Sensory deficits may significantly affect functional tasks such as balance. As noted earlier, balance is a complex interaction of cognitive, visual, perceptual, and motor skills. The PT needs to examine each of these systems individually to determine which may be contributing to a balance problem.

Both static (standing still) and dynamic (moving) balance should be examined. Tests and measures for examining **static balance** include the norm-referenced Unipedal Stance Test (UPST), which consists of timing the person standing on one foot with eyes open and eyes closed.[41] Another specific static balance test that can predict the likelihood of falling in healthy normal adults is the **Functional Reach Test**.[42] This test is a simple measure of how far the person can reach forward without losing balance or taking a step.

Dynamic balance is assessed in a number of ways. Gait and functional mobility are important aspects of dynamic balance. The PT may measure how long it takes the older person to walk a set distance using a measure such as the Timed Up and Go (TUG).[43] Other tests include the Berg Balance Scale, the Performance Oriented Mobility Assessment (POMA), and the Dynamic Gait Index.[44-46] The Gait Abnormality Rating Scale (GARS) looks at several components of gait and relates them to balance.[47] These are just a few of many tools available to assess balance. The PT selects an appropriate tool based on such factors as the individual's ability to follow directions, the person's living situation, and the specific features of the test. Gait examination should always include the use of any required assistive device and a description or consideration of the type of footwear the person uses. The type of sole or the weight of the shoe will affect the way the person ambulates. In Figure 13-9 the PT is performing an initial gait examination of a man approximately a month after hospital discharge after a stroke. The quadruped cane is needed at this time to assist with dynamic balance.

Information regarding balance and potential for falling is useful to the entire interdisciplinary team working with the older person. Another balance measure that may reveal information useful to the team is a self-efficacy measure entitled Falls Efficacy Scale (FES).[48] This type of test focuses on the individual's confidence regarding balance and provides useful information for program planning. The team will be able to develop strategies in fall prevention that range from exercise and environmental modification to teaching fall prevention skills.

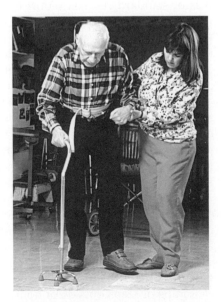

Figure 13-9 ■ Gait assessment using a quadruped cane after a stroke. (Courtesy Bruce Wang.)

Standard tests of cardiovascular and pulmonary function are used to assess individuals to determine if exercise programs should be modified. Measurements of cardiovascular and pulmonary function performed before and after treatment help the PT to determine whether goals to increase endurance are realistic and appropriate (see also Chapter 10).

Pain assessment is an important part of the examination of the older person. A description of its location, intensity, and circumstances that elicit or alleviate the pain is needed. It should be noted whether the pain is acute or chronic and whether it increases or decreases from one session to the next. Because pain is perceived differently from one individual to the next, it is important to assess how much discomfort the person is willing to tolerate to maintain independent function.

One simple means of measuring pain is on a visual analog scale (VAS).[49] The individual indicates the amount of pain being experienced along a 10-cm scale (see Figure 8-2). If an objective pain index such as this is used, decreasing pain from one measurable point to another on the scale may be an appropriate goal. Another approach is to set a goal for a specific functional task to be performed within a tolerable level of pain.

The tests and measures just described relate to specific impairments or functional limitations. It is also important for the PT to examine the older adult's overall function. For many years PTs have used checklists to indicate whether a patient can perform particular tasks. More recently, several standardized measures have been developed. Standardized measures allow health care professionals to compare a person's scores as the individual moves from one setting to another. They can also measure change at specific time intervals. Measures generally fall under the categories of self-report or performance measures. Examples of standardized self-report measures are the Functional Status Questionnaire (FSQ)[50] and the Functional Status Index (FSI),[51] in which the older person or the caregiver reports the person's ability to perform functional activities. In performance tests such as the Physical Performance Test (PPT), the therapist observes the older person performing tasks and scores the performance according to the instructions for the tool.[52]

Information about the environment in which the older person lives is essential. Whether the individual is in a nursing home or living at home (with or without a partner) several aspects of the environment must be considered. The physical layout of the living area, access to and from the residence, and access from the home to outside services are important. Ideally, prior to discharge, the PT should visit the residence rather than relying on reports from others.

The PT investigates access to and from the residence based on the individual's specific abilities and limitations. The following items are important in determining how much assistance the older person will require to be as independent in the living environment as possible:

- Ground surfaces—gravel, pavement, grass, sidewalks
- Curbs and curb cuts
- Ramps or steps outside of home
- Stairways within the home
- Presence or absence of handrails

- Size of door openings
- Door handles, latches
- Furnishings and floor coverings
- Arrangement of kitchen and bathroom fixtures
- Distance between rooms used most often

In addition to these, a thorough examination includes such items as lighting, doorways, floor plans, and adequate space for adaptive equipment. Because the clinician has so many items to consider a checklist with space for individual notation is most efficient for this assessment.

An environmental examination is equally important whether the older person is in a private home or an LTC facility. According to federal regulations, LTC facilities receiving federal reimbursement (such as Medicare or Medicaid) are obligated to ensure that residents are as free from the use of restraints as is practical. Such items as seat belts in wheelchairs, lap tables, and bedrails are not to be used for restraint without extensive evaluation. PTs in these settings are obligated to assess mobility skills and safety and make recommendations to the interdisciplinary team regarding the need, if any, for these devices. The team must attempt to modify the physical environment to meet individual needs for safety before considering restraints. Only when other options have been exhausted should the team recommend the temporary use of such supports.

As described earlier, few cognitive changes are solely the result of aging in a healthy older person. However, many of the conditions common in the elderly are associated with the potential for development of dementia. For this reason, the PT should either obtain information from other health care professionals or make observations during the physical therapy evaluation regarding cognitive function. The older person's cognitive abilities have great influence on how the PT provides instructions, the number of repetitions required when demonstrating, and how much practice is required when teaching a new skill. A standard, quick cognitive assessment tool such as the St Louis University Mental Status Examination (SLUMS) is readily available and can easily be used by PTs without extensive training.[53]

As with all patients, the PT must obtain psychosocial information as part of the complete evaluation of the older person. The person's success in adjusting to the present disability is important information that will help the therapist determine the individual's level of motivation and whether special strategies are necessary to increase that level. An older person may become depressed, viewing a problem such as stroke or heart attack as "the beginning of the end." The therapist benefits from knowing the significant people in the patient's life—spouse, family, friends, or caregivers.

The interprofessional team determines discharge disposition. Social workers or case managers are able to provide the PT with pertinent details regarding each patient's specific health insurance coverage and financial status so the impact on rehabilitation services can be considered. The health care team plans and prioritizes intervention for each individual, based not only on the findings of the examination, evaluation, and prognosis, but also on social supports.

PRINCIPLES OF EVALUATION, DIAGNOSIS, AND PROGNOSIS

Once information about the patient or client is obtained through the examination process, the next step in managing physical therapy for the older adult is to evaluate the findings of the examination. Evaluation is a dynamic process that requires the PT to use clinical judgment regarding the data from examination. The PT determines whether the patient is likely to benefit from physical therapy, as well as whether a referral to another practitioner is required. From the evaluation, the PT determines a diagnosis by identifying the functional impact that directs the course of rehabilitation. The diagnosis is a label or classification assigned to the cluster of findings related to a particular individual. It is important to remember that older adults frequently have multiple medical diagnoses. The PT considers these medical conditions, impairments in body structure and function, and functional limitations, and then evaluates how they affect the individual's ability to function. The diagnosis reflects the result of the evaluation process and determines appropriate interventions.

Weighing all variables allows the PT to arrive at a prognosis that will direct the planning and goal-setting process for the older adult. Prognosis involves determining the type, frequency, and duration of intervention necessary to reach the expected outcomes thus resulting in a plan of care.

Two 80-year-old individuals with identical medical conditions will not necessarily have the same prognosis or subsequent plans for physical therapy. Social supports, environmental factors, internal factors such as cognitive level, and other variables all contribute to determination of a prognosis.

PRINCIPLES OF INTERVENTION

Based upon data gathered from the evaluation, diagnosis, and prognosis, the PT focuses on problems identified from the evaluation and selects and implements relevant interventions for the individual to regain or maintain physical, psychological, and social well-being.[54] PT and PTAs who specialize in treating the older adult understand the aging process, therapeutic interventions, environmental factors, and social support systems to provide quality of life to this population.

In establishing goals for intervention, the first consideration is to set meaningful goals that address daily function. For example, a goal to have the person reach full shoulder flexion may not be meaningful if the person does not have the need to reach overhead. If the highest cupboards in the house require only partial shoulder flexion and the person does not put any clothing on over the head, perhaps valuable time for direct intervention should be spent on other activities. However, if this older adult is working part-time and must reach overhead, full shoulder flexion is important. Examples of interventions for older adults include, but are not limited to, therapeutic exercise, functional training, physical agents, manual therapies, and always, patient instruction.

PTs can achieve expertise in evidence-based exercise prescription through additional coursework and credentialing offered by the Academy of Geriatric Physical Therapy and the American Physical Therapy Association such as Certified Exercise Expert for Aging Adults (CEEAA).[55]

To set functional goals with measurable outcomes, the therapist involves the older person throughout the process. Measurable outcomes assist the PT with assessment and reassessment and serve to provide the client with specific feedback about what has been accomplished by physical therapy. This may require some encouragement from the professional, especially if the person believes that the role of the health care professional is to issue direction and wait for patient compliance. Older people may feel that determining treatment is not the patient's role. In this case the professional encourages the older adult to be more involved in decision-making regarding care.

The interdisciplinary approach mentioned throughout this chapter is important when goals are being set. The individual may have multiple medical and rehabilitative needs. The team, including the patient and family, examines all the problems and prioritizes short-term and long-term goals. The entire team is responsible for identifying functional outcomes to improve the older person's ability to participate in daily activities.

Effective instruction of the older person encompasses both general and specific information. General, factual information about the effects of aging on the various body systems gives the older person a good background and model from which to judge changes he or she is experiencing. This information helps the person appreciate the importance of achieving or maintaining an active lifestyle to prevent changes that are linked to inactivity. More specific information pertaining to the particular problem the older adult is experiencing is also important. Such topics as the typical course of the disorder, expected type and length of treatment, expectations for the home program, and impact on function should be clearly outlined for the individual and family members.

Education plays a role in motivating older adults, but other techniques can increase motivation as well. Often, older people enjoy therapy if social interaction is built into the process. Establishing a group of people with similar abilities for exercise may be beneficial and fun. Designing intervention in such a way that the person is competing, either with results of the last session or with peers, may also increase motivation to perform. Technologic developments, such as Wii Sports by Nintendo®, provide contemporary approaches to exercise that can easily be carried out at home and may even involve younger family members. Lists of activities, diagrams, charts with spaces to check off, or a notebook may be valuable in assisting older adults to take control of their routine.

Intervention for older adults focuses on improving daily function. Programs should incorporate movement patterns that normally occur during the person's routine. For example, treatment for balance problems is the most beneficial if it includes such activities as balance during transitional movements (sit to stand, in and out of bed) and on uneven surfaces. In Figure 13-10, the woman is engaged in resistive exercise to increase strength in hip and knee musculature. However, modification may be necessary in the presence of certain medical conditions. Cardiovascular and pulmonary conditions, arthritis, and diabetes are common in older individuals and may necessitate modifications of accepted approaches.

Some medications taken by older individuals also necessitate the modification of intervention. Certain medications affect the ability to perform physical activity. Older people commonly take multiple medications, both prescribed and over the counter. The PT should be aware of the medications taken by the individual, possible drug interactions, and side effects. For example, dizziness is a side effect of many drugs. A PT or PTA who is working with someone on getting out of bed,

13

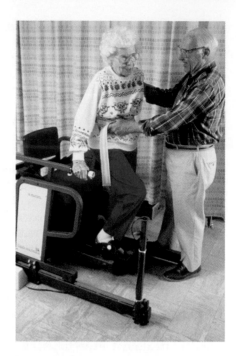

Figure 13-10 ■ Resistive exercises to increase strength, in this case in the hip and knee musculature, are effective in the older person. (Courtesy Bruce Wang.)

up from the floor, or performing more advanced balance activities must be alert to any signs of dizziness. If the person is taking medication that increases dizziness, the PT or PTA must take greater safety precautions during these activities.

When providing services to an older person, the PT considers the need for environmental modification and adaptive equipment. Simple changes in the environment (improved lighting, removal of throw rugs, or furniture rearrangement) make the individual safer, allow the patient to function optimally in the living environment, and may improve the person's quality of life. Appropriate adaptive equipment (a grab bar in the shower or a reacher) and training in its use enable the older person to be more independent. Training in adaptive equipment use should include demonstration and repeated opportunities to practice.

An important component of any physical therapy plan of care is to provide the patient/client with information about how to maintain or improve his or her health and prevent further problems that could limit physical function. Planning a health care team event (such as a "wellness fair") with a local senior center—assessing for fall risk, providing blood pressure screening, offering nutritional information, and teaching basic exercise (regardless of age)—provides an opportunity for PTs and PTAs to target a larger audience with wellness education. Strategies to improve balance or to modify the home environment to be safer are examples of teaching to prevent falls and fractures. Figure 13-11 is an example of a couple that chose to use the stairs as part of their wellness program.

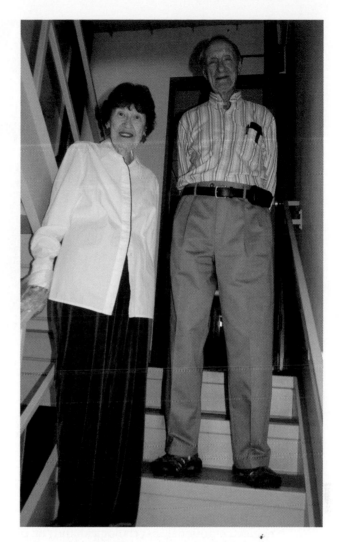

Figure 13-11 ■ Using stairs instead of the elevator is a much healthier choice. (Courtesy Terri Hoppenrath.)

A final consideration in determining the most appropriate intervention for an older person relates to the setting. Inpatient settings have multiple pieces of equipment available for use in improving strength and mobility or decreasing pain. The PT may have to be creative, however, to ensure that enhanced performance on objective tests in this setting will translate into improvement in daily function in the home environment. Physical therapy provided in the home setting provides the opposite challenge. There will be many opportunities in a home to improve functional skills, but it may be difficult for the PT or PTA to increase strength (owing to limited equipment) or endurance (owing to limited space). The therapist must keep these advantages and limitations in mind when planning programs for intervention. In Figure 13-12 parallel bars are used to assist

13

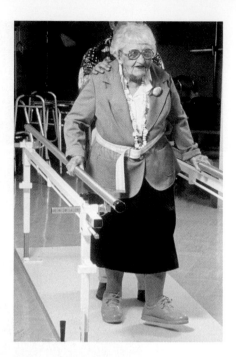

Figure 13-12 ■ Gait training is enhanced by using parallel bars in a clinical setting. (Courtesy Bruce Wang.)

a woman in gait training. When she is ready to return to a home environment, another device, such as a walker, may be necessary to increase the distance she is able to walk.

ETHICAL CONSIDERATIONS

The PT or PTA may be in a position to recognize elder abuse. Identified risk factors include age, cognitive impairment/dementia, low functional level, socioeconomic status, race, and caregiver stress.[56,57] Abuse can be seen in forms of neglect; emotional, psychological and/or physical abuse; or financial exploitation.[58] Abuse is most common in private homes, SNF, and LTC. A 2010 study indicated that 47% of persons with dementia had been mistreated.[59] Laws vary state by state; however, any suspected abuse must be reported. Abusers are often family members; therefore, referrals should be made to an outside agency such as Adult Protective Services or a social worker.[59,60]

SUMMARY

As the Baby Boomers age, the proportion of the U.S. population over 65 years of age, and especially over 85, will continue to grow. PTs and PTAs serve older adults in every type of setting, not solely in LTC facilities. Certainly, some therapists will choose to specialize in working with people over 65 years old, but almost all therapists and assistants will have contact with patients in this age group at some point. To provide high-quality services to the older population, therapists should recognize the similarities and differences between the older person and any other individual in need of physical therapy. PTs should be ready to modify interventions as needed to address documented normal and pathological age-related changes. PTs and PTAs should educate the older person who requires services and all significant others in methods that will enhance the person's function. Finally, the therapist must be able to communicate and cooperate with older individuals, their families, and team members to develop a meaningful and successful plan for intervention.

CASE STUDY

CASE STUDY ONE

This example is provided with the intent of demonstrating the complex medical, cognitive, psychosocial, and ethical issues facing the health care practitioner who works with older people and their families.

Margaret Sanford is an 81-year-old woman who has been hospitalized for 4 days after a total hip replacement. Her medical history includes RA, osteoporosis, and hypertension. She is also hearing impaired. The arthritis causes almost constant pain in her hips, knees, and hands. The surgery was performed to relieve pain in her right hip, which was the side with more severe pain. Mrs. Sanford lives alone in the home where she has resided for 40 years. Payment on her home mortgage was completed 6 years ago. Her husband is deceased, her son lives 250 miles away, and her daughter lives with her family about 10 miles away. Mrs. Sanford has a limited income (Social Security), and her medical coverage is Medicare.

Mrs. Sanford is considered medically ready for discharge from the hospital. She has been receiving physical therapy once a day, consisting of (1) range of motion and strengthening exercises in all extremities, focusing on hip and knee musculature; (2) bed mobility (teaching supine to sit following hip precautions); (3) transfer training (instructing in sit to stand and toilet transfers); and (4) gait training with a walker. The PT made a home visit and noted that (1) there are four steps into the house; (2) her bedroom is upstairs (13 steps with one railing); (3) there are many throw rugs on the hardwood floors; (4) there are bathrooms on both floors with bathtub/shower; and (5) the laundry facilities are in the basement.

Mrs. Sanford wants to go home as soon as possible. She has been very lonely for her neighbors while in the hospital. She sometimes awakes at night disoriented and confused about where she is. Her daughter, who works full time, is concerned about her mother's safety at home and is not sure whether her mother is ready to go home alone. She has also stated that she wants to be sure her mother has every opportunity for full rehabilitation and is advocating for daily physical therapy.

The team, including Mrs. Sanford and her daughter, meets to discuss a discharge plan. A short-term placement is proposed. In this plan, Mrs. Sanford would be discharged to an SNF where daily physical therapy could be provided. Mrs. Sanford is opposed to that move, although her daughter tries to convince her that it is a good proposal. The social worker suggests discharge to home and asks the team what other support services are necessary to ensure her success at home. The PT indicates that Mrs. Sanford should learn to navigate stairs safely with a cane, obtain adaptive equipment such as a bathing chair and a raised toilet seat, and modify the home environment for safety. Physical therapy (and occupational therapy) services could be provided two or three times weekly through a

13

home health care agency. The social worker suggests that a home health aide would be appropriate to assist Mrs. Sanford with personal care, housework, and laundry.

Should Mrs. Sanford be coerced into going to the SNF as the team feels this is the best/safest placement? Who should make the final decision? *The patient's goals must always be considered. The interdisciplinary team should weigh all viewpoints. Forcing any decision is not advisable. Education is the key! The team should come to consensus by reflecting on physical and psychosocial aspects of their final decision.*

What other options can you come up with that may help Mrs. Sanford go home? *Temporarily moving a bed to the first floor would initially avoid excessive stair climbing. The home PT would make this a therapy goal. An emergency call button can be worn around the neck when Mrs. Sanford is alone. Mrs. Sanford's daughter can speak with neighbors about making short visits with her mom throughout the day.*

Acknowledgment

The author wishes to acknowledge the staff and members of The Friendly Home and the clients, staff, and faculty at Nazareth College Physical Therapy Clinic, both of Rochester, New York, for their assistance.

REFERENCES

1. State and County Quick Facts. U.S. Census Bureau. http://quickfacts.census.gov/qfd/states/00000.html. Accessed September 2, 2014.
2. The Older Population in the United States: 2010–2050, U.S. Census Bureau. www.census.gov/prod/2010pubs/p25-1138.pdf. Accessed September 2, 2014.
3. Xu JQ, Kochanek KD, Murphy SL, Arias E. Mortality in the United States, 2012. NCHS data brief, no 168. Hyattsville, MD, National Center for Health Statistics. 2014.
4. *Health United States: with Health and Aging Chartbook,* Hyattsville, MD, 1999, National Center for Health Statistics.
5. Essential Competencies. www.geriatricspt.org/pdfs/Section-On-Geriatrics-Essential-Competencies-2011.pdf. Accessed September 15, 2014.
6. *Guide to Physical Therapist Practice 3.0.* American Physical Therapy Association. http://guidetoptpractice.apta.org/. Accessed September 15, 2014.
7. Fiatarone MA, Marks EC, Ryan ND, et al.: High intensity strength training on nonagenerians: effects on skeletal muscle, *JAMA* 263:3029–3034, 1990.
8. Doherty TJ, Vandervoort AA, Taylor AW, et al.: Effects of motor unit losses on strength in older men and women, *J Appl Physiol* 74(2):868–881, 1993.
9. Mosekilde L: Normal age-related changes in bone mass, structure, and strength consequences of the remodeling process, *Dan Med Bull* 40(1):65–83, 1993.
10. Christensen R, Astrup A, Bliddal H: Weight loss: the treatment of choice for knee osteoarthritis? A randomized trial, *Osteoarthr Cartil* 13:20–27, 2005.
11. Lewis CB, Bottomly JM: *Geriatric Rehabilitation: A Clinical Approach,* ed 3, Upper Saddle River, NJ, 2008, Pearson Prentice Hall.
12. Fear of Falling in Age-related Macular Degeneration. http://www.biomedcentral.com/1471-2415/14/10. Accessed September 17, 2014.
13. Older Persons Health, CDC. http://www.cdc.gov/nchs/fastats/older-american-health.htm. Accessed October 7, 2014.
14. High Blood Pressure Facts, CDC. http://www.cdc.gov/bloodpressure/facts.htm. Accessed September 19, 2014.
15. Older Persons Health: Hypertension, CDC. http://www.cdc.gov/nchs/fastats/older-american-health.htm. Accessed September 17, 2014.
16. Schneider EL, Rowe JW, editors: *Handbook of the Biology of Aging,* New York, 1990, Academic Press.

17. Tromp AM, Pluijm SMF, Smit JH, et al.: Fall-risk screening test: a prospective study on predictors for falls in community-dwelling elderly, *J Clin Epidemiol* 54:837–844, 2001.
18. Tinetti ME: Prevention of falls and fall injuries in elderly persons: a research agenda, *Prev Med* 23:756–762, 1994.
19. Alzheimer's Disease, CDC. http://www.cdc.gov/aging/aginginfo/alzheimers.htm. Accessed September 22, 2014.
20. Hebert LE, Weuve J, Scherr PA, et al.: Alzheimer disease in the United States (2010–2050) estimated using the 2010 census, *Neurology* 80:1778–1783, 2013.
21. Salthouse TA: Age related changes in basic cognitive processes. In Storundt M, VandeBos G, editors: *The Adult Years: Continuity and Change*, Washington, DC, 1989, American Psychiatric Association.
22. Norris MP, West RL: Activity memory and aging: the role of motor retrieval and strategic processing, *Psychol Aging* 8(1):81–86, 1993.
23. LGBT Older Adults: Facts at a Glance. http://issuu.com/lgbtagingcenter/docs/lgbtolderadultsfactsataglance?e=2766558/5287055#search. Accessed September 22, 2014.
24. Bruce ML, McNamara R: Psychiatric status among the homebound elderly: an epidemiological perspective, *J Am Geriatr Soc* 40:561–566, 1992.
25. Miller R, Zhang Y, Silliman RA, et al.: Effect of medical conditions on improvement in self-reported and observed functional performance of elders, *J Am Geriatr Soc* 52(2):217–223, 2004.
26. Barbour KE, Helmick CG, Theis KA, et al.: Prevalence of doctor-diagnosed arthritis and arthritis-attributable activity limitation-United States, 2010–2012, *MMWR* 6:869–873, 2013.
27. Centers for Disease Control and Prevention: Prevalence of Arthritis—United States, 1997, *MMWR Morb Mortal Wkly Rep* 50:334–336, 2001.
28. Metsios GS, Stavropoulos-Kalinoglou A, Veldhuijzen van Zanten JJCS, et al.: Rheumatoid arthritis, cardiovascular disease and physical exercise: a systematic review, *Rheumatology* 47:239–248, 2008.
29. America's Bone Health: The State of Osteoporosis and Low Bone Mass. National Osteoporosis Foundation. www.nof.org/advocacy/prevalence/. Accessed September 29, 2014.
30. Kanis JA, Melton LJ III, Christiansen C, et al.: The diagnosis of osteoporosis, *J Bone Miner Res* 9:1137–1141, 1994.
31. Meier D, Luckey M, Wallenstein S, et al.: Racial differences in pre- and postmenopausal bone homeostasis: association with bone density, *J Bone Miner Res* 7:1181–1189, 1992.
32. Palombara KM, Black JD, Buchbinder R, et al.: Effectiveness of exercise for managing osteoporosis in women postmenopause, *Phys Ther* 93:1021–1025, 2013.
33. Home and Recreational Safety, CDC. http://www.cdc.gov/homeandrecreationalsafety/falls/adulthipfx.html. Accessed September 29, 2014.
34. Injury Prevention and Control, CDC. http://www.cdc.gov/HomeandRecreationalSafety/falls/data/cost-estimates.html. Accessed September 29, 2014.
35. Jette AM, Harris BA, Cleary PD, et al.: Functional recovery after hip fracture, *Arch Phys Med Rehabil* 68:735–740, 1987.
36. Panula J, Pihlajamäki H, Mattila VM, et al.: Mortality and cause of death in hip fracture patients aged 65 or older: a population-based study, *BMC Musculoskelet Disord* 12:105, 2011.
37. STEADI Tool Kit, CDC. http://www.cdc.gov/homeandrecreationalsafety/Falls/steadi/about.html. Accessed September 29, 2014.
38. National Diabetes Statistics Report, 2014. http://www.cdc.gov/diabetes/pubs/statsreport14/national-diabetes-report-web.pdf. Accessed September 30, 2014.
39. Tuttle LJ, Sinacore DR, Cade WT, et al.: Lower physical activity is associated with higher intermuscular adipose tissue in people with type 2 diabetes and peripheral neuropathy, *Phys Ther* 91:923–930, 2011.
40. Kruse RL, Lemaster JW, Madsen RW: Fall and balance outcomes after an intervention to promote leg strength, balance, and walking in people with diabetic peripheral neuropathy: "feet first" randomized controlled trial, *Phys Ther* 90:1568–1579, 2010.
41. Springer BA, Marin R, Cyhan T, et al.: Normative values for the unipedal stance test with eyes open and closed, *J Geriatr Phys Ther* 30:8–15, 2007.
42. Duncan PW, Weiner DK, Chandler J, et al.: Clinical measure of balance, *J Gerontol* 45(6):M192–M197, 1990.

13

43. Podsiadlo D, Richardson S: The Timed "Up & Go": a test of basic functional mobility for frail elderly persons, *J Am Geriatr Soc* 39:142–148, 1991.
44. Berg KO, Wood-Dauphinee SL, Williams JI, et al.: Measuring balance in the elderly: validation of an instrument, *Can J Public Health* 83(Suppl 2):S7–S11, 1992.
45. Tinnetti M: Performance oriented assessment of mobility problems in elderly patients, *J Am Geriatr Soc* 34(2):119–126, 1986.
46. Shumway-Cook A, Woolacott MH: *Motor Control: Theory and Practical Applications*, Baltimore, 1995, Williams and Wilkins.
47. Wolfson L, Whipple R, Amerman P, et al.: Gait assessment in the elderly: a gait abnormality rating scale and its relation to falls, *J Gerontol* 45(1):M12–M19, 1990.
48. Tinetti ME, Richman D, Powell L: Falls efficacy as a measure of fear of falling, *J Gerontol* 45(6):P239–P243, 1990.
49. Scott J, Huskisson EC: Graphic representation of pain, *Pain* 2:175–184, 1976.
50. Jette AM, Davies AR, Cleary PD, et al.: The functional status questionnaire, *J Gen Intern Med* 1:143–149, 1986.
51. Jette AM: The functional status index: reliability and validity of a self-report functional disability measure, *J Rheumatol* 14:15–19, 1987.
52. Reuben DB, Sui AL: An objective measure of physical function of elderly outpatients: the Physical Performance Test, *J Am Geriatr Soc* 38:1105–1112, 1990.
53. SLUMS Examination. http://aging.slu.edu/index.php?page=saint-louis-university-mental-status-slums-exam. Accessed October 7, 2014.
54. Physical Therapy for Older Adults, APTA HOD. http://www.apta.org/uploadedFiles/APTAorg/About_Us/Policies/HOD/Practice/OlderAdults.pdf. Accessed October 7, 2014.
55. Academy of Geriatric Physical Therapy. https://www.geriatricspt.org/. Accessed October 7, 2014.
56. Marshall CE, Benton D, Brazier JM: Elder abuse. Using clinical tools to identify clues of mistreatment, *Geriatrics* 55:42–53, 2000.
57. Wiglesworth A, Mosqueda L, Mulnard R, et al.: Screening for abuse and neglect of people with dementia, *J Am Geriatr Soc* 58:493–500, 2010.
58. Collins KA, Bennett AT, Hanzlick R: Elder abuse and neglect. Autopsy committee of the college of American pathologists, *Arch Intern Med* 160:1567–1568, 2000.
59. National Center on Elder Abuse. http://www.ncea.aoa.gov/Library/Data/#abuser. Accessed October 7, 2014.
60. Elder Abuse State Laws. http://www.ncea.aoa.gov/Library/Policy/Law/State/index.aspx. Accessed October 7, 2014.

Glossary

Abuse Situations when a payment is made for services or items when there is no legal entitlement or right to that payment and when health care providers have not knowingly and/or intentionally misrepresented facts to obtain payment.

Acceptable standard of care Standards established by the APTA for the delivery of physical therapy services.

Access Ability for an individual to obtain health care services when needed.

Accessory motion Ability of the joint surfaces to glide, roll, and spin on one another.

Accountable Care Organizations (ACOs) Groups formed voluntarily by hospitals, doctors, and health care providers, including physical therapists and possibly physical therapist assistants, to provide coordinated high quality care to their Medicare patients. The purpose of coordinated care is to ensure that patients receive the right care at the right time, while preventing medical errors and avoiding unnecessary duplication of services.

Active assisted range of motion Joint movement in which the patient may be assisted either manually or mechanically through an arc of movement.

Active member Former membership category in the APTA for the physical therapist.

Active range of motion (AROM) Ability of the patient to voluntarily move a limb through an arc of movement.

Active resisted exercise Joint movement in which an external force resists the movement.

Activities of daily living (ADLs) Activities in which individuals participate daily to meet their basic needs. Examples include bathing, dressing, using the toilet, and eating.

Adaptive equipment Pieces of equipment that allow individuals to perform functional tasks with increased ease or independence.

Advisory Panel of Physical Therapist Assistants   Unit within the APTA consisting of five PTA members who provide advice and input to the APTA Board of Directors on matters that pertain to the PTAs.

Aerobic training   Exercise program that uses oxygen as the major energy source.

Affective domain   The domain of learning that deals with attitudes, values, and character development and that influences all other professional skills.

Affiliate assembly   Past component of the APTA that represented and was composed of physical therapist assistants; precursor to the National Assembly.

Affiliate member   Former membership category in the APTA for the physical therapist assistant.

Affiliate Special Interest Group   Past component of the APTA that served the interests of the physical therapist assistant; precursor to the Affiliate Assembly.

Affordable Care Act (ACA)   Health reform legislation passed by the 111th Congress and signed into law by President Barack Obama in March 2010. It is informally referred to as *Obamacare* and formally known as the Patient Protection and Affordable Care Act (PPACA). This legislation includes the following provisions: coverage extended to millions of uninsured Americans, measures implemented to lower health care costs and improve system efficiency, and practices eliminated that include the denial of coverage due to preexisting conditions.

American Board of Physical Therapy Residency and Fellowship Education (ABPTRFE)   Organization that accredits postprofessional residency and fellowship programs in physical therapy.

American Board of Physical Therapy Specialties (ABPTS)   Unit created by the House of Delegates to provide a formal mechanism for recognizing physical therapists with advanced knowledge, skills, and experience in a special area of practice.

American Council of Academic Physical Therapy (ACAPT)   A component of the APTA that exists to promote the highest standards of excellence in physical therapist education. Replaced the preexisting Academic Administrators Special Interest Group of the Education Section.

American Physical Therapy Association (APTA)   National organization that represents and promotes the profession of physical therapy.

American Physiotherapy Association (APA)   Organization (formerly called the *American Women's Physical Therapeutic Association*) responsible for maintaining high standards and educational programs for physiotherapists; precursor to APTA.

American Women's Physical Therapeutic Association   First national organization representing "physical therapeutics." Established in 1921 to maintain high standards and provide a mechanism to share information.

Americans with Disabilities Act (ADA)   Federal law that prohibits discrimination against persons with disabilities and requires government offices and private businesses to be accessible to persons with disabilities.

Amyotrophic lateral sclerosis (ALS)   Also known as *Lou Gehrig's disease*; rapidly progressive neurologic disorder associated with a degeneration of the motor nerve cells.

Anencephaly   A form of neural tube defect that results from a lack of the neural tube closure at the base of the brain. It is not compatible with life and results in fetal death or death shortly after delivery.

Angina   Condition in which chest pain occurs from ischemia.

Angiography   Technique in which radiopaque material is injected into the blood vessels to better visualize and identify problems such as occlusion (blockage) of blood vessels, aneurysms, and vascular malformations.

Aquatic physical therapy Therapeutic use of water for rehabilitation or prevention of injury.

Arterial insufficiency Deficiency or occlusion of blood flow through an artery.

Arteriosclerosis Hardening of the arteries.

Assembly Component of APTA whose purpose is to provide a means by which members of the same class may meet, confer, and promote the interest of the respective membership class.

Assistive device Device that provides individuals with assistance to perform tasks or during periods of mobility. Examples include canes, walkers, and adapted keyboards.

Autism A neural developmental disorder characterized by impairments in social interaction, communication skills, and repetitive behaviors.

Autonomous practice Services provided by physical therapists using independent, professional judgment within their scope of practice.

B

Balance Ability to maintain the body's center of gravity over the base of support.

Balanced Budget Act of 1997 (BBA) Federal legislation, passed by Congress and signed by President Clinton, that cut health care expenditures for Medicare and other government-sponsored programs to achieve a balanced budget.

Bariatrics Area of health care that deals with the origin, prevention, and treatment of obesity.

Beginning professional behaviors Professional behaviors that develop during the didactic (academic) portion of the physical therapy curriculum.

Beneficiary Individual who is covered by a health insurance policy; as a result of this coverage, the person can receive health care benefits.

Benign paroxysmal positional vertigo (BPPV) Refers to a non-life threatening disorder affecting the vestibular system which occurs suddenly and is associated with specific head positions; it causes symptoms of vertigo.

Blood gas analysis Assessment of blood (usually arterial) to determine the concentrations of oxygen and carbon dioxide.

Board of Directors (BOD) APTA unit consisting of six APTA officers and nine directors whose duty is to carry out the mandates and policies established by the House of Delegates.

Bradykinesia Slow of movement.

Bundled payment models Connect payments for multiple services received by Medicare beneficiaries during an episode of care. In contrast to separate payments to providers for each of the individual services they provide to beneficiaries for a single illness or course of treatment, which rewards the quantity of services offered by providers rather than the quality of care provided, bundled payments reward providers for coordinating care, preventing complications and errors, and reducing unnecessary or duplicative tests and treatments.

Bursitis Inflammation of bursae, fluid-filled sacs located throughout the body, which decrease the friction between two structures.

C

Capitation Method of payment (reimbursement) in some health maintenance organizations (HMOs). The HMO pays the health care provider a fixed dollar amount per member per month (PMPM) in advance (before services are delivered).

Cardiac catheterization   Passage of a catheter (a flexible tube) into an artery in the arm or leg, then along the artery to reach the heart and measure pressure, inject dye, or take a tissue sample.

Cardiac muscle dysfunction   Various pathologic conditions associated with heart failure.

Cardiac pacemaker   Electronic device that produces a pulse to control heart depolarization.

Career ladder   Employer's structure, creating levels within a specific field or position to enable promotion of employees in that category.

Case management   Process used to monitor and coordinate treatment delivered to patients, usually those requiring costly and extensive services.

Case-mix   Method used to measure the mix of cases (patients) being treated by a health care provider and the scope of resources needed to serve this combination of patients.

Centers for Medicare and Medicaid Services (CMS)   Government agency within the Department of Health and Human Services responsible for directing the Medicare and Medicaid programs.

Cerebral palsy (CP)   Group of conditions caused by a nonprogressive lesion on the brain. Most often CP has its origin during gestation (before birth), at birth, or immediately after birth and is caused by an interruption of oxygen to the brain of the fetus or newborn.

Certification   Process by which a state legally regulates the use of a professional title without creating a separate scope of practice. State law will not permit use of the title unless state standards are met. This differs from the private certification offered by private organizations for meeting the standards of that organization.

Chapter   Organizational unit of APTA that is defined by specific legally constituted boundaries such as a state, territory, or commonwealth of the United States or the District of Columbia. Membership is automatic and is based on location of residence or employment, education, or greatest active participation.

Children's Health Insurance Program (CHIP)   Program under the Centers for Medicare and Medicaid Services administered by the states for uninsured children. Matching funds are provided by the federal government to help states expand health care coverage.

Children's Health Insurance Program Reauthorization Act (CHIPRA)   This Act expands and extends the Children's Health Insurance Program by adding $33 billion in federal funds through 2013.

Chronic inflammation   Low-grade, protracted inflammatory process.

Chronic obstructive pulmonary disease (COPD)   Group of disorders that produce certain specific physical symptoms, including chronic productive cough, excessive mucus production, changes in the sound produced when air passes through the bronchial tubes, and shortness of breath (dyspnea).

Civil law   Law of a jurisdiction concerned with private rights and remedies; the administration of justice involving the violation of private duties owed by individuals.

Claims   Bills submitted by health care providers to health insurance and managed care companies for payment (reimbursement). Sometimes these claims are denied (not paid).

Client   Individual who seeks the services of a physical therapist to maintain health, or a business that hires a physical therapist as a consultant.

Clinical practice guidelines   Systematically developed evidence-based statements designed to help the clinician manage specific health conditions.

Clinical problem solving   Area of responsibility of the PTA that includes ability to adjust, modify, or discontinue an intervention within the plan of care established by the PT.

Closed kinetic chain exercise   Exercise incorporating several muscle groups through the use of several joints with the end segment fixed.

Clubfoot   Disorder in which the foot is turned inward and slanted upward.

Code of ethics   Principles set forth for the physical therapy profession by APTA for maintaining and promoting ethical practice.

Co-insurance   Cost-sharing obligation required by a health insurance policy. The subscriber assumes a percentage of the costs incurred.

Collaborative care models   Evidence-based approaches for integrating health services that can be implemented within a primary care-based Medicaid health home model, among other settings. Collaborative care includes care coordination and care management, ongoing and proactive monitoring and treatment using validated clinical rating scales, and regular consultation for patients or clients who do not show clinical improvement.

Collagen   Supportive, strong, and fibrous connective tissue protein that is found in the dermis, tendon, cartilage, fascia, ligament, and bone.

Combined Sections Meeting (CSM)   Annual meeting (February) of APTA sections' members to provide an opportunity for sharing information.

Commission on Accreditation in Physical Therapy Education (CAPTE)   Unit responsible for evaluating and accrediting professional (entry level) physical therapist and physical therapist assistant education programs.

Common law   Law created by court decision rather than by legislative action.

Components   Organizational units within APTA currently limited to chapters, sections, and assemblies as established by APTA bylaws.

Computed (axial) tomography (CAT or CT)   Computer synthesis of X-rays transmitted through a specific plane of the body.

Conducting airways   Passageways and tubes that allow air to pass into or out of the lungs.

Congestive heart failure (CHF)   Condition in which the heart muscle is compromised to the point that it cannot move blood volume effectively.

Constraint-induced movement therapy   A training technique involving intense practice and use of the involved upper extremity while limiting use of the lesser involved arm.

Consumer-driven health plans   Range of health insurance plans designed to allow different degrees of employer and employee responsibility. A common design allows for catastrophic (high severity, low incidence, high deductible) coverage combined with a health care spending account.

Contract   Agreement between two or more persons that creates a legal obligation to do, or not do, a particular thing.

Copayment   Fixed amount of money stipulated in the health insurance plan paid to the health care provider by a beneficiary at the time of service.

Core values   Seven characteristics that define and describe professionalism in physical therapy: accountability, altruism, compassion and caring, integrity, professional duty, and social responsibility.

Coronary artery bypass grafting (CABG)   Grafting (attaching) a small artery or a leg vein to a point beyond the blockage or plaque. This bypasses the blockage, reestablishing blood flow to the heart.

Coronary heart disease (CHD)   Arteriosclerosis, or a hardening of the arteries, affecting the coronary vessels.

Covered services   Services covered by a health insurance plan.

Criminal law   Administration of justice, through the enforcement of the criminal code of a state or of the United States; involves violations of duties owed to society at large.

Cryotherapy   Application of cold agents to cause decreases in blood flow and metabolism, which result in a decrease in swelling and pain.

Cultural continuum   Theoretical model that describes six stages of culturally related behaviors, including cultural destructiveness, incapacity, blindness, pre-competency, competency, and proficiency.

Culture of medicine   Beliefs, attitudes, and behaviors unique to the practice of medicine. Biomedical Western medicine operates primarily through low-context assumptions. These assumptions may conflict with those of practitioners, patients, and families who operate from more high-context assumptions.

Current procedural terminology (CPT) codes   Standardized list of five-digit codes assigned to medical services and procedures.

Cystic fibrosis (CF)   Most common inherited chronic pulmonary disease among white children, characterized by the production of thick mucus with progressive lung damage.

D

Deductible   Amount of money that must be paid by the insured before a health insurer will assume any liability for covered services.

Dermatitis   Inflammation of the skin indicated by any one or all of the following: redness, rash, itching, irritation, and possible skin lesions.

Dermis   Portion of the skin directly under the dermis; it is made up of fibrous connective tissue and supports sweat glands, sebaceous glands, nerves and nerve endings, blood and lymph vessels, hair follicles, and their allied smooth muscle.

Developing professional behaviors   Professional behaviors that develop during the first half of each clinical internship of an education program.

Developmental coordination disorder (DCD)   Motor condition in children encompassing a wide range of dysfunctions, including gross or fine motor coordination problems such as awkward running, frequent falling, slow reaction times, immature balance reactions, poor handwriting, and difficulty with activities of daily living such as dressing.

Developmental delay   Failure to attain predictable movement patterns or behaviors associated with children of a similar chronologic age.

Developmental dysplasia of the hip (DDH)   Dislocation resulting from the abnormal development of some of the structures surrounding the hip joint, allowing the head of the femur to move in and out of the hip socket. The cause is unknown.

Developmental milestone   Movement pattern that appears at a certain stage of growth and development.

Diagnosis   Final interpretation of findings based on examinations.

Diagnostic related groups (DRGs)   Classification scheme developed by the federal government as a means to establish uniform reimbursement for a variety of diagnostic conditions.

Direct access   Availability of the physical therapist to anyone seeking physical therapy services without stipulation of a referral by another health care provider.

Direct supervision Presence on-site and immediate availability of a PT when supervising a PTA.

Disablement model Conceptual approach to health care based on the functional abilities of the patient/client that result from a medical condition. As applied to physical therapy, includes impairment, functional limitation, and disability.

Disablement process Examination process that focuses on the individual's impairments, functional limitations, disability, and resultant restrictions in activities.

District Most local organizational unit in the structure of APTA. Membership is automatic and may be based on location of residence or employment, as provided in the bylaws of APTA.

Down syndrome Congenital developmental disability caused by a defect of chromosome 21; sometimes called *trisomy 21*. Characterized by low muscle tone, a flat facial profile, upwardly slanted eyes, short stature, varying levels of intellectual ability, slowed growth and development, a small nose with a low nasal bridge, and congenital heart disease.

Duchenne muscular dystrophy (DMD) Progressive pelvic muscle weakness and wasting in the male child, combined with enlarged, yet weak, thigh muscles and tight heel cords.

Durable medical equipment Medical equipment prescribed by a medical provider for a patient's extended use.

Dynamic balance Balance maintained with the body in motion.

Dynamical systems theory Treatment approach in children that incorporates all of the body's systems with the environment to facilitate or inhibit movements. It emphasizes the process of moving rather than the product of a movement.

Dysfunction Any functional disability.

Dyspnea Shortness of breath.

E

Echocardiography Technique using high-frequency ultrasound to assess the size of the heart chambers, the thickness of the chamber walls, and the motion of the chamber walls and heart valves.

Eclectic approach Combination of therapeutic approaches used by the physical therapist and thought to be useful for treatment of a given client.

Electrical stimulation Application of electricity at specified locations to stimulate nerves, muscles, and other soft tissues to reduce pain and swelling, to increase strength and range of motion, and to facilitate wound healing.

Electrocardiogram (ECG) Readout produced by placing electrodes on the anterior chest wall to record depolarization or contraction of the heart muscle; assesses the heart's rate and rhythm.

Electroencephalography (EEG) Technique for recording the electrical potential or activity in the brain by placing electrodes on the scalp.

Electromyography (EMG) Technique for recording the electrical activity in the muscle during a state of rest and during voluntary contraction.

Electronic health record Health-related information on an individual that conforms to national standards and is entered and stored electronically. It can be accessed by different health care organizations.

Episode of care Care provided for a specific condition over a period of time.

Embolus Clot formed by a substance detached from elsewhere.

Employer-sponsored health insurance Health insurance offered to employees by employers; offered as a benefit of employment.

Enablement process   Examination process that focuses on the individual's structural body and concurrent abilities while addressing age-appropriate movement patterns and activities.

Entitlement   Right or privilege.

Entry level professional behaviors   Professional behaviors that develop during the second half of each clinical internship of an education program.

Epidermis   Outer layer of the skin.

Essential Health Benefit (EHB)   Health care service categories that must be covered by certain health insurance plans starting in 2014. The Affordable Care Act ensures that health plans, offered both inside and outside of the Health Insurance Marketplace and in both the individual and small group markets, offer this comprehensive package of services and items (essential health benefits) within *at least* the following 10 categories: ambulatory services, emergency services, hospitalization, rehabilitative and habilitative services and devices, preventive and wellness services, chronic disease management, maternity and newborn care, mental health, substance abuse, and behavioral health services, prescription drugs, laboratory services, and pediatric services (including oral and vision care).

Evaluation   Judgment based on an examination.

Evidence-based practice   Interventions used in physical therapy, based on research that demonstrates the reliability and validity of the procedures.

Exacerbation   Refers to a relapse or flare-up of a disease such as Multiple Sclerosis; this causes new symptoms or the worsening of old symptoms.

Examination   Process of gathering information about the past and current status of the patient/client.

Exercise stress testing   Noninvasive method of determining how the cardiovascular and pulmonary systems respond to controlled increases in activity; most frequently used to diagnose or assess suspected or established cardiovascular disease.

Expiration   Breathing out.

Expressive aphasia   Impaired ability to express oneself.

Extrinsic factors   Factors outside of the individual.

F

Family assessment   Family interview, survey, or discussion used to obtain the family's insights regarding a patient, especially a child; includes family history, relationships, concerns, needs, and resources.

Federalism   The division of governmental authority between the federal and state levels of government.

Federation of State Boards of Physical Therapy (FSBPT)   National organization through which member state boards work together to promote and protect the health, welfare, and safety of the American public by identifying and promoting desirable and reasonable uniformity in physical therapy regulatory standards and practices.

Fee-for-service (FFS)   A method of health care reimbursement in which a health care provider bills the health insurer a fee for each service provided.

Fee schedule   A listing of health care services in which a specific amount of money is associated with each service.

Fetal alcohol syndrome (FAS)   Most severe condition in a continuum of alcohol-induced disabilities related to high levels of maternal alcohol consumption during pregnancy.

FITT principle of exercise prescription   Exercise prescription used to establish guidelines for exercise. Frequency describes how often to exercise. Intensity describes how hard to exercise. Time describes the duration of exercise. Type describes the mode or type of exercise.

Flexibility   Ability to move a limb segment through a range of motion.

Flexibility exercise   Exercise performed over time, using stress, to change the length and elasticity of soft tissue such as muscle; usually performed for postural or ROM enhancement.

Fluidotherapy   Use of a self-contained unit filled with sawdust-type particles heated to the desired temperature and circulated by air pressure around the involved body part.

Foundation for physical therapy   Organization, separate from APTA, that promotes and provides financial support for scientific research, clinical research, and health services research in physical therapy.

Fracture   Break in a bone.

Functional capacity evaluation   Examination of a worker's physical abilities to perform required tasks.

Functional exercise   Exercise that mimics functional movements and activities. Functional movements incorporate strength, flexibility, balance, and coordination.

Functional limitation   Decreased ability of a person to perform a task, without regard to the context or environment.

Functional reach test   Specific balance test that can predict the likelihood of falling.

G

Gatekeeper   Health care provider who provides the consumer with access to the health care system. Historically, this has been the primary care physician.

General supervision   Level of supervision in which the PT is not required to be on site when supervising a PTA. Availability must be at least by telecommunications.

Goal-directed movement approach   Treatment approach that emphasizes the importance of both task and environmental features as a primary impetus for movement.

Goals   Measurable, functional objectives that are linked to a problem identified in a patient evaluation.

Goniometer   Instrument used to measure and document ROM.

Goniometry   Methods to measure and document ROM.

Ground substance   Supportive, amorphous gel-like substance secreted by fibroblasts; fills space between connective tissue fibers and cells.

Guide to Physical Therapist Practice 3.0   Extensive description of the roles and scope of practice of a physical therapist. Describes tests and measures and interventions for patients/clients for musculoskeletal, neuromuscular, cardiovascular/pulmonary, and integumentary conditions.

Guillain-Barré syndrome (GBS)   An acquired neuromuscular condition resulting from the inflammation of a peripheral nerve. Often follows a viral infection and presents with symmetric, progressive weakness, usually beginning in the lower extremities.

H

Habilitation service   Health care services that help individuals retain, maintain, learn/relearn, or improve skills and functioning for daily living. Services may include physical therapy, occupational therapy, speech-language pathology, and other services for people with disabilities in a variety of inpatient and/or outpatient settings.

Hand-off communication   Procedures to maintain effective communication among caregivers to ensure accurate description and coordination of services.

Haptics   The use of touch in communication between people. The use of touch varies depending on cultural norms.

Health insurance   Financial protection against health care costs arising from disease or injury.

Health Insurance Marketplace   Resource available for individuals, families, and small businesses to help them learn about health insurance options; compare health insurance plans based on costs, benefits, and other features; and then, choose and finally enroll in a plan. The Marketplace also provides information on programs that help individuals with low to moderate income and resources pay for coverage as well as information about other programs, including Medicaid and the Children's Health Insurance Program (CHIP).

Health Insurance Portability and Accountability Act (HIPAA)   Wide-ranging federal law that includes sections on access to and storage of confidential patient information, ability to maintain health insurance coverage when changing jobs, and strengthening federal efforts to combat fraud.

Health maintenance organization (HMO)   Prepaid health insurance that may provide all health care services needed within one facility.

Heart failure   Decrease in the pumping capability of the heart muscle.

Hemiparesis   Weakness or partial paralysis affecting one side of the body.

High-context assumptions   Assumptions found in cultures in which the group is more important than the individual. Communication is indirect; meaning is based on implicit cues. Nonverbal aspects such as posture, eye contact, and gesture are considered.

History   Description of the past and current health status of the patient/client.

Hot pack   Pouch filled with silica gel and soaked in thermostatically controlled water.

House of delegates (HOD)   Highest policymaking body of APTA, consisting of voting chapter delegates and nonvoting section and assembly delegates and members of the Board of Directors.

Hydrotherapy   Use of the therapeutic effects of water by immersing the body part or entire body into a tank of water.

Hypermobile joint   Joint with excessive motion.

Hypertonia   High muscle tone.

Hypertrophic scar   Excess of collagen deposited at the site of a healing or healed wound that is noticeably different from the normal skin; scar remains within the boundaries of the original wound.

Hypokinesis   State of decreased activity or movement.

Hypomobile joint   Joint with less motion than is considered functional.

Hypotonia   Low muscle tone.

I

Indemnity   Health insurance plan-defined maximum amounts that will be paid for covered services.

Independent practice association (IPA) model   Organized form of prepaid medical practice in which participating providers remain in their own (independent) practice settings yet negotiate contracts with health insurers as a group (organization).

Individualized education plan (IEP)   Model using collaboration of therapists, family members, educators, and other health care team members to provide direct intervention in the classroom setting.

Individualized family service plan (IFSP)   Detailed total plan of care for the child in the context of the family unit.

Inflammatory phase   Phase of wound healing encompassing vascular reactions that decrease blood loss and initiate vessel repair, and cellular responses that moderate blood loss, fight infection, and provide nutrition and oxygen to initiate and sustain tissue repair.

Inflammatory skin diseases   Diseases of the skin whose causes invoke an inflammatory response (causes for these diseases commonly include immune reactions and contact irritants or allergens).

Inspiration   Contraction of the muscles of respiration, resulting in an increase in the space contained within the thoracic cavity. This expansion causes the air pressure to drop inside the lungs, resulting in movement of air into the lungs.

Instrumental activities of daily living (IADLs)   Activities that individuals must perform to function in the community. Examples include shopping, driving, and paying bills.

Insured   Individual covered by a health insurance plan.

Insurer   Organization that offers health insurance plans.

Integument   Skin.

Internal dialog   Communication within an individual ("silent talking" to oneself) that may affect nonverbal communication with other people.

Interprofessionalism   Patient-centered care provided by an interdisciplinary team. This approach also promotes interdisciplinary education.

Intervention   Procedure conducted with the patient/client to achieve the desired outcomes.

Intrinsic factors   Personal characteristics of the individual.

Ischemia   Insufficient oxygenation of tissues resulting from a blocked blood vessel.

J

Joint mobilization   Technique used when a patient's dysfunction is the result of joint stiffness or hypomobility (loss of motion); applies to joint-specific passive movements, either oscillatory (rapid, repeated movements) or sustained.

Juvenile rheumatoid arthritis (JRA)   One of the many rheumatic diseases characterized by an inflammation of the connective tissue that manifests as a painful inflamed joint (arthritis); begins in childhood.

K

Keloid scar   Excess of collagen deposited at the site of a healing or healed wound that is noticeably different from the normal skin; scar commonly extends beyond the boundaries of the original wound.

L

LAMP document   Document created by the Section on Health Policy and Administration of the American Physical Therapy Association that describes behaviors for the development of Leadership, Administration, Management, and Professionalism in Physical Therapy (LAMP).

Law   Formal rule having binding legal force laid down, ordained, or established by a governing body.

Learned nonuse   Phenomenon by which a patient learns through trial and error that it is easier to use his lesser involved limb to complete an action, rather than attempting to use a weaker extremity.

Licensure   Process by which the state grants permission to practice a profession to an individual who has met state standards and grants legal recognition to a particular scope of practice.

Low-context assumptions   Assumptions found in cultures in which the individual is considered more important than the group. Communication is direct; meaning is based on explicit verbal cues. Communication is less dependent on cues or nuances and is influenced by what the speaker is saying.

Lumbar puncture (LP)   Injection of a hypodermic needle into the lumbar subarachnoid space.

M

Magnetic resonance imaging (MRI)   Creation of a computer image by placing the body part in a magnetic field.

Malpractice   Failure to do (or avoid doing) something that a reasonably prudent member of the profession would do (or would not do), with subsequent injury to a patient/client.

Managed care   Arrangement in which an insurance company contracts with health care providers to provide health care to the consumers who subscribe to the insurance plan.

Managed care organization (MCO)   Health insurer that offers managed care plans.

Manual muscle testing (MMT)   Test allowing the therapist to assign a specific grade to a muscle, based on whether the patient can hold the limb against gravity, how much manual resistance can be tolerated, and whether there is full range of motion at a joint.

Massage   Systematic use of various manual strokes designed to produce certain physiologic, mechanical, and psychological effects.

Maturation phase   Phase of wound healing that includes collagen synthesis and lysis, as well as reorientation of the collagen fibers that remain at the wound site; this phase may also be referred to as the *remodeling phase.*

Medicaid   Reimbursement system established at the state level to provide health care for those with limited financial means.

Medicare   Reimbursement system established at the federal level for individuals older than 65 years of age.

Medicare advantage (Medicare Part C)   Medicare program developed under the 1997 Balanced Budget Act that offers more flexibility for beneficiaries. Persons eligible for Medicare Parts A and B are also eligible for this program.

Medicare fee schedule   Physician fee schedule (payments) allowed by Medicare to those who provide services to Medicare beneficiaries.

Medicare modernization act (MMA)   Legislation (Medicare Prescription Drug Improvement and Modernization Act of 2003) that provides a prescription drug benefit, more choices, and better benefits to Medicare beneficiaries.

Medicare Part A—Hospital Insurance   Hospital insurance covered under Medicare. This program helps to pay for inpatient care in hospitals, care in critical access hospitals (small facilities that give limited outpatient and inpatient services to people in rural areas), care in skilled nursing facilities, hospice care, and some home health care. Most people get Part A automatically when they turn age 65. They do not have to pay a monthly premium for Part A because they or a spouse paid Medicare taxes while they were working.

Medicare Part B—Supplementary Medical Insurance   Medical insurance covered under Medicare. This program helps to pay for doctors' services, outpatient hospital care, and some other medical services that Part A does not cover, such as the services of physical and occupational therapists, and some home health care. Part B helps to pay for these covered services and supplies when they are medically necessary. Enrollment in part B is voluntary, and individuals pay a Medicare Part B monthly premium.

Meningocele   Benign herniation of the meninges manifesting as a soft tissue cyst or lump that surrounds a normal spinal cord and produces no neurologic deficits.

Meningomyelocele   Open congenital spinal cord lesion with minimal to no skin protection covering the deeper nerve roots. Most severe of the spinal closure defects that usually results in loss of motor function and sensation of the lower part of the body.

Minimum data set (MDS)   A specified collection of data that is documented and used to measure the amount of care provided to a patient at a skilled nursing facility.

Mirroring and matching   One method of developing rapport. It may include mirroring the body language or using similar verbal pacing, tonality, intent, or speed of communication of the person with whom one is communicating.

Motor control   Ability to manipulate movement and nonmovement of the body's musculoskeletal components.

Motor learning   Body's mechanism for acquiring or learning voluntary motor control.

Multiple sclerosis (MS)   Disease in which patches of demyelination occur in the nervous system, leading to disturbances in conduction of action potentials along the nerves.

Muscle endurance   Ability to produce and sustain tension over a prolonged period of time.

Muscle power   Amount of work produced by a muscle in a given period of time.

Muscle strength   Maximal amount of tension an individual can produce in one repetition.

Muscle tone   Inherent resistance that is felt when a muscle is passively stretched.

Myocardial infarction   Heart attack resulting from blockage by an embolus (clot) of one of the coronary arteries.

Myofascial release   Manual stretching of the layers of the body's fascia (connective tissue that surrounds muscle and other soft tissues in the body).

N

National Assembly of Physical Therapist Assistants (National Assembly)   Former component of APTA that consisted of all affiliate (physical therapist assistant) and life affiliate (retired) members. Included officers and regional directors who represented the interests of its members.

National Foundation for Infantile Paralysis (the Foundation)   Foundation established in 1938 in response to repeated polio epidemics. Established to provide research, education, and patient services. Provided substantial support for the profession and practice of physical therapy.

Negligence   Failure to do something that a reasonably prudent person would do, or behavior that would normally not be done under similar circumstances.

Neoplastic skin diseases   Cancers affecting the skin.

Nerve conduction velocity (NCV) study   Study that records the rate at which electrical signals are transmitted along peripheral nerves.

Nerve entrapment   Pressure on a nerve.

Neural tube defect   Condition in which the neural tube fails to close completely during the first month of gestational development.

Neuropathic (neurotropic) ulcer   Skin lesion caused by a decreased cutaneous sensation that disallows protective responses such as weight transfer; these ulcers are commonly associated with diabetes mellitus.

Neuroplasticity   The ability of neurons in the brain to compensate for injury or disease.

NEXT conference and exposition   Yearly (usually June) meeting of APTA, which includes an extensive program of educational presentations, meetings, and activities.

Norm referenced   Type of assessment based on a large number of participants to create a comparison group for the assessment. In children, norm-referenced assessments can be used to compare a child's functional abilities or activities with those of other children of the same age.

Normal developmental theory   Model asserting that therapy goals and objectives are designed to follow the progression of normal motor development. Assumes that children with central nervous system damage will acquire motor skills in a similar fashion as children with normally developing nervous systems do.

A Normative Model of Physical Therapist Assistant Education   Approved by the House of Delegates, this document is a guide for physical therapist assistant education programs to ensure that the academic program meets the quality and comprehensiveness established by the members of the profession.

A Normative Model of Physical Therapist Professional Education   Approved by the House of Delegates, this document is a guide for physical therapist education programs to ensure that the academic program meets the quality and comprehensiveness established by the members of the profession.

O

Objective examination   Quantitative or qualitative measurements that are taken by the physical therapist or physical therapist assistant or by use of a mechanical device.

Obstructive lung disease   Pathologic abnormality in airflow through the bronchial tubes.

Oculesics   The use of eye contact or gaze aversion or a combination of both between people. This varies according to cultural norms.

Open enrollment   Specific period of time each year in which a health insurer must accept all who apply for health insurance coverage.

Open kinetic chain exercise   Exercise in which the end limb segment is free.

Osteoarthritis   Condition characterized by degeneration of cartilage as a result of many years of use. Hands, spine, knees, and hips are most commonly affected.

Osteogenesis imperfecta (OI)   Common and severe bone impairment of genetic origin. Affects the formation of collagen during bone development, resulting in frequent fractures during the fetal or newborn period.

Osteoporosis   Decreased mineralization of the bones caused by decreased production of new bone cells and increased resorption of bone.

Outcome measure   Standardized instrument used to measure an individual's actual or perceived limitations and participation restrictions, and/or quality of life or health status.

Outcomes   Measurable results from the interventions provided during an episode of care.

P

Palpation An examination technique using light touch with your hand and fingers to the surface of the body to determine the quality of tissue structures.

Paraffin treatment Use of a mixture of melted paraffin wax and mineral oil maintained at a specific temperature to promote relaxation and pain relief and allow greater comfort during range-of-motion exercises.

Paraplegia Impairment of sensory and motor function affecting the lower extremities as a result of injury to the spinal cord.

Parkinson's disease Progressive condition caused by a lack of the neurotransmitter dopamine, characterized by a classic triad of symptoms: tremor, rigidity, and bradykinesia.

Passive range of motion (PROM) Amount of movement at a joint that is obtained by the therapist's moving the segment without assistance from the patient.

Patient Individual who has a disorder that requires interventions to improve function.

Patient-centered medical home (PCMH) Model or philosophy of primary care that is based on accessible, comprehensive, and coordinated patient-centered care provided by a team of practitioners who focus on quality and safety. Ideally, this model provides an approach for how primary care could be organized and delivered throughout the entire health care system; an approach in which providers and care teams are encouraged to engage patients across a wide spectrum of conditions.

Per diem Method of health care reimbursement; a set payment per day.

Perception Ability to integrate various simultaneous sensory inputs and to respond appropriately.

Percutaneous coronary intervention Process of mechanically dilating a blood vessel.

Pervasive development disorder (PDI) A group of disorders of neural development characterized by impairments in social interaction and communication and the presence of unusual behaviors such as repeating actions and poor play skills.

Pharmaceutical formularies Usually a list of generic drugs and their indications for use.

Physiatrist Title given to physicians who specialize in physical medicine.

Physical therapist (PT) Professional who works to evaluate, treat, and/or prevent physical disability, movement dysfunction, and pain resulting from injury, disability, disease, or other health-related conditions.

Physical therapist assistant (PTA) Health care provider who assists the PT in the provision of physical therapy and has graduated from an accredited physical therapist assistant associate degree program.

Physical therapist assistant member Membership category in APTA for the PTA.

Physical therapist assistant special interest group (PTA SIG) A subunit of a component of APTA, such as a chapter, that serves the unique professional interests of the members.

Physical therapist member Membership category in APTA for the PT.

Physical therapist of record The PT who assumes primary responsibility for patient/client management and is accountable for coordination, continuation, and progression of the plan of care.

Physical therapy Assessment, evaluation, treatment, and prevention of physical disability, movement dysfunctions, and pain resulting from injury, disease, disability, or other health-related conditions.

Physical therapy aide or technician Support personnel who performs designated tasks that do not require the clinical decision making of the physical therapist or the clinical problem solving of the physical therapist assistant.

Physical therapy political action committee (PT-PAC) An organization that raises funds to support federal legislation favorable to the profession and practice of physical therapy.

Physician quality reporting system (PQRS) This program uses a combination of incentive payments and payment adjustments in order to ensure quality information is reported. Beginning in 2015, the program also applies a payment adjustment to eligible professionals who do not satisfactorily report data on quality measures for covered professional services.

Physiotherapist Synonym for physical therapist, commonly used outside the United States.

Physiotherapy Synonym for physical therapy, commonly used outside the United States; used by the first national organization, American Women's Physical Therapeutic Association.

Plagiocephaly Deformation of the skull during development caused by prolonged positioning in utero or in the first few months of life.

Plan of care Goals, interventions (including duration and frequency), desired outcomes, and criteria for discharge.

Plaques A lesioned area of the nervous system that has become inflamed or has lost its myelin covering.

Point-of-service (POS) plan Health insurance plan in which subscribers can select the type of health care at the time of need; allows more subscriber choice, usually at a higher cost.

Policy Plan or course of action designed to influence and determine decisions. APTA further defines this as "Association directives defining operational or administrative activities."

Post entry-level professional behaviors Professional behaviors that develop once the physical therapist is working in the profession of physical therapy.

Postural drainage Use of gravity through appropriate positioning and chest wall percussion to promote removal of excessive secretions from the tracheobronchial tree.

Practice act State's official statement or document of definition and regulation of a specific profession, setting down guidelines for those practicing the profession within its jurisdiction.

Preferred provider organization (PPO) Organization formed by hospitals and other health care providers that provides health care services to purchasers, usually at discounted rates.

Premium Money owed to the health insurance company upfront to guarantee future health insurance coverage.

Prenatal cocaine exposure Fetal exposure to cocaine in utero resulting from maternal cocaine use during pregnancy. Infants often show clinical signs of exposure after birth such as hyperirritability, poor feeding patterns, high respiratory and heart rates, increased tremulousness, and irregular sleeping patterns.

Presbycusis Decreased ability to perceive higher pitches and to distinguish between similar sounds.

Pressure ulcer Skin lesion caused by ischemia of the integument secondary to pressure; these ulcers are generally located at bony prominences.

Prevention Services designed to avoid the occurrence of pain and dysfunction or to limit or reduce those that exist.

Primary care   Level of health care delivered by a member of the health care system who is responsible for the majority of the health care needs of the individual.

Primary care provider (PCP)   Generalist physician who provides primary care; commonly a family practice, internal medicine, or general pediatric physician.

Profession   Career or means of employment demonstrating five characteristics: commitment to field, a representative organization, knowledge in a specific area, social service, and recognized autonomy.

Professional behaviors (formerly known as *generic abilities*)   Behaviors essential for physical therapy professionals that are not explicitly part of the profession's core of knowledge and technical skills but are required for success in the profession.

Professional misconduct   Violation of the state statutes and/or regulations that define competent professional practice by those professionals regulated by the state.

Prognosis   Prediction of the level of improvement and time necessary to reach that level.

Proliferative phase   Phase of wound healing that involves increased activity of fibroblasts, instigation of aggressive wound contraction, and epithelialization.

Prospective payment system (PPS)   Establishment of a reimbursement rate to be paid in advance of the delivery of care. It is often based on the diagnosis and level of care needed.

Provider contracting   The process used by managed care companies to negotiate contracts (formal, legal relationships) with providers for the future provision of health care services.

Provider network (panel)   Formal affiliations of health care providers with third-party payers.

Proxemics   The distance between two people in a formal interaction. The distance varies depending on cultural norms.

PT/PTA team   PTA(s) working under the direction and supervision of a designated PT to provide physical therapy services. Maximum ratios of PTs to PTAs vary depending on the setting and laws and regulations.

PT:PTA ratio   Maximum number of PTAs who can work under the direction and supervision of a PT as defined by policy, law, or regulation.

PTA Caucus   A body consisting of one physical therapist assistant representative from each chapter of the American Physical Therapy Association. It meets annually just before the House of Delegates meeting and provides input to the latter through five delegates from the Caucus.

Pulmonary function test   Assessment of the effectiveness of the respiratory musculature and the integrity of the airways and lung tissues to help classify the lung disease pattern as obstructive or restrictive.

Q

Quadriplegia   See *tetraplegia*.

R

Range of motion (ROM)   Movement at a joint.

Range-of-motion exercise   Exercise for mobility of a joint. Falls into two categories: active or passive. Active ROM exercise involves voluntary movement of a limb through an arc of movement; passive ROM exercise involves the therapist's moving the limb without patient assistance.

Rapport—cultural, verbal, and behavioral Communication that is characterized by mutual collaboration and respect but does not necessarily indicate agreement. It occurs at the cultural level (style of greeting and form of dress), verbal level (verbal pacing, tonality, speed), and behavioral level (body language and gestures).

Receptive aphasia Diminished ability to receive and interpret verbal or written communication.

Recognition of advanced proficiency for the PTA Formal recognition of advanced clinical skills of the PTA awarded by APTA.

Reconstruction aide Aide (exclusively a woman) responsible for providing physical reconstruction to persons injured in war; forerunners of the profession and practice of physical therapy in the United States.

Registration Process by which the state tracks regulated professionals by requiring updated listing of names, addresses, and qualifications. This generally does not involve a review of whether standards of practice are met.

Regulation Administrative or departmental rules issued to carry out the intent of the law.

Reimbursement The process of payment for the provision of health care services. Typically, health care providers are reimbursed by third-party payers that insure patients.

Representative body of the national assembly (RBNA) Former deliberative body for the physical therapist assistant with representatives from each chapter. Replaced by the PTA Caucus.

Resistance exercise Form of active movement in which some form of resistance is provided to increase muscular strength and endurance.

Resisted test Test that allows the therapist to determine the general strength of a muscle group and assess whether any pain is produced with the muscle contraction.

Resource-based relative value scale (RBRVS) Medicare payment rules for physician services established as part of the Omnibus Reconciliation Act of 1989. Fees determined based on work completed, costs to practice medicine, and malpractice insurance expense.

Resource utilization groups (RUGs) The Balanced Budget Act (1997) changed Medicare reimbursement for skilled nursing facilities (SNFs) from a cost-based system to a prospective payment system (PPS). Under the PPS, SNFs are required to assign residents to 1 of 53 resource utilization groups that are calculated based on a clinical assessment tool.

Respiration Process of exchanging oxygen and carbon dioxide between the air a person breathes and the cells of the body.

Restrictive lung disease Pathologic reduction in the volume of air in the lungs.

Retrospective reimbursement Payment made to providers after health care services have been rendered.

Rheumatoid arthritis Chronic inflammation of the joints, of unknown cause.

Rigidity Disturbance of muscle tone; manifests as a resistance when the limbs are passively moved.

Risk Probability of a financial loss.

Risk management Process by which coordinated efforts are made by an organization to identify, assess, and minimize the risk of harm and loss to the organization, employees, and clients.

S

Sarcopenia Loss of muscle mass associated with aging.

Scar contraction Dynamic movement of the edges of a scar (wound boundaries) toward each other.

Scar contracture   Permanent or relatively permanent lack of mobility of the scar tissue that results in functional and/or cosmetic impairment.

Scoliosis   Lateral curvature of the spine; may be idiopathic (of unknown origin), neuromuscular, or congenital (present at birth).

Scope of work   A term used to refer to the selected interventions, tasks, and documentation of care provided by the PTA under the direction and supervision of the physical therapist. State practice acts define the specific activities permitted by law within each jurisdiction, and may vary. The practice of physical therapy is conducted by the physical therapist.

Screening   Procedure to determine if there is a need for further services of a physical therapist or other health care professional.

Secondary care   Services provided by individuals on a referral basis.

Secondary condition   Condition that is potentially preventable and is a direct or indirect consequence of inadequate attention to (or inadequate amelioration of) an impairment or disability.

Section   National level of organizational unit of APTA for members of all classes to promote similar interests. Membership is voluntary.

Self-assessment   Ability to critically examine and evaluate one's own cognitive, affective, and psychomotor behaviors in the professional setting.

Sensation   Ability to receive sensory input from within and outside the body and transmit it through the peripheral nerves and tracts in the spinal cord to the brain where it is received and interpreted.

Sensory integration (SI)   Technique based on the theory that poor integration and use of sensory input (feedback) prevent subsequent motor planning (output). Providing controlled vestibular and somatosensory experiences enables the child to integrate the sensory information to evoke a spontaneous, functional response.

Shared savings program   A program to facilitate the coordination and cooperation among health care providers, ultimately to improve the quality of care for Medicare Fee-For-Service beneficiaries and to reduce unnecessary costs. This program will reward Accountable Care Organizations that meet performance standards on quality of care, lower their growth in health care costs, and demonstrate patient-centered caret.

Short-wave diathermy   Use of electromagnetic energy to produce deep therapeutic heating effects.

SOAP note   Documentation format taken from the Problem-Oriented Medical Record System; its components are (1) Subjective (what the patient or family member describes), (2) Objective (what the physical therapist observes or measures), (3) Assessment (clinical judgment based on evaluation; includes goals), and (4) Plan (of care).

Soft tissue mobilization   Variety of "hands-on" techniques, including massage and myofascial release, designed to improve movement and decrease pain or swelling.

Sole extender of the physical therapist   Affirmation by APTA that the PTA is the only individual recognized to assist the PT in providing selected interventions under the direction and supervision.

Spasticity   Velocity-dependent hypotonia.

Special interest group (SIG)   One of the many groups existing at multiple levels of tAPTA to enable members at all levels to organize into smaller specialty areas.

Special tests   Tests designed for examination of specific joints to indicate the presence or absence of a particular problem.

Spina bifida   Congenital incomplete closure of a vertebra.

Spina bifida occulta   Congenital incomplete closure of a vertebra (separation of the spinous process) that is not associated with disability.

Spinal cord injury (SCI) Damage to the spinal cord that results in neurologic dysfunction.

Spinal muscular atrophy (SMA) Genetic disorder characterized by severe muscle weakness in infancy and progressive respiratory failure.

Spirometer Instrument measuring various volumes and airflow rates; findings are then compared with a normal scale.

Sprain Overstretching of a joint ligament accompanied by a tearing of the fibers, causing pain and instability of the joint.

Staff model (of HMO) A managed care organization (MCO) model in which the health care providers are employed by the MCO.

Standardized testing Type of formal test in which the evaluation procedures remain the same when administered by different therapists and at variable test locations.

Standards of Ethical Conduct for the Physical Therapist Assistant Principles set forth by APTA for maintaining and promoting high standards of professional conduct among affiliate member physical therapist assistants.

Standards of Practice for Physical Therapy Document approved by the House of Delegates of APTA that identifies conditions and performances essential for the provision of high-quality physical therapy.

Static balance Balance maintained while standing still.

Statute Formal written enactment by the legislative department of government.

Stereognosis Ability to perceive, recognize, and name familiar object through touch.

Strain Tearing of muscle fibers caused by a sudden contraction of a muscle or excessive stretch to the muscle.

Strength Amount of force produced during a voluntary muscular contraction.

Stroke or cerebrovascular accident (CVA) Neurologic dysfunction as a result of disruption of blood flow in the brain.

Student assembly Component of APTA whose members are physical therapist and physical therapist assistant students; provides a forum in which physical therapist and physical therapist assistant students can better understand their roles.

Subjective examination Interview of the patient about the extent and nature of an injury; a qualitative measurement based on the patient's perception of the problem.

Subscriber Individual who makes an advance payment for something; specifically, an employee who pays a health insurance premium through his or her employer to purchase a health insurance policy.

Systems approach Intervention techniques used for neuromuscular conditions that consider the interplay of perceptual, cognitive, and action systems, as well as the specific intended task.

Systems review Brief examination to provide information about the general health of the patient/client, including the physiologic, anatomic, and cognitive status.

T

Tachypnea Increase in rate of breathing.

Target heart rate (THR) Appropriate heart rate to be maintained during the peak period in aerobic training; calculated as a percentage of the individual's maximum heart rate.

Tendinitis Inflammation of a tendon, a structure that is located at the ends of muscles and attaches muscle to bone.

Tendinopathy Disorder of a tendon.

Tendinosis Degeneration of a tendon from overuse.

Tertiary care   Service provided by specialists who are commonly employed in facilities that focus on particular health conditions.

Tests and measures   Specific procedures selected and performed to quantify the physical and functional status of the patient/client.

Tetraplegia   Impairment of sensory and motor function affecting all extremities as a result of injury to the spinal cord.

Thermal agent   Agent used to modify the temperature of surrounding tissue, resulting in a change in the amount of blood flow to the injured area.

Third-party administrator or payer   Organization that pays (or insures) health and medical expenses on behalf of beneficiaries.

Tort   Civil injury for which the injured party can seek legal relief from the courts.

Torticollis   Condition when the head and neck are bent to one side. If the sterno-cleidomastoid muscle is shortened in utero, the head and neck are bent to that side, and this results in congenital muscular torticollis at birth.

Training zone   Individual's ideal range of minimum and maximum heart rates (see target heart rate) that must be achieved for that individual to experience an aerobic training effect.

Total body surface area (TBSA)   The extent of the surface of the body covered by skin. The percent of TBSA is used to describe the size of a skin injury (routinely used to estimate the size of a burn injury).

Traumatic brain injury (TBI)   Damage to the brain caused by physical means resulting in neurologic dysfunction.

Tremor   Alternating contractions of opposing muscle groups.

U

Ultrasound   Therapeutic application of high-frequency sound waves that penetrate through tissue and cause an increase in the tissue temperature to promote healing and reduce pain.

Unilateral spatial neglect   Failure to attend to sensory stimuli on the side of the body opposite to a brain lesion.

Usual, customary, and reasonable (UCR)   Range of fees allowable for physician reimbursement based on typical charges that fall within a reasonable cost of service.

Utilization   Use of services.

Utilization review (UR)   An evaluation of the need, correctness, and efficiency of health care services and procedures.

V

Values-based behaviors for the physical therapist assistant   An APTA document that describes the core values of the PTA, those values that most significantly influence PTAs in the provision of patient/client care, and include sample indicators for each value. The values are Altruism, Caring and Compassion, Continuing Competence, Duty, Integrity, PT/PTA Collaboration, Responsibility, and Social Responsibility.

Vancouver burn scar scale   Clinical method for assessing scar tissue. The characteristics of scar that are examined include pigmentation, vascularity, pliability, and height.

Venous insufficiency   Deficiency or occlusion of blood flow through a vein.

Ventilation   Process of inspiration and expiration; results in an exchange of oxygen and carbon dioxide between the air found in the lungs and the pulmonary circulation.

Vertigo   Sensation of spinning or whirling that occurs as a result of a disturbance in balance.

Vicarious liability   Principle by which one individual may be held indirectly liable legally for the acts of another—for example, the liability of an employer for the acts of an employee during the performance of job responsibilities.

Vision 2020   A statement (and sentence in abridged version) adopted by the American Physical Therapy Association House of Delegates in 2000 that establishes expectations for the practice of physical therapy in the year 2020. It addresses six components: autonomous practice, direct access, practitioner of choice, doctor of physical therapy, evidence-based practice, and professionalism.

Vision statement for physical therapy   A statement adopted by the APTA in 2013 that replaced Vision 2020. It reads, "Transforming society by optimizing movement to improve the human experience."

W

Waste   Overutilization of services or other practices that, directly or indirectly, result in unnecessary costs to the health care system. In general, waste is more common than fraud.

Whirlpool   Tank of water used in hydrotherapy for immersing a body part or the entire body.

Work hardening/conditioning   Intervention program for an individual designed to restore the capacity and function for return to work.

World Confederation of Physical Therapy (WCPT)   International organization that represents physical therapy on a global level and consists of physical therapy organizations in member nations.

Index

Page numbers followed by *f* indicate figures, *t* indicate tables and *b* indicate boxes.